D1559887

INTERPERSONAL THEORY
IN NURSING PRACTICE
Selected Works of
Hildegard E. Peplau

Anita Werner O'Toole, R.N., C.S., Ph.D. received her master's degree in psychiatric nursing from Rutgers University, New Brunswick, NJ and her doctoral degree in sociology from Case Western Reserve University, Cleveland, OH. She is currently Professor and Director of the Graduate Program in Psychiatric Mental Health Nursing at Kent State University, Kent, OH. She also maintains a part-time private psychotherapy practice with adults and families. Dr. O'Toole has published extensively in both nursing and sociology. Her recent research publications are in the areas of family violence and development of a classification system for psychiatric nursing diagnosis.

Sheila Rouslin Welt, R.N., M.S., received her master's degree in psychiatric nursing from Rutgers University, New Brunswick, NJ. As a psychotherapist working with children and adults, she is currently in private practice of psychotherapy and clinical supervision in New York and New Jersey. She has presented lectures and workshops throughout the U.S. and abroad and has an extensive list of publications to her credit. In 1963, she coauthored *Group Psychotherapy In Nursing Practice,* the first book on group psychotherapy by a nurse. Her coauthored book, *Issues in Psychotherapy,* received the 1982 American Journal of Nursing *Book of the Year* award. Her 1983 coauthored book, *A Collection of Classics in Psychiatric Nursing Literature,* was chosen the 1983 Book of the Year by the American Journal of Nursing. Volume II of *Issues in Psychotherapy,* tentatively renamed *Narcissism And The Therapist-Patient Relationship,* will be published by Guilford Publications in 1989.

INTERPERSONAL THEORY IN NURSING PRACTICE
Selected Works of Hildegard E. Peplau

Anita Werner O'Toole, R.N., C.S., Ph.D
Sheila Rouslin Welt, R.N., M.S.
Editors

SPRINGER PUBLISHING COMPANY • NEW YORK

Springer Publishing Company, Inc.
536 Broadway
New York, NY 10012

89 90 91 92 93 / 5 4 3 2 1

Library of Congress Cataloging-in-Publication Data

Peplau, Hildegard E.
    Interpersonal theory in nursing practice : selected works of
  Hildegard E. Peplau / edited by Anita Werner O'Toole and Sheila
  Rouslin Welt.
        p. cm.
    Bibliography: p.
    Includes index.
    ISBN 0-8261-6060-3
    1. Psychiatric nursing. 2. Nurse and patient. I. O'Toole, Anita
  Werner. II. Welt, Sheila Rouslin. III. Title.
  RC440.P423   1989
  610.73'68—dc19   89-5870
                                                          CIP

Printed in the United States of America

Contents

Foreword by Grayce Sills   ix

Acknowledgments   xiii

Introduction   xv

PART I: Interpersonal Relations Theory

Introduction

1. Interpersonal Relationships in Psychiatric Nursing   5
2. Theory: The Professional Dimension   21
3. Interpersonal Relationships: The Purpose and
   Characteristics of Professional Nursing   42
4. Interpersonal Constructs for Nursing Practice   56

PART II: Therapeutic Milieu

Introduction

5. The History of Milieu as a Treatment Modality   75
6. Psychiatric Nursing: The Nurse's Role in
   Preventing Chronicity   80
7. General Application of Theory and Techniques of
   Psychotherapy in Nursing Situations   99
8. Pattern Interactions   108
9. Psychiatric Nursing: Role of Nurses and Psychiatric
   Nurses   120

PART III: The Teaching of Psychiatric Nursing

Introduction

10. What Is Experiential Teaching?   139
11. Interpretation of Clinical Observations   149
12. Clinical Supervision of Staff Nurses   164

PART IV: Psychotherapy

Introduction

13. Interpersonal Techniques: The Crux of
    Psychiatric Nursing   173
14. Psychotherapeutic Strategies   182
15. Therapeutic Nurse-Patient Interaction   192
16. Investigative Counseling   205
17. Professional Closeness   230
18. Themes in Nursing Situations   244

PART V: Concepts

Introduction

19. Loneliness   255
20. Theoretical Constructs: Anxiety, Self, and
    Hallucinations   270
21. Thought Disorder in Schizophrenia: Corrective
    Influence of Nursing Behavior on Language
    of Patients   327
22. An Explanatory Theory of the Process of Focal
    Attention   338
23. Process and Concept of Learning   348
Editors' Summary   353
Index   367

INTERPERSONAL THEORY IN NURSING PRACTICE
Selected Works of Hildegard E. Peplau

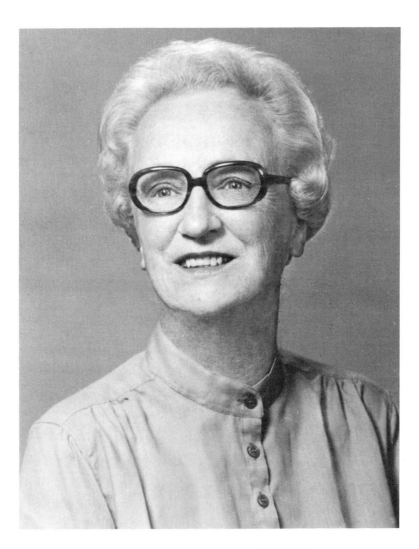

HILDEGARD E. PEPLAU

Foreword

I have known Hilda Peplau for over forty years. I count myself as friend, colleague and student. Not a student *of* Peplau, but a student with Peplau. When one studies with Hilda the study is *of* the data. This wise, caring, and gentle person is one of the finest and best scholars the profession has known. Someone has said that scholarship requires the discipline of the examined life. Hilda is the epitome of scholarship. For over sixty years her scholarship has been evocative, informative, and provocative. The present work is no exception.

In the early 1950s Peplau introduced an interpersonal relations paradigm for the study and practice of nursing (Peplau, 1952). The paradigm held that nurse and patient participate in and contribute to the relationship and, further, that the relationship itself could be therapeutic. This relationship could be examined, and through that examination would come teaching and learning. Since 1952 Peplau has extended many of her ideas. She continues to work with the issues generated by the paradigm.

The collective thinking of nurses about the practice of nursing has only recently become readily accessible to the professional community. Until the last decade, scholarship in nursing was more often than not shared with audiences through the spoken word. Many of Peplau's formulations, therefore, have not been accessible to the nursing profession at large. Many of her early contributions were published in obscure places—difficult to find or impossible to retrieve in current computer-based literature searches. Thus, this volume affords access to select segments of Peplau's work. These papers, compiled and edited by O'Toole and Welt, are a joy to behold as well as a delight to read. It is a boon to psychiatric nursing that these editors have diligently worked to make Peplau's ideas viable and available for use in practice, teaching, and research.

Pragmatism suggests that we are obliged to test knowledge by asking what we would be required to do if we believe the paradigm to be true (Kaplan, 1964). Responses to that question can be generated from this volume. If the Peplau paradigm is to be believed, then nursing will be practiced differently from practice based on earlier models; nursing will be taught and learned differently from the modes currently prevailing; and nursing will be researched differently.

But in what ways would nursing be different? To practice nursing using the paradigm of interpersonal relations requires the development of new norms: norms that govern the conduct of practice. The papers in the volume devoted to the characteristics of social versus professional relationships are classic. Herein, guidelines are provided for therapeutic relationships that honor the integrity and self-worth of both nurse and patient. Given the recent spate of reported abuses by therapists in the course of treatment, these thoughtfully reasoned papers on the normative structure of the professional practice of the nurse are needed additions to the field of psychiatric nursing. I expect that nurses will integrate these ideas into their practice, as well as recommend these chapters to colleagues in other mental health disciplines.

A second major difference to be evidenced if one accepts the Peplau paradigm concerns the teaching and learning of relationship skills and processes. In this area the editors have chosen some of the very best of Peplau's work. The experiential mode of teaching and learning has been central to Peplau's thinking. Her basic thrust is that people will grow and change when they can learn to sustain the discomfort connected with examination of the experience, while utilizing new ideas and new responses.

The third area that would be conducted differently from the perspective of the Peplau paradigm is the study of clinical phenomena of concern in nursing practice. This volume includes classic papers demonstrating both the development of theoretical constructs from clinical data and the testing of theoretical constructs using that data.

No one does it better than Peplau! In these chapters one feels the excitement derived from operationalizing clinical phenomena, for instance, loneliness. Also evident is the thoughtful, systematic, and disciplined approach to the work of assisting patients to learn through the examination of their experiences.

Macmillan of London has reissued Peplau's 1952 book, *Interpersonal Relations in Nursing*. That seminal text and this volume together bring Peplau's ideas to nursing at a time when the field has the capacity to receive and use the work in substantive ways. In the 1990s there are the scholars, the well prepared researchers, and indeed the collective intellectual energy available to advance Peplau's ideas in the service of both the profession and society. As the reader embraces this volume, in the spirit of interpersonal relationships, and to paraphrase Kaplan (1964), I say: "May it do you much good and may you do it much good."

GRAYCE SILLS, R.N., PH.D., F.A.A.N.
Ohio State University
Columbus, Ohio

References

Kaplan, A. (1964). *The conduct of inquiry*. New York: Chandler.
Peplau, H. E. (1952). *Interpersonal relations in nursing*. New York: Putnam. Reissued by Macmillan, London, 1988.

Acknowledgments

This book has been germinating in our minds for much of our professional lives. Until we seriously considered the project, historical research was merely an impressive term. For two years, however, we have labored and learned a great deal about the historical research process and have admiration for those hearty souls who pursue it. We were helped immeasurably by Dr. Patricia King and her staff at the Arthur and Elizabeth Schlesinger Library on the History of Women in America at Radcliffe College, where the Hildegard E. Peplau Archives are housed. This research was supported in part by funds given by Radcliffe College for research at the Schlesinger Library. We are also grateful for financial support from Kent State University Research and Sponsored Programs, and Kent State University School of Nursing.

Without Hilda, of course, there would be no book. We can no longer complain to her that much of her work that we had wished were in print remains unpublished. Although there is much more where this came from, we have made a start. In a way, our considerable effort is a tribute to her as our mentor. As our teacher, our supervisor, our scholarly clinical role model, she taught us about logical thinking, the scientific method, and perseverance. As our mentor, her "tender (and sometime not so tender) cooperation" assured that our clinical and theoretical needs took precedence, that our learning was primary, that the development of our selves was paramount. We thank her for her unflagging concern, for her knowledge and desire to share it, and for her discipline that surely we have internalized. Her marvelous intellect and wonderful mind, always seeking knowledge and encouraging others in their quests, have inspired us to question—and certainly because we were free to do so, we have had some moments together far apart in our opinions. We have grown up with Hilda, personally and professionally. She is now our mentor, our colleague, and our friend and we cherish our relationship and her legacy. Our lives would not have been the same without her.

Without each other it is doubtful we could have produced this book. When one of us doubted, wavered, or faltered, the other held up. And without similar obsessional minds, complementary styles, and humor, cooperation and collaboration would have been impossible. Our relationship with Hilda and each other has deepened through the experience of so carefully studying our professional roots. The experience is indelibly with us.

To our husbands, Richard and Aaron, we give extended thanks and many rainchecks for time apart. Their support of our intellectual activity and appreciation of the need for and commitment to the project got us through the difficult times more easily than we would have otherwise. Their companionship, love, humor, and appreciation of Hilda was there more often than we knew we needed it.

To little William Philip Rouslin Welt—son of Sheila, and godson of Anita—who arrived near the end of the project, we give thanks for inspiring the much-needed creativity for the finish line. He surely has the longest record for a newborn of time spent in a bassinet in a study! Certainly this baby will go into the 21st century having internalized Peplau by proxy.

We sincerely thank Monika Ineman, who prepared the manuscript, for her excellent work. She had to decipher Peplau, O'Toole, and Welt—and that was no mean feat. We also thank Wendy Lewandowski for her assistance in the initial library search of published papers. The publishers and editors were there when we needed them, and let us proceed on our own when we did not. We hope this is the beginning of a fruitful Springer, Peplau, O'Toole, and Welt interpersonal relationship.

Introduction

In 1952 the nursing world was formally introduced to interpersonal theory by Hildegard E. Peplau. Nursing has never been the same since. Peplau's influence on nursing and particularly psychiatric nursing has been enormous. She is often referred to as the mother of psychiatric nursing, a designation that is well deserved, because she spawned a new generation of psychiatric nurses who learned to use theory, specifically interpersonal theory, in their therapeutic work with patients.

This book presents a selection of Peplau's best clinical and theoretical papers written between the years 1953 to 1988. We decided to collect and edit her papers because most summaries of her theory encountered in nursing literature are based primarily, and often singularly, on her 1952 landmark book, *Interpersonal Relations in Nursing*. Although that work presented the most complete exposition of her theory of interpersonal relations, it was followed by decades of work to refine and elaborate upon that beginning. Unfortunately, many of the post-1952 papers were not published or are not readily available, having appeared in journals that are no longer available or in texts that are now out of print.

Fortunately, Peplau is a prodigious saver of her work. Her papers were solicited for an archival collection by the Arthur and Elizabeth Schlesinger Library on the History of Women in America at Radcliffe College, Harvard University. The Hildegard E. Peplau Archives consist of 46 cartons containing personal letters and documents; papers, notes, and records from her college years; professional correspondence, lectures, unpublished papers, and workshop materials; correspondence and papers related to her positions in professional organizations; and publications. All but the personal documents are open to researchers.

The method for selecting the papers to be published involved several steps. (1) We obtained a copy of all Peplau's published papers through interlibrary loan services and reviewed the published works. (2) Peplau contributed papers from her personal files that had not been published or contributed to her archives. (3) The archive collection at Schlesinger Library was reviewed during two periods: July 20 to 25, 1986 and October 5 to 10, 1986. (4) Papers were selected for copying from the collection if they met predetermined criteria: papers not previously published, papers that contributed to theory development in psychiatric nursing, and letters or notes that provided background information about the papers. That part of the collection open for researchers was reviewed, including: Series II: School, College, Career; Series III: Professional Activities; Series IV: Organizations; and Series V: Writings (Knowles, Dolan, King, & Fraser, 1984). The contents of 32 cartons were surveyed and 138 documents were selected for copying and further review. (5) Papers were sorted by content category (clinical/theoretical, professional issues, and educational methods) and reviewed by both editors for clarity, value of contribution, and repetition. Papers selected for this publication were limited to those related to clinical and theoretical issues, and educational methods. Peplau was consulted to verify the professional and historical context of the papers noted in the introductions to each section.

The book is divided into five major sections: Part I includes papers related specifically to interpersonal relations theory. Part II addresses therapeutic milieu and includes concepts such as pattern interaction, pattern maintenance, and prevention of chronicity. Part III contains three papers on the teaching of psychiatric nursing: experiential teaching, techniques of interpretation, and clinical supervision. Part IV is about psychotherapy and addresses interviewing techniques and other aspects of the nurse-patient relationship including thematic abstraction. And Part V includes papers on the major concepts that form the backbone of Peplau's interpersonal theory: loneliness, anxiety, self, hallucinations, thought disorders, focal attention, and learning. The final chapter, Editors' Summary, is a synopsis of Peplau's major ideas.

In order to place Peplau's work in context it is important to review aspects of her personal and professional biography. Hildegard E. Peplau was born on September 1, 1909 in Reading, Pennsylvania, the second daughter of Gustav and Ottylie Peplau. Both of Hilda's parents were immigrants to the United States; they were of German origin, although born in Poland (H. E. Peplau, personal communication, August 5, 1988). Hilda was one of six children, three girls and three boys. As a child she witnessed the major flu epidemic of 1918, an event that had a profound influence on her understanding of the impact of illness and death on families.

Peplau graduated from Pottstown, Pennsylvania Hospital School of Nursing in 1931. She received a B.A. in psychology from Bennington College, Vermont in 1943. She received her M.A. in psychiatric nursing in 1947 and Ed.D. in nursing education in 1953, both graduate degrees from Teachers' College, Columbia University. She was certified in Psychoanalysis for Teachers by the William Alanson White Institute of New York City in 1954 (Knowles et al., 1984).

After graduating from nursing school in 1931, Hilda worked as a private duty and general staff nurse in Pennsylvania. During summers she served as a camp nurse for the New York University summer camp. In an interview for *Geriatric Nursing* (1986) Hilda recounted the significance of the summer camp position to her subsequent education. She was recommended for the camp position by a female physician, for whom Hilda served as a tennis partner during her student years. The camp director recommended her for the position of College Health Service Nurse at Bennington College, where she came into contact with the president of the college who, recognizing her ability, offered her a full scholarship. She had her first exposure to interpersonal theory while a student at Bennington where she studied with Erich Fromm and later with Frieda Fromm-Reichman in a field study experience at Chestnut Lodge, Rockville, Maryland (Knowles et al., 1984). There she attended lectures by Harry Stack Sullivan and began her lifelong endeavor to interpret and extend Sullivanian theory for use in nursing practice.

She served in the U.S. Army Nurse Corps from 1943 to 1945 and was assigned for most of that period to the School of Military

Neuropsychiatry in England, where she came into contact with the top psychiatrists of the world (Peplau, 1981). After receiving her master's degree from Teachers' College, she taught there from 1948 to 1953 as an instructor and director of the Advanced Program in Psychiatric Nursing. It was during this period as a faculty member at Teachers' College that Peplau formulated many of her theories. The book *Interpersonal Relations in Nursing* was completed in 1948. It was not published until four years later because it was considered too revolutionary for a nurse to publish such a book without a physician as coauthor. Peplau developed the classes for graduate level psychiatric nursing students at Teachers' College, with a strong emphasis on direct clinical experience with psychiatric patients. She began as early as 1948 to require that students interview patients, record those interviews, and study them for recurring themes and patterns of interaction. From these notes and her own clinical experience she formulated operational definitions of concepts: for example, anxiety, learning, conflict, and frustration.

She was a private duty nurse in New York City from 1953 to 1955; from that experience came data for her work on loneliness (H. E. Peplau, personal communication, August 5, 1988.) In 1954 she was employed part time and then full time in 1955 by the College of Nursing, Rutgers University, where she became chairperson of the Department of Psychiatric Nursing and Director of the Graduate Program in Psychiatric Nursing. There she developed the first graduate program devoted exclusively to the preparation of clinical specialists in psychiatric nursing. She was promoted to professor in 1960 and retired as professor emerita in 1974. She maintained a part-time private psychotherapy practice from 1958 until her retirement.

During her tenure at Rutgers she became widely known for the summer clinical workshops she conducted for nurses (mostly in state psychiatric hospitals) throughout the country. She taught interviewing techniques, personality theory, family and group therapy, and advocated that nurses become educated so they could provide therapeutic care and reverse the trend toward chronicity characteristic of state mental institutions. Through these clinical workshops and her frequent presentations at professional meetings she became an ambassador for advanced education for nurses and an advocate for the plight of the mentally ill. Most nurses who experienced a Peplau workshop came away changed for life; many went on to further their education and make significant contributions to psychiatric nursing. As one nurse said, "Peplau has a way of stretching your intelligence."

Peplau's influence on students who studied with her at Teachers' College and Rutgers was profound. She is a mentor in the truest sense of the word, one who respects the autonomous development of a learner and provides a model of a disciplined scholar to emulate. She is one of the early nursing educators to recognize and develop teaching methods for intervening in the self-concept problems women experienced as learners in higher education in a time and culture that discouraged women and particularly nurses from pursuing careers as scholars. Many of the nurses who studied with her went on to become leaders in nursing.

Peplau was executive director of the American Nurses' Association from 1969 to 1970, president from 1970 to 1972, and second vice-president from 1972 to 1974. She served as third vice-president and board member for the International Council of Nurses from 1973 to 1981. After her retirement from Rutgers in 1974, she served as a World Health Organization consultant and visiting professor at the University of Leuven in Belgium for two periods, 1975 and 1976 to 1977 (Knowles et al., 1984). Hilda now resides in Sherman Oaks in Los Angeles and continues to lecture and write, heeding her own advice, "If you don't use it, you'll lose it."

REFERENCES

Geriatric Nursing (Interview). (1986, November/December). Hildegard E. Peplau: Grande dame of psychiatric nursing (pp. 328–330).

Knowles, J. S., Dolan, M., King, S., Fraser, C. L. (1984, October). *Hildegard Elizabeth Peplau papers.* Unpublished preliminary inventory, Schlesinger Library, Radcliffe College, Cambridge, MA.

Peplau, H. E. (1952). *Interpersonal relations in nursing.* New York: Putnam. (Reissued, 1988. London: Macmillan)

Peplau, H. E. (Speaker). (1981). *Peplau on Peplau.* Cassette Recording. Schlesinger Library, Radcliffe College, Cambridge, MA. No. 84-M107 Hildegard E. Peplau Archives, carton 31, volume 1151.

Through ambition alone you cannot reach your goal. You must have assistance from trained minds. Minds who like yours craved knowledge and found it.

HILDEGARD E. PEPLAU
Circa 1927

From "The Goals of Our Lives and the Paths That Lead to It." Writings of E. H. Peplau and Selected Articles. Schlesinger Library, Radcliffe College, Cambridge, MA. No. 84-M107, Hildegard E. Peplau Archives, carton 8, volume 264. Copyright 1986 by Schlesinger Library. Reprinted by permission.

PART I Interpersonal Relations Theory

Introduction

During the 1950s and 1960s, a time when some psychiatric nurses were focusing attention on their "uniqueness" by virtue of their ubiquitous presence and ability to physically touch the patient, Hildegard E. Peplau was well into developing interpersonal theory as the crux of psychiatric nursing and the core of all nursing practice. Although she advanced no formula for interpersonal relationships, she was never vague. Her concerns were to determine the crucial elements in a nursing situation and to scrutinize those elements so as to better understand and improve the interpersonal process. While other nurses talked and wrote about theory, Peplau did so in such a way that theory was inextricably bound to clinical practice. The first nurse to use operational theory creatively, she gave form to interviewing, thereby catapulting psychiatric nursing into the health field as an applied science.

What had been nebulous, kindhearted, well-intended, but theoretically weak interviewing skills of nurses now had theoretical concepts: ways to understand concepts and ways to use them in the interpersonal relationship of nurse and patient, as well as in the interest of the patient's problems in living.

A clinician/scholar in the true sense of the combination, Peplau pointed out that phenomena derive from clinical practice—thus they are observed, collected, ordered, analyzed, formulated, and ever refined on the basis of new data. Surely this is a capsule of the psychotherapeutic process; it is also in the highest order of scientific inquiry.

CHAPTER 1

Interpersonal Relationships in Psychiatric Nursing

The crucial elements in nursing situations are obviously the nurse, the patient, and what goes on between them. Although there are of course other elements in nursing situations, it is useful for learning purposes to scrutinize carefully what goes on between the nurse (as a person) and one patient with whom the nurse has continuing contacts. If you learn well what the interpersonal relations are like in this basic unit of interaction, the learning can be generalized to other relationships between nurses and patients. These three crucial elements appear deceptively simple. Both the nurse and the patient are human persons with all of the characteristically human experiences that go on intrapersonally in each one of us—thoughts, feelings, and actions. Each one of us experiences interacting expectations, preconceptions, wishes, and desires, as well as feelings when we are in situations with other persons. It is the interaction of the thoughts, feelings, and actions of nurses and patients that constitutes what goes on between them. There is, therefore, a need to be able to characterize the quality of the interaction.

Paper presented at Annual Institute, Psychiatric and Mental Health Section, Illinois State Nurses Association, Chicago, IL, November, 1954. Schlesinger Library, Radcliffe College, Cambridge, MA. No. 84-M107 Hildegard E. Peplau Archives, carton 20, volume 675. Copyright 1986 by Schlesinger Library. Adapted and edited by permission.

QUALITIES OF INTERACTION

There are a number of ways to indicate qualities of interaction. We refer for example to the nursing problem, that is, the problem of the relationship between nurse and patient, which is a shared concern. The nursing problem is different from the nurse's problem or the patient's problem, although there may be an interpretation of the problems of nurse and patient or there may be a unique way in which the nurse and patient work together on the patient's problem. In psychiatric nursing situations, then, there are these elements: nurse, patient, and whatever goes on between them that can be characterized either as a nursing problem, a patient's problem, or a theme of the relationship.

The ability to recognize and validate themes in nursing situations is difficult. I call your attention to some common problems and then discuss one aspect of interpersonal relations in psychiatric nursing that requires study on-the-job by each practicing or student nurse.

Some time ago a pediatric nursing teacher commented to me how she missed opportunities to see children because her administrative activities kept her away from clinical contact. "I love to see the children's faces light up for me," she said quite innocently, "I go around and hug them every chance I get." At about the same time a male nurse commented to me, "I have a patient on my ward and he is giving me a hard time. He is constantly complaining of feeling nervous and begging for medication. How can I keep him out of my hair?" Now, these nurses had failed to observe what was going on in the relationship of nurse to patient. Their recitations were like dreams told glibly and easily, events for which each of these two nurses took no responsibility. Their participant roles with the patients were not noticed. The needs of one nurse to "give love" and of the other nurse "to be free of the complaints of patients" seem self-evident, yet they did not notice them. Nor was the pediatric nurse aware of the way in which children served as a potential audience for her; nor did the male nurse see the implication that he was seeking a more reliable management technique, as if he thought the patient perpetrated complaints merely to annoy the nurse. The needs of these two nurses, to have a love object and to have patients who would not make demands, were important elements in their interpersonal contacts and integrations with patients.

A nursing student walked into a patient's room one day and observed that the patient looked worried. Immediately, the patient commented to the nurse, "My, what lovely hair you have." The student did indeed have very attractive, neatly groomed red hair. The student replied, "Do you think so? I am glad you like it." Then the patient continued, "It is so lovely, how do you take care of it?" Whereupon the student discussed how she cared for her hair—shampoo, shampooing technique, setting procedure—all were gone into at length while she bathed the patient. The patient seemed interested. Afterward, the student thought she had done a good job of "health teaching" with reference to care of the hair. Somewhere along the line a nursing arts instructor had given out a list of subjects to be taught to patients, and care of the hair was on that list.

Some months later I asked this student to describe a health teaching situation in which satisfaction had been experienced. The nurse described the foregoing event with glowing pride and immense satisfaction. Then I asked the simple question, "What happened about the worries which apparently concerned the patient and you when you entered the situation?" The student was aghast; she blushed and mumbled hastily, "I never thought of that." Now, what had happened was not a great crime in this instance, but it is one step in a long series of steps in nursing education by which nurses begin more and more to fail to notice what goes on in a situation that is significant. It was obvious that the student, months later, was for the first time noticing how her own needs got in the way of serving the needs of the patient, how the patient had been permitted to operate as an audience for the nurse, and how the needs of the patient went unnoticed and unattended in this situation.

All three situations were reduced by the nurses to a deceptively simple level. One result was that important interpersonal events went unnoticed. What took precedence was the need of each nurse either to show love; to have an orderly quiet situation; to talk about herself. If these seem like appropriate nurse actions to you, then interpersonal theory will not make any difference in your practice. Interpersonal theory is a body of knowledge that can assist nurses to observe more intelligently and to intervene more sensitively in nursing situations—more intelligently and more sensitively than the nurse would without it.

MECHANISTIC VERSUS DYNAMIC THEORY

At the present time, psychiatric nurses are caught between two different types of theoretical knowledge offered to explain human behavior and to treat human difficulties in living. Psychiatric nurses are caught between mechanistic and dynamic ways of looking at nursing situations where they work. This affects the entire work role of psychiatric nurses.

The mechanistic views include several variations that I mention briefly. You are all familiar with descriptive psychiatry in which clusters of symptoms are labeled and diagnosed. You are no doubt familiar with typological psychiatry in which aspects of persons, their body build, and some "personality traits" are clustered, and the individual then typed. In nursing we have gone along with typological psychiatry to the extent of discussing "the overactive patient" and "the underactive patient." In these two typings one grossly observable aspect of the person becomes the label, thereby suggesting how the patient is to be "handled." Mechanistic theory, from my point of view, includes such treatment procedures as electroshock therapy (which you may know was first observed in use in a slaughterhouse to stun pigs before decapitating them). Lobotomy and insulin coma are also treatments that constitute doing something to the patient, in a way more mechanical than would be found in participant interpersonal experiences occurring in situations with the patient.

A more dynamic orientation to the understanding of human problems in living began largely with the work of Sigmund Freud. His theoretical statement on "unconscious motivation" and the work in biology by Walter Cannon, gave us the beginnings of a new orientation, a new way to look at psychiatric problems. The merging of these two streams of knowledge now makes it possible to study mind-body relationships, to see relations between feelings, thoughts, actions and sickness within, between and among persons and in communities. The social sciences have more recently contributed to an evolving body of theory that renders human experience more understandable. In some quarters, the new term *socio-psychosomatic* is used to indicate the three methodologies used for a comprehensive understanding of the sick person and of the contexts in which illness and recovery occur. Sullivan, among others, has taken his own clinical observations and generalized from them, leading to the development of a body of knowledge he called a "theory of interpersonal relations." I might add, too, that his earlier work at Sheppard Pratt was carried out on the wards because the information he secured from nurses was not adequate for understanding his patients. The term *interpersonal relations* can be changed to *human relations, social interaction,* or whatever one wants to use to refer to the objects of study, namely, the relations between persons in a situation.

This body of theory, which makes use of biological, psychological, and social science theory, offers assistance and explanation for the meaning of interactions, of reciprocal relations among people in a situation. It is therefore more contextual and whole than the more mechanistic theories, which are nihilistic or segmental. A mechanistic theory is largely partial, one-sided. It depends for its data on spectator observations made by an individual who presumes detachment from the individual studied. In contrast, dynamic theory requires participant observation. Data collected come from all relevant participants in a situation including the nurse-observer and the patient.

Mechanistic theories have led psychiatric nurses down some dead-end streets. Interpersonal theory sharpens the significant differences between co-acting and interacting. It points up the differences between proximity or contacts with a patient and getting in touch with the patient, that is, coming to understand the situation the way it looks to the patient rather than from the standpoint of preconceived notions familiar in descriptive and typological theory. It points up the difference between parallel play and interplay. It clarifies the significant concept of relatedness that is so essential to an understanding of all psychiatric patients.

NURSING THEORY

Apart from the theories currently presented in literature by other professional workers (M.D.s, social scientists, psychologists) psychiatric nursing must have a dynamic theory of its own. Conceptual models clarifying nursing situations are needed. Every nursing student ought to be assisted to develop her or his own operational concepts and to compare them with what is available in psychiatric nursing literature. Such is the route toward the development of professional thinking. Operational concepts that are useful in clinical nursing situations will have to be on four different levels:

1. Concepts that help the nurse understand the *generic roots* of the current patterns of living that nurse and patient use
2. Concepts that help the nurse grasp the *structural aspects* of situations
3. Concepts that make it possible for nurses to formulate and validate the *dynamics,* that is, the meanings and purposes operating in current nurse-patient integrations
4. A body of directional concepts is also needed as *guides* to nurses in moving from proximity, to contact, to "intouchness" or relatedness in situations with patients.

A useful body of psychiatric nursing theory assists nurses to understand the experiential nature of the helping process in psychiatric nursing. It is, of course, unique to the nursing situation and to no other professional work situation. It ought not to be lifted from any other professional literature, although statements by others are useful in helping nurses to interpret the uniqueness of the work situation and the work role.

Comprehensive study of nurses and patients in psychiatric facilities is just beginning. Not all nurses appreciate such study. I noticed in an October, 1954 issue of *Nursing Research* that one reader complained, "These were interesting studies but they seem to weight [the journal] too heavily in psychiatric nursing." I, for one, would like to see more studies pertaining to actual care of patients. A study of what goes on between psychiatric nurses and psychiatric patients in the ward as a social context is needed in every psychiatric facility. What goes on in "the other twenty-three hours a day" in the situation of inpatients who are fortunate enough to have an hour of daily psychotherapy is not actually known. The nurse, theoretically, is closest to the patient, over the longest period of time; therefore, the nurse has unlimited possibilities for observation and intervention favorable to patients. Psychiatric nurses have dimly known this for a long time. It is my hope that each nurse who feels responsibility about it will seek needed training to make himself or herself competent for the complex but vastly interesting task that is ours. The role of psychiatric nurse is crucial; the variations of this work role are crucial: the way nurses in psychiatry carry out customary nursing procedures; the way they execute managerial functions; the pattern of socialization they set up in relationships with patients; the educational experiences they provide for patients; and their therapeutic intervention in situations of anxiety, panic, dread, loneliness, terror, hallucinatory experiences, and the like.

The role of psychiatric nurse is not only crucial in what happens to patients, it is also exceedingly complex. Specifically, it involves many roles and movement from one to another based on the nurse's judgment of what is needed. Nurses work in an interpersonal situation and in a hospital social system and this demands shifts in the nurses' responses. Nurses need to be aware of what is gong on in nurse-patient interpersonal situations, and alert to what that situation calls for. They need to know the particular role well enough to assist the patient in receiving the help inherent in the various roles. I have been working in private practice for nearly a year and one-half, studying the movement in psychiatric nurse participation in nursing situations, but it will be another year before I am prepared to say anything significant about it. In the meantime, however, I am learning a good deal about the use of interpersonal theory in developing nursing theory and practice.

UNDERSTANDING INTERPERSONAL PRACTICE

Two major problems of psychiatric patients are communication and relatedness difficulties. The nurse can offer a patient an experience leading toward a feeling of being understood and of being respected, of being related to another human being. How this works out in practice can be seen from the following examples.

On the first day I spent with one patient I was observing I tried to be generally helpful in responding to her requests. The patient spent a good deal of time calling "help," saying "I'm dying," or crying softly to herself. About four hours after my arrival the patient said, "Hold my hand." Now, this, as you know, is a seductive maneuver that in our culture can have a great many meanings, including a childlike pleading for maternal closeness, a gesture of friendship, or a wish for physical closeness to another individual. Obviously the patient and I were strangers so I could not know what this request really meant. Nor is the nurse a mind reader. So I asked, "May we talk about how my holding your hand would help you?" The patient immediately became more anxious, as indicated by restlessness. I commented, "You can talk about what you are thinking or feeling." The patient replied, "If you must know, I have the feeling I am slipping, slipping off the bed, and I have never told that to anyone before." The nurse asked, "Now that you have brought it into the open, how do you feel?"

The patient, it would seem, was suggesting she experienced a sense of deterioration, for she was not literally slipping off the bed. She had already been sick some 15 years and had many exposures to outpatient and institutional efforts at getting well. After this feeling was revealed and talked about, as the object of inquiry by nurse and patient, the patient dropped off to sleep.

Several days later the patient again started crying, then commented directly about a feeling of "slipping." Immediately she became so anxious that visual and auditory hallucinations were employed to convey what was going on intrapersonally. A hallucination is an inner event expressed as though it were an outer event. The nurse moved closer toward the bedside and said, "You can describe what you are seeing and hearing; you can talk about your experience." This statement had to be repeated in voice tones that communicated the nurse was not terrorized, as was the patient. The need for repetition is understandable if you consider the concept of anxiety that indicates that the perceptual field narrows in the greatly anxious individual. The patient truly could not grasp what the nurse said because anxiety restricted what she could notice. However, the patient finally described, in a fairly vivid way, the nature of her hallucinatory experience, first the present one and then one similar to it she underwent several years prior. After describing, the patient felt more able, more powerful, more respectful of her own capacities. Her anxiety therefore lessened. The nurse then asked, "What does the content mean to you?" The patient said, as many nurses would say concerning their dreams, "It doesn't mean anything to me as it stands." The nurse replied, "Well, talk about it and perhaps together you and I can make some sense out of it." Then the patient began to speculate about and discuss various aspects of the hallucinatory content. Eventually, the obvious meaning occurred to her. In this way it was possible to use an immediate experience of the patient, undergone in a nursing situation, to help the patient to unveil a truth about herself.

The patient said that people had always given her orders, which she followed uncritically, and when the orders turned out to be nonsense, she followed them anyway. The tendency to follow directions uncritically was elaborately represented in the hallucination as described by the patient; the interpretation of the hallucination, linking her life experiences with the hallucinatory content, was made by the patient. The patient sighed, knowingly, after formulating this truth about her living, and dropped off to sleep. After three more such hallucinatory experiences in the following weeks the patient not only stopped using hallucinations as the initial mode of experience and communication with the nurse but she was also no longer terrorized by the possibility of hallucinating. This is to say that hallucinating was now an experience about which she knew something; therefore she was not powerless, not the unwitting victim. She recognized that hallucinations do not just happen; rather, they have meaning and have purposeful use. Initially, the patient said repeatedly, "I know it means a hospital or sanitarium when this starts," a combination that spelled a double terror, for she did not get well in her several hospitalizations. Perhaps this is why the experience of hallucinating and "slipping" were combined with the statement about hospitals.

Because the nurse did not participate with the patient in the search for immediate relief, thereby avoiding squarely facing the immediate nursing problem, the patient's immediate experience became understood. The nurse assisted the patient toward clarification of an immediate event in which both had participated. Needless to say, in a situation of this kind, if the nurse is made anxious by her preconceptions of her role or by the patient's condition or the eventual disruption of the patient, he or she is not able to be helpful. Instead, an anxious nurse (who probably does not know she is anxious, only angry or upset) will contribute to the anxiety of the patient. The interpersonal communication of anxiety is one of its outstanding features.

Some months later the patient was vomiting. The nurse gave medication as prescribed by the physician, but this was regurgitated. The patient became increasingly anxious, as indicated by restlessness and agitation, and then asked the nurse to read from the newspapers as a diversion. While the nurse was reading from the Sunday papers the patient said, "Don't read any more of that, I have heard it all before." On the surface, this sounded like a smug, arrogant remark. The nurse, sensing the general theme, commented, "You mean it all seems familiar?" The patient said, "It is familiar, read something else." So the nurse selected another section of the paper, and again the patient commented that everything seemed familiar. Then the patient said, "Get that new book over there; I haven't read that; I want to test whether that will be familiar too." The nurse read a portion of the book. The patient, obviously more anxious than before, as shown by exasperation, said, "That is familiar too." The nurse realized there was a similarity between this and hallucinatory experience, that is, the patient was dealing with an inner experience in a highly disguised way. The nurse then said quite directly, "It obviously is not the reading material that is familiar. The newspaper just came. The book is new. It must be something in this situation of you and me that is familiar." The patient asked, "What could it be?" The nurse replied, "We can find out. Have you ever been sick in this way before?" The patient commented, "The only thing that comes to my mind was the time I had my tonsils out. My mother came and she brought me some lemonade and said, 'This will make you better.' But it didn't; it hurt my throat." The nurse said, "So what is the connection with this situation of you and me?" With some further discussion the patient was able to formulate that what was familiar was a feeling of being in a situation with a trusted person who is counted on for help that fails to effect relief from discomfort and instead makes that discomfort worse. This was what the nurse represented to the patient when the medication failed to work as expected. The vomiting ceased with the formulation of this "inner truth" about the patient's experience. These instances of nurse-patient interpersonal relationships suggest several generalizations. However, these are merely suggested inasmuch as data presented here are brief and insufficient to support statements of principle. The instances mentioned suggest that:

The feelings of a patient regarding an immediate experience in a nursing situation, in which nurse and patient participate, are objects of mutual inquiry that leads to favorable improvement for the patient.

The meaning of an immediate experience of the patient in a nursing situation can be interpreted by the patient, with assistance of the nurse who aids the patient to formulate meanings by use of intelligent, alert listening, raising crucial questions, and other related forms of nurse participation.

An immediate experience of the nurse and/or nursing situation by a patient may be representative of older experiences the patient has undergone in the past. The meaning of the immediate experience and its connections with generically older events can be grasped by the patient and stated with the assistance of a nurse. The formulations made by the patient lead to relief of a symptom or some other form of nonrational experience and communication such as hallucinatory experiences.

FAVORABLE CHANGE

The three situations I described earlier, of the pediatric nurse, the male nurse, and the nursing student, indicate how the needs and preconceptions of the nurse function as barriers that interfere with the quality of nursing service. I am assuming that qualitative nursing service has as its goal improvement favorable for the patient. It is possible to interpret favorable change in a number of ways. For some nurses, favorable change is interpreted when the patient conforms to most of the patterns of behavior that are familiar to the nurse or generally acceptable in a ward situation. In the situation with the male nurse indicated earlier, it is likely that he would interpret favorable change when the patient no longer volunteered complaints to him. There is a good deal written in psychiatric nursing literature about "habit training" (Noyes, 1947; Steel, 1938). A nurse who subscribed to this opinion about "what should be done" would regard tidiness, for example, as a favorable change in an untidy patient. In contrast, it is possible to interpret favorable change by how the patient handles immediate experiences, particularly in regard to qualitative shifts in the patient's thinking. For example, in the instance I discussed earlier where the patient was experiencing "familiarity" in the nursing situation, recall that, in the course of my inquiring as to what was actually going on, the patient asked the nurse to read from a new book "to test" whether that too would be familiar. Here then was a favorable improvement. The patient herself was taking an active part in collecting data needed to understand an immediate experience. This was a favorable improvement over the abilities shown in the first instance, where even simple description of an immediate experience was most painstaking.

ROLE EXPECTATIONS IN THE NURSE-PATIENT RELATIONSHIP

As you can see then, role expectations are a complicated, complex matter. Consider what the nurse and patient expect of themselves and of each other in psychiatric situations if the general hospital view of nurse and patient are held. In the general hospital, complicated technical functions and customary nurse performances, such as bathing, feeding, medicating, and carrying out procedures often lead to satisfaction responses in both nurse and patient. Shorn of these performances in psychiatric facilities the nurse feels lost, useless, and the patient feels neglected, deprived. In the psychiatric situation, a whole new series of interpersonal techniques is needed. The problem, however, is that the nurse has not learned them in the professional program. If the nurse does not initiate techniques, the patient cannot expect them. In fact, the patient has no reason to believe the nurse's proper role includes anything other than custodial responsibilities. Nurses generally have not prepared themselves for situational interviewing, marginal counseling, consciously executed experiential relationships with patients, and other interpersonal techniques that would be useful. That is, we are just beginning to build a new set of expectations of the role of nurse in psychiatry.

An emergency situation in a general hospital means a call for an intern, the hurried preparation of a hypodermic, an oxygen tank, a respirator, or blood plasma. Something dramatic happens that calls out a response to affect the patient favorably. Emergency situations in psychiatric hospitals include such disruptive social events as panic, terror, loneliness, isolation-withdrawal, and hallucinations. They do not necessarily or always merit a call to the physician. Often they lead to seclusion, restraint, sedation, or electric shock, to experiences the patient might interpret as abandonment, punishment, or further social isolation. Ideally, these emergency situations require alert nurse participation over long periods of time with skilled specialists in psychiatric nursing. Psychiatric patients are persons in serious trouble unable to extricate themselves. They are not unlike patients, then, in general hospitals. But the expectation of help may not be fulfilled. Perhaps because psychiatric emergencies with psychiatric patients are more nebulous, less technically oriented, they therefore generate feelings of helplessness, fear, and loss of power on the part of both nurse and patient. Emergency situations represent crucial elements of nurse-patient role interaction in psychiatric facilities and encompass good points for further study. How do nurses and patients relate to each other when the patient's behavior is disruptive? What actually goes on?

What goes on between nurses and patients seems to be related to the expectations that each hold of the sick role and nurse role. When nurses are aware of what some of these interacting expectations are, then the nurse-patient relationship can be reviewed and perhaps transformed to a more useful therapeutic one. I have been reviewing data I collected in nursing situations in private practice in terms of the expectations that nurses and patients hold in experiences they have had with nurses or hospitals. There is some consistency in my data on the following:

If the patient is physically helpless, the nurse is expected to take over; both nurses and patients agree on this. Also, they both view the physical helplessness as largely temporary. What the nurse is doing for the patient, he or she will at some future date do. Both are aware of and know a good deal about the customary activities of bathing, feeding, bed making, dressing, and cleanliness. These are cultural preoccupations, as any series of magazine advertisements will let you know. On the other hand, most often, what is expected of a psychiatric nurse beyond care for physical incapacitation is not clearly formulated. As one patient put it, "I expected help from them but I don't know just what kind. It is hard to think back to where I discovered through testing that I couldn't find out. So I moved from expecting help to seeing if they knew as much as I did about psychiatry and if they didn't, then there was no point in expecting anything anyway."

One feature stands out in my work with patients, at least to me. All the patients had to work at developing new expectations of the nurse, as represented by me. They gave recognition to this with various comments that signified "You are different; you work differently from other nurses; you must be a psychologist." The patient is more aware of the nurse as a person, and as a professional worker who ought to have specialized knowledge useful to the patient, than is ordinarily realized. One patient put it this way: "The incompleteness of Miss Jones carries out in her body, in the way she moves, sings, stoops down; and her hair was most becoming but she was an incessant, a ridiculous person who strewed hairpins. There her awareness stopped." Or another patient, who commented, "The nurse ought to see the patient as a person whose opinions and feelings she is looking for, not somebody to classify according to cultural or moral significance. She should be here only to help the patient see better for himself." This patient continued, "When the nurse isn't interested in me then I show interest in her and this can be anything from a minor extraction of her opinions to getting her to reveal her life history to me." Or still another patient, "We used to try to get the gist of the framework of what the nurse wants to put things in and then take on the game of fitting the facts of life, our life on the ward, into what she wanted but we knew all the time that what we got out of it was nothing, just zero."

Often, in psychiatric inpatients, perception is focused on one thing or at the most a few things. In general, that one focus is "to get out; to get home." More often than not it is this expectation rather than anticipation of help that governs the patient's behavior. In this regard, psychiatric patients tend to view the nurse as a "go-between who gives information to the doctor." Several patients described to me how they spent time determining what to tell the nurse so that convincing information about their improvement reached the doctor who would discharge them. Everyone knows that it is the doctor's decision to discharge patients, but the patients also know that the information that gets to the doctor helps determine that decision. Consequently, the patients communicate among themselves about "what gets you out," and the nurses unwittingly participate. All the patients I worked with commented that they expected the nurse to "be fun," "good company," or "to give the right information to doctors," but none thought of her as a source of constructive help, or therapeutic assistance, only as an ally who could help the patient "to get out." One patient commented, "We had sort of a scale of all the useful people, from the most to the least powerful persons, who had something to do with our getting out and saw to it that we weren't disagreeable. We didn't fight with them." The patient who is so disturbed that he or she cannot share this common focus is a rarity but even these patients, eventually, come to see the nurse as a stepping-stone to discharge. Health as a goal is subordinate, yet it sometimes glimmers.

In the spring, when the Rutgers students were at Greystone State Hospital, we heard patients comment to one another, "Those nurses in gray, if you can get to talk with one of them, they can really help you." In general, however, patients recognize fairly soon that nurses expect them to behave, not to quarrel, to eat, to go to bed nicely, and to stay clean. If patients act on these nurse expectations the chances of getting out are better, even though their thinking disorders have not in any way been touched upon during hospitalization. Patients know that it is their behavior that is watched and that how they act determines if and when they will get out. Interestingly, all the patients with whom I have worked knew there was no relation between actual favorable improvement in them and in their getting out. As one patient put it, "The courageous patient can ignore the 'maze' aspect and persist in revealing his problems in the hope of getting help, but then he is sent to the back wards or given a lobotomy." Or another, "What a thousand patients say makes no difference because the nurses wouldn't notice it anyway. They have a prescribed method and it tells them what they will see, and so they are no longer free to see anything else about the patient, and when the patient catches on to this he has to choose between getting out or staying forever where nobody really listens."

These statements from patients suggest direction. It is possible for psychiatric nurses to better understand nurse-patient and nurse-patient-system interactions and integrations. Each nurse has a contribution to make in the definition of sick role and nurse role in psychiatric situations, and of what should go on in the interpersonal nurse-patient situation. If you remember just one message, I hope that it will be to recognize the importance and great need to study the role of nurse and the role of patient in psychiatric nursing situations and the interaction of expectations regarding these roles in your ward and in the hospital in which you work. I hope that you will make time for study of this aspect of your everyday work. Unless you find out what actually goes on, what expectations of nurse and patient now interact, you will not be in a position to facilitate changes. This is one area in which interpersonal theory can be of help to you; it can assist in identifying for yourself the baseline of all change by truly understanding what goes on currently.

REFERENCES

Noyes, A. P., & Haydon, E. (1947). *Textbook of psychiatric nursing.* New York: Macmillan.
Steele, K. McL. (1938). *Psychiatric nursing.* Philadelphia: Davis.

CHAPTER 2

Theory: The Professional Dimension

One of the most important tasks before the profession of nursing is to establish the nature and uses of theory in professional nursing practice. It is not an easy task. Similarly, to present a paper on an aspect of this task to this group of nurse scientists is not exactly the most comfortable experience. Recently, Merton (1969) published an illuminating essay in which is included a description of the climate of scientific communities similarly at work on the task of clarifying and validating scientific theories that are proposed:

> The organization of science operates as a system of institutionalized vigilance, involving competitive cooperation. It affords both commitment and reward for finding where others have erred or have stopped before tracking down the implications of their results or have passed over in their work what is there to be seen by the fresh eye of another. In such a system, scientists are at the ready to pick apart and appraise each new claim to knowledge. This unending exchange of critical judgement, of praise and punishment, is developed in science to a degree that makes the monitoring of children's behavior by their parents seem little more than child's play. Only after the originality and

Reprinted from *Proceedings of the First Nursing Theory Conference*, pp. 33–46. University of Kansas Medical Center, Department of Nursing Education, March 20–21, 1969. Publication of the Conference Proceedings was supported by PHS, Division of Nursing, Research Grant No. NU 00309-01. Copyright 1969 by Hildegard E. Peplau. Reprinted with permission.

consequence of his work have been attested by significant others can the scientist feel reasonably confident about it. Deeply felt praise for work well done, moreover, exalts donor and recipient alike; it joins them both in symbolizing the common enterprise. That, in part, expresses the character of competitive cooperation in science. (p. 220)

There are many forms of theory. In this paper, the use of established theoretical concepts and processes, and the development of knowledge from observations in nursing situations will be described. These are but two small aspects of the larger task—clarifying the nature and uses of scientific knowledge in nursing.

USES OF ESTABLISHED THEORETICAL CONCEPTS AND PROCESSES

Nursing, like other professions, is primarily an applied science. It uses established knowledge for beneficial purposes. One such use is the application of known concepts and processes to observations made in nursing situations. Such application serves the purposes of interpretation of observational data and the derivation of theory-based nursing actions (Peplau, 1968).

In nursing practice, the starting point is something observed during a contact with a patient. The name of a particular concept, relevant to that particular observation—or to a selection of the more crucial among diverse phenomena observed at a particular moment—"flips up" in the mind of the professional. Thus naming, categorization, or classification of observed phenomena is a first step in application of theory in nursing practice. It occurs at the point of observation especially for the most effective nursing interventions in instances of crucial observations. Thus, the nurse who observes blood in some amount on the body and sheets of the bed of a patient, "flips up" a concept such as "bleeding" or "hemorrhage"—i.e., choosing this concept—nursing interventions deriving from this concept are likely to follow. It is this point—of using available concepts to name and thus to begin to explain observed phenomena and to derive theory-based nursing actions—which is glaringly omitted in two recent publications on the subject of nursing theory (Dickoff & James, 1968; Sarosi, 1968).

Naming the phenomena observed, however, is only the first step. The professional goes beyond mere naming (although in some fields, such as psychiatric work, it is not uncommon to note concepts used in a "name-calling," derogating sense). A second step in the application of a selected concept to observation is to use the concept definition as a structured format for obtaining more information, by observation or interviewing (see Table 2.1; see also Bullough & Bullough, 1966; Mereness, 1966; Peplau, 1962). Such data collection may widen the base of information obtained. Thus, a concept selected initially may be discarded and still other concepts, which arise in the mind of the professional in relation to observations of data being obtained, provide a basis for a new selection of a concept for application. As data being obtained becomes clearer, a particular explanatory concept tends to be selected and its definitional format ultimately serves a third step, which is to consider options for resolution of the difficulty and to judge which option to use.

Known concepts, defined in operational terms—by stating in serial order of emergence those behaviors generally associated with that concept—thus serve several purposes: (1) naming observed phenomena; (2) providing a structure for obtaining more information; and (3) suggesting resolution options relevant to the particular phenomena that were noticed. A professional encounter—whether the nurse–patient contact is for a duration of ten or one hundred minutes—is a very fluid interaction in which the professional uses observation, then interpretation of observed phenomena, and then responds with theory-based interventions.* Such encounters thus

---

* There is also a fourth step in the total process of professional thought at the "bedside" and that is: evaluation of effects of interventions on the phenomena observed and interpreted. Such continuing evaluations, over time, lead to standardization of practices in relation to observation of known phenomena. Such standardized practices can then be developed into manuals for technical nursing practice. Such manuals would (1) point out what to look for—what can be observed under certain circumstances; (2) what to do when such observations are noticed; and (3) a reason or rationale for the action—which, in effect, is a simplified restatement of the theory used by the professional as described above. Thus, technical nursing has to do with known or standardized nursing practices as these have been evolved by professional nurses through repeated use of the four steps described in relation to particular phenomena seen in nursing situations.

TABLE 2.1 Format for Definition and Application of Theoretical Concepts in Nursing Practice.

Serial order of emergence of observable behaviors associated with the concept	Structure for obtaining more information about a specific problematic situation by further observation or interviewing, inherent in concept definition	Structure of resolution options inherent in concept definition for choice of theory-based nurse actions based upon professional judgment of which option to use first
A. Concept of Frustration		
1. A Goal is set.	What Goal? Is it attainable? When set? Was it clearly formulated? Expressed to others?	Identify the goal. Give up the Goal. Revise the Goal. Discuss Goal with others.
2. There is movement toward the Goal.	What strategies? Were these reasonable? Were these clearly related to Goal?	Change strategies. Acquire new ones if needed
3. An Obstacle prevents goal achievement.	What obstacle? External or internal? Can it be removed or bypassed?	Remove or bypass the obstacle.
4. Aggression is felt and expressed. Directly toward the obstacle. Indirectly away from the obstacle.	Was the relation of Aggression to Goal, movement, and/or obstacle recognized?	Formulate the relation.
B. Anxiety		
1. An expectation (wish, desire, goal, etc.) becomes operative.	What expectations? Is it attainable? Was it communicated to the other(s) in the situation?	Connect the anxiety and expectations. Give up the expectation. Revise the expectation in relation to what is possible. Communicate the expectation.
2. The expectation is not met.		
3. Extreme discomfort and internal tension is experienced.	Discomfort experienced where—what part of the body?	Name the experience as anxiety.

TABLE 2.1 *(Continued)*

Serial order of emergence of observable behaviors associated with the concept	Structure for obtaining more information about a specific problematic situation by further observation or interviewing, inherent in concept definition	Structure of resolution options inherent in concept definition for choice of theory-based nurse actions based upon professional judgment of which option to use first
4. The energy from the tension is converted, more or less automatically (without thought) into "relief behavior."	What pattern of behavior is used? Is there a series of relief behaviors that are used? Does the series recur in the same order in subsequent anxiety-producing behaviors. The amount of anxiety is also inferred from the relief behaviors.	Connect the anxiety and relief behavior. Name the relief behavior.
5. Relief is felt and justified or rationalized.		

require the professional to have in mind readily available to recall, the definitional components of those concepts crucial to the recurring phenomena pertinent to nursing situations, conscious and well-disciplined use of procedures of theory applications of different types, and critical judgment so as to discriminate and select well from among resolution options that are available.

There are, of course, conceptions—ideas, generalizations—which cannot be used in the manner described, which do not have the specificity, but which are useful in other ways. Whorf's idea that "language influences thought" (and with rare exceptions, not the other way around) can be extended by stating that: (1) language influences thought; (2) thought then influences action; (3) thought and action taken together evoke feelings in relation to a situation or context. The only specificity, then, is in terms of nursing actions—the suggestion that impact upon language behavior of patients is the major point of corrective impact for disturbance of action and feeling. In psychiatric work, that is an important testable hypothesis rather than an explanatory concept at this time.

A concept, as used narrowly in this paper is explanatory of a fairly small amount of behavior. On the other hand, a process represents many concepts, which, taken together, provide explanations of a broader range of behavior. The processes of development, socialization, learning, hallucinations, provide instances (Peplau, 1963). A process is, in effect, an organization of concepts into larger components—called phases, stages—each of which includes a series of separate concepts arranged in a serial order showing the emergence of particular behaviors. Thus, the process of development shows concepts explanatory of some behaviors seen in such phases as infancy, childhood, juvenile era, et cetera—both phases and concepts being arranged in the order in which such behaviors ordinarily evolve (see Appendix, this chapter).

A process provides a somewhat different definitional format for application in professional practice. Each concept can, of course, be used separately as described previously. The definitional format of the entire process, however, provides a structure for observations of several kinds. The process of personality development provides an instructive instance. (1) The professional can place observed behavior within the established structure. Thus, the behavior of a 30-year-old may be recognized as more compatible with an 8-year-old, at a given moment of observation. (2) The process definition can be used to anticipate subsequent behavior that should follow observed behavior (as in the case of a healthy child observed *vis-a-vis* the process of development). (3) The process definition can be used to place current behavior *and* to identify "next-step" behavior that should be stimulated. Thus, a patient who uses competition recurringly, may need help to learn behaviors that tend to evolve subsequently such as compromise and cooperation. The process-definitional structure for development can be used to map out age-related interpersonal competencies that are observable in a patient, those that are lacking, and the serial order of development of such competencies can be followed to design a nursing care plan. Such a plan should help patients to gain interpersonal competencies lacking by reason of unfortunate experience, lacks in growth opportunities, or the effects of disease processes upon human functioning.

To this point, this paper has suggested some important uses for established theory in the clinical practice of nursing. It might be useful to keep in mind Stainbrook's noteworthy observation that "some professionals use theory the way a drunk uses a lampost—for support rather than for illumination." What has been suggested here is the use of known concepts and processes for illumination of clinical observations in nursing, a purpose that requires considerable development of intellectual competencies in professional nurses through collegiate education.

DEVELOPMENT OF KNOWLEDGE FROM OBSERVATIONS IN NURSING SITUATIONS

Theory represents a formulation of the meaning of observed phenomena in an order or form that enables the formulation to be used to explain similar phenomena, observed in other situations of like kind, and to guide the professional in choosing interventions relevant to the phenomena observed. Theoretical concepts, therefore, are a shared explanatory language—a shortcut language—of particular use to professionals in the field to which those concepts pertain and from which they were derived. Nursing situations provide a field of observations from which unique nursing concepts can be derived and used for the improvement of the professional's work.

Concepts generally derive first from empirical observations—an astute clinician noting a phenomenon about which there is a question. In another context, Davis gives a description of this process of "the irrepressible and cyclical gropings of intent minds to *solve a puzzle* that has resisted solution." (1969, pp. 53–56) He says:

> In his description of the quest for a solution, Watson makes us intimate witness to the frailties, opportunities, and unsuspected resources of the creative thinker, be he scientist, artist, or man of affairs; the false starts, the moody setting asides and quirkish picking ups, the imaginative though empirically unsubstantiated leaps forward, the profoundly deflating collapse of an apparently promising line of inquiry, the ego-massaging rehearsals of fantasized future fame, the long-neglected clue thrust suddenly and inexplicably into consciousness and last, though not least, the serendipitous chance remark of a colleague working on seemingly unrelated problems. Instead of some simple-minded cognitive linear progression from problem to solution, Watson gives us

a much richer, multi-level, and emergent rendition of the discovery process; a kind of dialectical backing and filling in which concept, data, and empirical focus constantly interact upon each other until some convincing, internally consistent explanation is finally achieved.

And that is pretty much how it will be in delineating concepts relevant to phenomena seen in nursing practice. To name them, as was suggested earlier, is to have at least the name of the concept in mind. As yet, there is not available an organized nomenclature of such phenomena. A second, very important task of the profession of nursing is to develop a nomenclature of nursing problems and to define these concepts in ways that serve to explain the phenomena and to guide nursing actions. In order to do this, the parameters of the field of nursing—in relation to other disciplines—may need to be clarified. Nursing can take as its unique focus *the reactions of the patient or client to the circumstances of his illness or health problem,* thus overlapping medicine only when dealing with disease processes more directly (Mereness, 1966; Peplau, 1955). Assuming that illness provides an opportunity for learning and growth through exposure to professionals, the stress of the event providing the energy, the profession could stake a *claim to a focus on helping patients to gain intellectual and interpersonal competencies beyond that which they have at the point of illness, by gearing nursing practices to evolving such competencies through nurse-patient interactions* (Gregg, 1954; Mereness, 1966).

In order to derive nursing concepts, then, professional nurses would take note of reactions of patients—to illness, hospitalization, effects of these upon life and living—observing those behaviors for which no explanatory concepts are as yet available. Such observations would be sought in other patients, under similar circumstances (Rouslin, 1963). As observations continued, certain regularities would begin to appear—concerning the nature of the data being observed. Thus, a name for the phenomena would occur to the professional. Subsequently, with further observations the concept of the phenomenon would become clearer—and thus be defined and tested against still other patients. Eventually, useful interventions would be derived from the explanation of the phenomenon and the effects of these interventions upon it also tested.

Nursing concepts, thus, are the result of a search for recurring phenomena seen in nursing situations. These regularities are then observed in greater detail and their variations and dimensions made more explicit. Initial formulation of the concept then serves as a format for more systematic observations in many similar situations and perhaps even by other observers. Thus a system to record recurring instances of like kind or similar to the phenomenon in question would have to be devised. The initial concept becomes a structured matrix for subsequent observations, and for locating the scope of variations in the particular phenomenon. The initial concept also provides the name (i.e., the concept of) of the phenomenon, while subsequent observations assure identification of all of the behaviors associated with that particular concept.

There are, to be sure, some reactions of patients about which much is already known and concepts are available in the literature (Burd & Marshall, 1963). Denial of illness is one such reaction. But denial is a concept used by other professions. Consequently, what may be needed at this time is a survey of published nursing literature to locate those concepts, if any, which are solely used by nurses and those shared with other disciplines in the health field. Meanwhile, the search for new concepts derived from nursing situations must and will go on.

SUMMARY

In this paper the use of theoretical concepts and processes already known has been described. An approach to obtaining nursing concepts has been discussed.

REFERENCES

Bullough, B., & Bullough, V. (1966). *Issues in Nursing* (pp. 232–242). New York: Springer Publishing Company.

Burd, S.F., & Marshall, M.A. (1963). *Some clinical approaches to psychiatric nursing.* New York: Macmillan.

Davis, F. (1969). *The double helix* by James Watson (book review). *Transaction, 6*(5), 53–56.

Dickoff, J., & James, P. (1968). A theory of theories: A position paper. *Nursing Research, 17*(3), 197–203.

Gregg, D. (1954). The psychiatric nurse's role. *American Journal of Nursing, 54*(7), 848–851. (Reprinted in D. Mereness, work cited, Vol. 1; pp. 178–185.)

Mereness, D. (1966). *Psychiatric nursing* (2 vols.). Dubuque, IA: Brown.

Merton, R.K. (1969). Behavior patterns of scientists. *The American Scholar, 38*(2), 197–220.

Peplau, H.E. (1955). Loneliness. *American Journal of Nursing, 55*(12), 1476–1481. (Reprinted in D. Mereness, work cited, Vol. 2; pp. 66–76.)

Peplau, H.E. (1962). Interpersonal techniques: The crux of psychiatric nursing. *American Journal of Nursing, 62*(6), 50–54.

Peplau, H.E. (1963, October–November). Interpersonal relations and the process of adaptation. *Nursing Science*, pp. 272–279.

Peplau, H.E. (1968). Operational definitions and nursing practice. In L.T. Zderad & H.C. Belcher, *Developing behavioral concepts in nursing* (pp. 12–15). Atlanta, GA: Southern Regional Education Board.

Rouslin, S. (1963). Chronic helpfulness: Maintenance and intervention. *Perspectives of Psychiatric Care, 1*(1), 25–28.

Sarosi, Grace M. (1968). A critical theory: The nurse as a fully human person. *Nursing Forum, 7*(4), 349–363.

Appendix

The "Tools and Tasks Outline" that is attached was prepared by a group of graduate students in partial fulfillment of requirements for the Master's degree at Teachers College, Columbia University, 1951. The title of the study was: *A Shift in Thinking: Instrument and Manual for Understanding Behavior.* Regrettably, the work was not published. The psychiatric nurses who participated in the preparation of this outline were Mrs. Elrose Daniels, Helen D. Johnson, E. Katherine LeVan (Fountain House, New York City), Claire Mintzer Fagin (Faculty, New York University), Janesy B. Myers (V. A., Northport, Long Island), Naomi Perry, Catherine M. Thilgen, and Gwen Tudor Will.

This instrument was constructed following a review of published literature of 26 authors; 13 of these were selected for study and synthesis and for development of the outline which shows developmental eras and two types of behavior (Tools and Tasks) characteristic of these eras. The outline was then used to classify behavior described in 184 situations—selected according to preestablished criteria. Validation of placement was secured by a panel of experts including Dr. Barbara Biber (Bank Street School), Dr. George Devereaux (anthropologist), Esther Garrison, R.N. (NIMH), Dr. Arthur Jersild (educator, Teachers College), Dr. Norman Kelman (psychoanalyst), Emmy Lanning Schockly, R.N., Dr. Irving Lorge, Jeannette Regensburg (Community Service Society, New York), Dr. Morris Schwartz (sociologist), Dr. Ellen Simor (psychoanalyst), and Dr. Otto Will (psychoanalyst). The results from the placement of 184 situations by graduate students and 29 situations by the jury of experts proved the instrument to be valid and reliable for categorizing presenting behavior according to guides provided in the Tools and Tasks Outline.

The outline was developed as an educational tool to indicate a common frame of reference regarding behavior characteristic of eras of development and constructive capacities that can be released for growth.

The outline has been used in clinical workshops for nurses as a basis for discussion of "tools" and "tasks" that emerge, and can be observed in the behavior of persons, during the process of normal growth and development. Discussion of each tool and task—its definition, its manifestation and variations shown in presenting behavior—leads to understanding of phenomena to be observed. When a variation of a particular tool or task is observed, in the presenting behavior of a patient hospitalized in a psychiatric facility, the outline can then serve to indicate the current "tools and tasks" used by a patient and the next steps in that patient's development which require the help of nursing services if the patient's growth is to be promoted.

HILDEGARD E. PEPLAU

DEFINITIONS

Tool: The instrument by which learning is effected or accomplished. Each individual has capacities that usually ripen and are available at each era of development.

Task: A learning experience that arises at or about a certain period in the life of an individual, as a result of biological maturation, cultural pressures, and level of aspiration. Each task that has been learned becomes a tool for the next era.

Learning: A process where capacities are actualized in the direction of growth or forward movement. This formulation is particularly oriented toward learning to live with people.*

Era: A period in time distinguished by certain criteria of a physiological or psychological nature. Each era usually has some

---

* Different from conditioning, i.e., adapting behavior to the situation merely in terms of tension reduction.

characteristics of preceding eras, but is sufficiently different quantitatively and qualitatively to differentiate it from other eras.

NOTE: Mastery of task plus movement toward a next task requires the exercise of the capacities of tools available. This leads to development of skill in their use.

Tools and Tasks Outline

Infancy: The period of living that starts with the birth of the individual and proceeds to emergence of the capacity for communication through speech, i.e., when child uses Mama or Dada in the mother–child relationship or father–child relationship. (0–1 1/2 years)

Tools	Tasks
1. *Cry and other prespeech* vocalizations are powerful tools available to the infant to call to the attention of the adults the infant's feelings and/or needs and, thus, to communicate with them.	1. *Learning to count on others to gratify needs and satisfy wishes.* a. Struggling to express needs. b. Accepting what is given with a feeling of comfort. c. Recognizing objects in immediate environment, i.e., significant people and things. d. Directing emotional expression to indicate needs and wishes. e. Beginning to see himself as separate from others.
2. *Mouth* is the tool for taking in (sucking), cutting off (biting), pushing out (spitting) and holding on to objects (mouthing or sucking) introduced by others in the situation.	
3. *The satisfaction response occurs* when the infant's biological needs are met and when a mutual feeling of comfort and fulfillment is emphasized by both. This is used by the infant as a tool in future relationships. . . . The needs of the infant are for nourishment, care and comfort. . . . The needs of the mother are to give these warmly to her infant.	
4. *Empathic observation* is a capacity arising in the infant that	

Tools and Tasks Outline *(Continued)*

Tools	Tasks

enables him to perceive the
feelings of others as his or her
own immediate feelings in the
situation.

5. *Autistic invention* is a primary
unsocialized state of symbol
activity that makes the infant
feel that he or she is master of
all he or she surveys. It is a
tool with which the infant sees
his or her environment in a
highly personal way.

6. Experiments, exploration, manipulation are tools infants use
to get acquainted with themselves and the things about
them. These activities are directed toward making the environment more familiar and less
threatening by the use of the
mouth, eyes, arms and legs in
reaching out, holding on, strik-
ing, feeling, rooting, playing,
etc. Masturbating may start as
an exploration of the body. Anxiety and autistic invention may
enter in—becomes habit with
comfort sought through oneself.

7. Emergency reactions arise in response to situations perceived
as threatening by the infant because they lead to reinforcement of feelings of helplessness
and powerlessness. The infant
responds by crying, increased
motor activity or apathy. Patterns of behavior arise to communicate greater striving for
help through increased struggle
or greater dependency. The infant responds with.

Tools and Tasks Outline *(Continued)*

Tools	Tasks
a. *Fear* that is called out by external events such as a sudden loud noise, sudden movements (falling) or sudden changes in the situation.	
b. *Rage* that is called out by external obstacles that limit efforts of expression.	
c. *Anxiety* that is the discomfort felt in infancy, which later becomes known as anxiety. It is empathized by the infant's experiencing contact with the mother or mother surrogate who is tense or generally uneasy. Anxiety is communicated between people in relation to internal events that may lie outside of their awareness, i.e.:	
1. One anxious person can make another person feel anxious.	
2. An individual may become anxious by concerning himself with an illusory image who makes the individual feel anxious.	

Childhood: The period of living that begins with the capacity for communication through speech and ends with a beginner need for association with compeers, i.e., when the child begins to form relationships with people of his or her own level who share his attitudes toward authority, activities, and the like. (1¹/₂–6 years)

Tools	Tasks
1. *Language* is a tool consisting of meaningful sounds used for verbal communication of needs and wishes.	1. *Learning to accept interference to his wishes in relative comfort.* a. Identifying and accepting self.

Tools and Tasks Outline *(Continued)*

Tools	Tasks
2. *Anus* is a tool of childhood used for giving or withholding a part of oneself to control significant people in his environment. It is used to express feelings (satisfaction-dissatisfaction, comfort-discomfort, power-powerlessness) in response to the present situation.	b. Seeing to own wishes in relation to the wishes of others.
	c. Recognizing that he has the power to stand alone to some degree.
3. *Self* is a tool made of reflected appraisals. The self-dynamism grows as it functions. The self perceives, organizes and uses experiences in terms of approval and disapproval, and in-attends or dissociates experiences not in accord with awareness.	d. Beginning to separate from parent and associate with agemates with interest.
	e. Awareness that postponing or delaying gratification of own wishes, in deference to others, may bring satisfaction.
4. *Autistic Invention* in childhood is the tool through which thoughts, feelings, and words have a magical power of fulfilling needs, wants, and wishes.	
5. *Experimentation, exploration, and manipulation.* In childhood there is a refinement of these tools. The child's aggressive behavior, his pushing forth in the world, his exhibitionism, imitation, curiosity, increased locomotion (walking), masturbation, and parallel play are his ways of becoming further acquainted with oneself and the things about one.	
6. *Identification* is a tool the child uses in an attempt to be like a person who is significant to him.	

Tools and Tasks Outline *(Continued)*

Tools	Tasks

7. *Emergency reactions* (as defined in infancy) which are used in this era are anger, shame, guilt, and doubt.

8. *Anxiety* is now recognized as anxiety rather than discomfort. It disciplines attention and restricts personal awareness. With the aid of significant adults this energy can be used to focus on learning.
   a. *Anger*—destructive feeling—thoughts which arise in response to a frustrating situation.
   b. *Shame*—feeling of self-consciousness and/or embarrassment that arises because the child feels that there is something unacceptable about his or her thoughts, feelings, or actions.
   c. *Guilt*—feeling state made up of shame and anger directed against oneself.
   d. *Doubt*—makes the child hesitate and/or question what he should or should not do. It helps the child through consistent experiences, to see relationships and lays the groundwork for later consensual validation and critical thinking.

Juvenile: The period of living that begins with the need for association with compeers and ends with the capacity to love, i.e., "When the satisfaction or the security of another person becomes as significant to one as is one's own satisfaction and security, then the state of love exists." (6–9 years)

Tools and Tasks Outline *(Continued)*

Tools	Tasks
1. *Competition* is a tool of the juvenile era used in contesting for affection and/or status with others. It is comprised of all activities that are involved in getting to a desired goal first.	1. *Learning to form satisfying relationships with compeers.*
	a. Loving from family to compeers for gratification.
	b. Testing sharing activities, attitudes, values, and beliefs of the peer group.
2. *Compromise* is a tool of the juvenile era that enables the child to give and take in a reciprocal relationship in order to maintain his own position.	c. Distinguishing different roles in the various social and authoritative situations.
	d. Acting out selected roles in different situations.
3. *Cooperation* is a tool of the juvenile era the child uses in maintaining his own position by adjusting and adapting to the wishes of others.	
4. *Experimentation, exploration, and manipulation.* In the juvenile era there is further refinement of these tools. The juvenile is experiencing learning as fun through cooperative play, recreation and sexual curiosity. These are his ways of becoming more aware of oneself and the world about one.	

Preadolescence: The period of living that begins with the capacity to love and ends with the first evidence of puberty, i.e., characteristic sexual changes. (9–12 years)

Tools	Tasks
1. *The capacity to love* is a tool in the preadolescent era that enables the individual to express oneself freely and naturally because he thinks as much of someone else as he thinks of himself. Tolerance, sympathy, generosity, and optimism flow	1. *Learning to relate to a chum of the same sex.*
	a. Identifying himself with peers of the same sex to the exclusion of peers of opposite sex.
	b. Being more loyal to chum than to family members.

Tools and Tasks Outline *(Continued)*

Tools	Tasks
out of this. (This capacity has its beginning in infancy with the satisfaction response.)	c. Becoming creative through expression of self.

2. *Consensual validation* is a tool in the preadolescent era that consists of talking things over, comparing notes with others and coming to a way of action. In this way, the preadolescent gets clear about the self and the world and is relieved of guilt feelings and anxiety.

3. *Collaboration* is a tool in the preadolescent era that is a step forward from cooperation. Achievement is no longer a personal success in terms of "we." He moves from his desire to maintain his position in the group to derive satisfaction from group accomplishment.

4. *Experimentation, exploration, and manipulation.* In the preadolescent era there is still further refinement of these tools. The preadolescent is experiencing an interest in learning as a way of implementing future living. He shows signs of rebellion through restlessness, hostility, irritability, taking less responsibility and becoming less obedient. These are ways of moving from "egocentricity toward a fully social state."

Early adolescence: The period of living that begins with the first evidence of puberty and ends with completion of psychological changes associated with primary and secondary sex changes. (12–14 years)

Tools and Tasks Outline *(Continued)*

Tools	Tasks
1. *Lust* as a tool of early adolescence "is a state of dissatisfaction that orients awareness toward the tendency to integrate situations chiefly affecting the genital zone." 2. *Experimentation, exploration, and manipulation.* In the early adolescent era there is continued refinement of these tools. The early adolescent is showing an intense interest in becoming an adult by actively rebelling against authority, engaging in fantasies, and over-identifying with heroes, cliques, and crowds. This results in a further realization of oneself as an individual in relation to other individuals. 3. *Anxiety* as used by the adolescent is a tool which restricts awareness so that he may function productively despite feelings of inadequacy and insecurity in this new role (guilt, shame, fears of not measuring up, or achieving full development). This is evidenced by his frequent moods of depression and exaltation.	1. *Learning to become independent.* a. Evaluating own limitations and powers. b. Examining and anticipating the consequences of own decisions. c. Evaluating critically ideals, beliefs, attitudes and values. 2. *Learning to establish satisfactory relationships with members of the opposite sex.* a. Accepting oneself as a sexual object. b. Finding suitable sex objects.

Late adolescence: The period of living that begins with the completion of the physiological changes and ends with the establishment of durable situations of intimacy, i.e., choice of love objects of opposite sex. (14–21 years)

Tools	Tasks
1. *The genital organs* are tools of the late adolescent era that are used for release of emotional tension through coitus in order	1. *Learning to become interdependent.* a. Tolerating anxiety and using it constructively.

Tools and Tasks Outline *(Continued)*

Tools	Tasks

that sexual satisfaction and procreation may take place.
 	
2. *Experimentation, exploration, and manipulation.* In the late adolescent era there is a special use of these tools in the sexual-social situation, i.e., in dating, dancing, sex play, socialized speech (repartee, "lines," jokes, etc.). Through these the late adolescent learns to pattern genital and social behavior.
	b. Establishing reciprocal relationships with his parents.
	c. Assuming responsibility for others.
	d. Making decisions and choices of far reaching importance for the future.
	e. Becoming economically, intellectually, and emotionally self-sufficient.
	
	2. *Learning to form a durable sexual relationship with a selected member of the opposite sex.*
	  a. Learning to verbalize consciously and to act out sexual interest.
	  b. Patterning of genital behavior.
	  c. Wooing and winning a mate with whom one develops
	    1. Willingness to share a mutual interest
	    2. Mutuality of orgasm
	    3. Willingness to share procreation
	    4. Willingness to regulate cycles of work and recreation.

CHAPTER 3

Interpersonal Relationships: The Purpose and Characteristics of Professional Nursing

Interpersonal relations is a developing body of scientific knowledge that can be used to explain observations and guide interventions. The knowledge pertains to observable phenomena that go on in an interaction between two or more people. A nurse-patient relationship is a specific kind of interaction that can be experienced, observed, interpreted, and regulated in accordance with useful theories. There is some effort toward and considerable interest in understanding nurse-patient relationships to make the participation of the nurse in them more meaningful and useful to the patient participants. Interpersonal theory, as a body of knowledge, therefore, is of great interest to nurses. It is not the only area of knowledge relevant to nursing practice; knowledge of anatomy, physiology, biochemistry, physics, microbiology, nutrition, and many other areas are also relevant to

Paper presented at Council of Hospital Services, District of Columbia-Delaware Hospital Association, Washington D.C., February, 1965. Schlesinger Library, Radcliffe College, Cambridge, MA. No. 84-M107, Hildegard E. Peplau Archives, carton 24, volume 834. Copyright 1986 by Schlesinger Library. Adapted and edited by permission.

nursing. For purposes of discussion, then, it is useful to single out one such area of scientific knowledge and to talk about its relevance to the practice of professional nursing.

THE PURPOSE OF PROFESSIONAL NURSING

I submit that the purpose of the nurse-patient relationship is somewhat different from the purpose of the nurse-doctor relationship, the doctor-patient relationship, the relationship between friends, chums, husband and wife, and so on. It is this purpose of the nurse-patient relationship that suggests many of the interpersonal characteristics of the nurse's participation in the nurse-patient situation. The purposes of the practices of a professional nurse are more than merely helping to heal the physical ailments of the patient, although of course this is one important activity of the nurse. The nurse, more than the physician, must relate meaningfully to the reaction of the patient to his or her illness, including the psychological and social changes that illness forces upon the patient. The nurse spends more time with the patient than does the physician, and therefore, has more opportunity not only to observe but also to talk with and come to know the patient. This time factor gives the nurse an opportunity to help the patient become aware of and make some sense out of his or her reactions to the current condition so that these can be more or less understood by the patient in light of long-range personal consequences.

The nurse has the opportunity to help the patient to learn something important about the self because illness forces a stock-taking that can lead to greater personal awareness. The nurse has an opportunity to convey health information because the patient needs it in order to make sense out of the experience of illness. These two items, awareness of self and health information, when promoted artistically and relevantly by the nurse, can strengthen the patient psychologically as a product of the physical or mental or psychosomatic illness. To implement a purpose of this nature requires that the professional nurse know a great deal about the theory and technique of interpersonal relations.

Let me add a word of caution. I am not suggesting that every professional nurse should be "omnipotent" and, therefore, able to bring about major sociopsychological changes in every patient with a few minutes of nurse–patient interaction. Instant personality change is not what is suggested here. What is suggested is utilization of available opportunities through the application of known theory and techniques of interpersonal relations. The opportunities are many. The nurse gives intimate and more total body care to patients than does the physician. Physical care of the body of another human being provides for a kind of "interpersonal intimacy," a closeness if you will, that more often than not cues off in the mind of the patient connections between the present circumstances and many earlier experiences that are somewhat similar. Indeed, merely showing interest, as for example when a public health nurse regularly visits a patient, gives an injection, and then tarries or talks, stimulates dormant memories of times when this happened—or should have—in the previous experience of the patient. In fact, "showing interest" is a powerful growth-provoking interpersonal competence about which nurses should know a great deal. A professional nurse sees patients under many types of informal conditions: at home with family members, in the hospital interacting with other patients who initially were strangers to the patient, in clinics interacting with other waiting clients, in schools and in industry.

All of these nurse–patient contacts provide openings for the nurse to implement the purpose of nursing—to find the ways to come to know a person, as a human being in difficulty—and to help that person to stretch his or her capabilities (if only one-quarter of an inch) and exercise innate capacities. For the patient, illness can be a source of new learning, leading to learning products that have immediate utility and carry-over effects into subsequent life situations. Seen in this light, the professional nurse provides a type of relationship that is special—unlike that of other professional disciplines and unlike relationships the patient may have with friends of his own choosing. In order, however, to provide this kind of more meaningful relationship, the nurse must be a sensitive observer and have a matrix of theory within which to interpret and extend observations, and on which to base the interpersonal actions of the nurse.

CHARACTERISTICS OF PROFESSIONAL NURSING

The foregoing purpose of professional nursing suggests relevant characteristics of the nurse's participation in the nurse-patient situation. I propose some of these characteristics, discuss them, and present further considerations of interpersonal relations in nursing.

The first characteristic of professional nursing is that the focus is on the patient. This characteristic, I believe, is the most difficult to maintain because it requires the nurse to attend to, relate herself to, and aid the patient in exploring his or her concerns and observations. Concerns of the patient are of two types: (1) those concerns having to do with the immediate situation, that is, the illness and the personal reaction to it, as well as its impact on the family and work; and (2) those concerns having to do with external events such as television or world affairs as events in the hospital situation that the patient has noticed or heard about and the like. To say that the focus is on the patient is to suggest that the focus is not on the nurse; that is, the nurse-patient situation is not an opportunity for the nurse to ventilate about her difficulties, anticipations, and hopes, or her concerns and workload. In working with nurses in a graduate program in psychiatric nursing, I am always struck by the enormous difficulty nurses have in shelving those personal nurse concerns and focusing on the experience of the patient. Of course, patients come to the nurse–patient situation with social skills along with the automatic expectation that these will be required in order to gain and retain the approval of the nurse. Patients, erroneously I believe, tend to have the notions that the nurse must be pleased with them, that the nurse will judge them in social terms, that the nurse's time is not really the patient's but is instead a test of the nurse's ability to make friends among patients. I think we ought to change these notions. I have found also that, when the nurse can focus exclusively on the needs and concerns of the patient, useful patient learning seems to happen.

Consider this clinical situation: The nurse asked a patient, "When did your husband last take you home for a visit from the hospital?" The patient replied, "I don't need to tell you anything about that;

if you ask questions like that I will go back to the ward." In this instance, the nurse said, "Very well, I won't require that you answer." In other words, the patient's intimidating tactic worked: The nurse felt intimidated and backed away. The focus at that moment was on the nurse's need to retain the patient regardless of the significance of the interaction. The significance was that this patient had many such seemingly innocuous intimidating maneuvers by which she prevented any exploration of the reality of her situation. Through recurrent use of these tactics the patient managed to keep herself sick and, in this instance, did so with the nurse's help.

It is of interest that in subsequent nurse–patient interactions the patient became increasingly uncomfortable with the nurse, that is, she must have dimly perceived that the nurse was vulnerable and could therefore be of little help to her. In fact, some sessions later, when finally the nurse did persist by saying, "This is information I must have if I am to grasp what you are up against in your life," the patient not only answered the question, but at long last began some substantial work on her difficulties. Similar situations come up in the nursing of general hospital patients.

Keeping the focus on the patient, thereby dealing out the personal and social needs of the nurse, is by no means an easy task. It requires that the nurse distinguish clearly between her behavior in rendering a professional service and her behavior as a social person in a social situation with friends of her own choosing.

The aim of the exclusive focus on the patient is to get to know the patient's view of self and the predicament—the way it looks to the patient—so that the patient can see it too.

A second characteristic of professional nursing is that the nurse uses participant observation rather than spectator observation. Spectator observation is the kind that you might use with an anesthetized or comatose patient, although even here, the nurse's reaction to the patient is an important factor to be taken into account. Participant observation requires the nurse to notice not only the behavior of the patient but her own as well. An interaction is an ongoing drama; the nurse enters the patient's room and says something, the patient responds to the nurse, the nurse then reacts to the patient, and so on. The behaviors and words of both nurse and patient have three aspects: (1) They tell something; that is, they contain a message that is sent to the other. (2) They ask for something; that is, they contain a question such as "Do you approve of me?" "Do you think I am important?" And (3) they evoke a feeling. For example, the patient may evoke in the nurse the feeling of anger or disgust, a response the nurse must then manage in one way or another. Participant observation is not a particularly easy kind of observation to learn. It is easier to teach new students to pay attention to their own response to patients than it is anytime thereafter. Concealment of negative responses, particularly, gets all tied up with pleasing teachers who give grades, and this makes more difficult the refinement of the student's competence as a participant observer.

A *third characteristic of professional nursing has to do with awareness of role.* The professional nurse must observe and draw inferences about the role she is taking and the role into which the patient is casting her. Professional nursing has, in the work role of staff nurse, a number of subroles: mother-surrogate, technician, manager, socializing agent, health teacher, and counselor or therapist. At any given time in working with a patient, the nurse is in one or the other of these subroles, perhaps with occasional overlap between the technical and health teacher subroles. Awareness of the role the nurse is taking helps her to distinguish what is going on in the work situation. The patient, on the other hand, will cast the nurse into many other roles—but the nurse chooses whether the professional service is enhanced or reduced when one or the other of these roles is taken by the nurse. The patient may cast the nurse into the role of chum, friend, parent, protagonist, sex object, and the like. In my view, none of these is a useful role for the nurse to take in rendering nursing services to patients.

A *fourth characteristic of professional nursing is that it is primarily investigative.* The nurse spends the bulk of her time observing and collecting data, which is then available to the patient. She does this by noticing, by asking questions, by pursuing remarks by the patient. There is often too hasty an effort on the part of nurses to make pronouncements, to reach conclusions, to give advice, to reassure and close off situations rather than to find out, to seek to know, to leave situations open to further discussion not yet neatly pinned down, even with relevant or good answers.

Although a high degree of technical efficiency and a matter-of-fact, or "this I must do" attitude, are useful in carrying out "medical orders," speed and dispatch are not characteristics of investigating or inquiring into the patient's reaction to his or her present situation. There is not much room for efficiency in talking over with another person his or her circumstances, especially when these are concerned with illness. It requires time for both elaboration and formulation of thought. Whenever possible, the professional nurse should find time to pull up a chair, sit down with patients, and say, "Tell me about yourself," "Give me more information about that impression," and so on. Talking with a professional person who has no particular stake in your future, who is not going to give you a grade, or decide if you are unfit for a job, has benefits all its own. This often happens on trains, buses, and planes: The anonymous stranger to whom one has no enduring commitment is often put into the position of listener, so that the person doing the talking can clarify something he cannot think through privately nearly as well. And I have noticed, when I get put into the position of listener, which frequently occurs on planes, that if I attempt to make it a two-way social relationship (I really don't think I should work in transit) that the effort of the individual dissolves in quite the same way that a therapeutic interview situation dissolves into something far less than that, when social and personal needs of the therapist are insinuated into the situation.

Furthermore, to be inquiring about the reaction of a sick person to his or her illness requires full attention of the nurse. The nurse must listen not so much for the details of what is said, but rather for the nuances of hidden meaning. In order to ask questions that help the patient provide a basis for self-solutions to interpersonal difficulties the nurse observes relations between what the patient is saying and doing, and relations between this and a range of possibilities, only some of which are suggested by a theoretical matrix the nurse might have. There is an artistic, intuitive aspect about asking the "right questions" in a particular situation, and these questions can neither be decided in advance nor generalized to all nurse–patient situations. Questions arise in the situation. Moreover, what the nurse observes is a rapidly shifting morass of signs from which he or she must note and discriminate the crucial material while simultaneously raising useful questions. Actually, it is not possible for the nurse—or any other health professional for that matter—to observe and attend totally to what is going on, for the field is constantly shifting. In this sense, objectivity in clinical work is very difficult to achieve, if possible at all, and especially with respect to interpersonal data.

With professional education and subsequent experience, development of self-awareness in the nurse makes it possible to rule out more and more of the subjective element, slowly creating a sensitive observer of interpersonal phenomena in which the nurse is a participant. I want to emphasize again this matter of the nontotality of observation and of the slowness with which sensitive observation can evolve in a particular nurse, for I think within the profession we too often make global claims and hold unreal expectations of ourselves and nursing students. The nurse can only see and do what she can see and do, within the time she has and the competence she has evolved as a result of education and experience. Take this as a principle.

There are, of course, some very simple guidelines for the novice. Cliche prompters like "tell me," "then what," "go on," "give me an example," "tell me about the last time that happened," will often serve the novice in good stead until comfort obtains in the nurse-patient verbal exchange wherein the nurse is freer to use rich variety in her own language behavior. Consciousness of language used by the nurse, and relevance of what she asks for from the patient, are exceedingly important ingredients in any nurse-patient verbal exchange. However, the nurse needs to hear what she says "automatically" to patients in order to be able to consider alternative wording that might elicit different responses from patients. An attitude of inquiry and an investigative approach, however, are absolutely essential ingredients in the interpersonal aspect of the nurse-patient situation.

A fifth and most important characteristic of professional nursing is the use of theory. Every nurse in all nursing situations uses three principal operations: observation, interpretation, and intervention. What is observed or noticed must be interpreted; that is, the raw data must be transformed into some meaningful explanation. There are several ways to interpret data—especially interpersonal data, namely, decoding (which is to put something that is said into other words), applying theory, and drawing inferences. In working with interpersonal data inferences play a large part; that is, the professional person observes and listens and then gets hunches, impressions, and general ideas about the meaning of what is going on. Such inferences then require checking or validation—and in the patient situation this can be done by saying "Is this what you meant?" or "Let me put it into other words to see if I understood the main idea," or "I get the impression you are saying thus and so, is this correct?" This is validating an inference with the patient. On the other hand, validation of inferences can occur by reviewing data with another observer and asking, "What is your impression?" then comparing this with one's own impression. Validation of inferences drawn from data is important simply because of the difficulties of observer bias, namely, the tendency to hear and notice in terms of one's own preconceptions of what went on rather than to grasp the essence of the patient's own description of the situation. The patient also may not give sufficient description of an event for the correct inference to emerge. In such instances it is better to utilize follow-up questions to get more complete descriptions: "Give me a blow-by-blow account of what happened" or "Tell me again everything that happened starting at the beginning," might be suitable questions.

An inference is a generalization drawn from a particular experience or descriptive data about that experience. When such generalizations tend to emerge recurringly from wide experience they become crystallized into a form of theory.

One kind of theory that is particularly useful in nursing practice consists of *explanatory concepts*. These are ideas that have been identified in unique situations, then in many situations of like kind, and finally emerge as *concepts* that explain similar situations. A concept is a term defined in such a way as to show the behaviors associated with it, and to which the term refers. A concept defined in this way can be said to have *structure* and *function*. The structure of the concept is the steps or behaviors stated in a serial order of their emergence. For example, the concept of frustration is defined as having four major behaviors: (1) a goal is set; (2) there is movement toward the goal; (3) an obstacle blocks goal achievement; and

(4) aggression is expressed indirectly (away from the obstacle) or directly (toward the obstacle). You will notice the serial order of the behaviors associated with this concept. A concept also has a function, that is, it can be used for something. Concepts can be used to explain what has been observed in a situation. The behaviors serve also as a structure for getting more information. For example, a nurse might notice behavior of a patient that classifies as aggression. The nurse might then realize that the concept of frustration offers some help or explanation regarding this situation. That is, however, the extent of the application of the concept to what has been noticed initially by the nurse. However, by recalling the concept the nurse now has a "structure" for considering other observations that have significance she might have overlooked had she no sequential "format" for asking questions. For instance, the nurse can inquire: What was the goal? When set? Why set? The strength of the goal? The meaning of the goal? There is the question of whether the goal must be reduced or given up by this individual, that is, whether it is an attainable goal. There is the question of movement: What steps were taken to achieve the goal? Were the tactics or strategies effective or ineffective? The nature of the obstacle can be investigated: Was it an internal or external obstacle? Can it be gotten around? Does the patient have what is required to remove the obstacle? and so on. In other words, resolution of the situation results from application of the concept as a structure for making available to the patient more complete information than was in his awareness at the time the aggression was expressed.

There are other explanatory concepts that can serve in the same way; some are well defined in operational terms while others are not. The concepts of conflict, self, anxiety, and identification, are particularly important in clinical work. The advantage of utilizing concepts is that they provide a ready-made structure for use in clinical work. This saves the professional person from using inferences exclusively. Considerable work needs to be done in clarifying concepts, ruling out overlap where it is present. For example, what is the essential difference between such concepts as identification, introjection, and imitation? Then we have the task of identifying the bare minimum of interpersonal concepts essential to interpersonally safe nursing practice. Then comes the task of teaching these to students and checking out their ability to recall and utilize such concepts in their actual encounters with patients. If nursing is to get beyond its present ad hoc intuitive state, it must develop in clinicians greater awareness and use of theory in clinical work.

One concept that nurses should know and be able to use in clinical work is anxiety. As Sullivan has pointed out, it has a profound role in interpersonal relationships. Anxiety is an energy, and therefore its presence is inferred from the behaviors into which anxiety is transformed. It occurs in degrees ranging from mild and moderate to severe and panic (awe, terror, dread, horror, uncanny sensation). The nurse must be able to distinguish the presence of these various degrees, for interventions are based on discrimination of the degree of anxiety. In mild and moderate anxiety the nurse continues to work toward learning products; in severe anxiety or panic the survival of the organized (i.e., not-split-into-a-million-pieces) personality is far more important. In other words, in mild and moderate anxiety the nurse is not so concerned with immediate reduction of the anxiety as she is in severe and panic degrees. Anxiety is also transmitted by empathic observation, whereby one anxious person in a situation evokes anxiety in others in that situation. Therefore, the nurse must be most observant of increased discomfort in herself, being particularly alert to empathized anxiety from the patient. Otherwise, the anxiety of both nurse and patient increases, moving in the direction of severe anxiety.

Sullivan defines needs as integrating tendencies, that is, tendencies to pattern behavior so that needs are satisfied. He defines anxiety as a disjunctive force, an energy transformed into behavior that has a disintegrating tendency. In other words, patterns of behavior used to relieve anxiety do not move in the direction of satisfaction of needs. This seems to me to be an important concept for professional nurses. Nurses ought to become sensitized to the security operations of patients, namely, the behaviors used recurringly to avoid what is not wanted. Security defined in this way suggests the nurse should be making observations not only of the behaviors used by the patient to feel safe, but she should also be sensitized to notice or infer what it is the patient is avoiding. Then the nurse is in a position to decide to what extent such matters can be opened up for discussion.

The concept of self, or the *self-system* as Sullivan calls it, is another important theoretical consideration of professional nurses. The behavior and statements of the patient constantly reflect the self-appraisals inherent in his or her self system. The self, as Sullivan defines it, is the anti-anxiety system made up of reflected appraisals and personifications. In other words, in the process of growing up, and as a result of experiences the child has had, particularly with parents, the child organizes his or her experience in terms of a concept of self. These conceptions are organized at first in terms of "good me" which is a reflection of experiences with a non-anxious, feeding mother, capable of expressing tenderness. Then "bad me" components enter, reflecting disapproving appraisals and "forbidding gestures" utilized by significant persons such as parents. These components become incorporated as personifications of self. Finally, as a result of experiences of extreme pain and punishment, "not me" experiences are organized. These are dissociated or not noticed components of experience related to the self-system. Later on, supervisory personifications become included; these are "illusory" straw men who represent previous experiences with significant people. A person brings a supervisory personification of mother into the bedroom when one says, "Wow, if my mother saw this room she'd have a fit." Recall of mother as supervisor of early life operates as an active ingredient in an ongoing, current, adult self-system.

In working clinically with patients, who are of course vulnerable to the authority of others, dependent on others for direction and feeling helpless, the patient more often than not organizes his or her behavior to get approval from the nurse (in contrast to learning something useful) and in terms of components already within the self-system. Nurses alert to such maneuvers can encourage more direct discussion in contrast to replication of previous mother–child relationships.

Another aspect of Sullivan's theory that has considerable usefulness is the concept of *modes of experiencing.* By this, Sullivan means that all experience occurs in three modes: prototaxic, parataxic, and syntaxic. It is particularly important for nurses to understand the dynamics of prototaxic and parataxic modes for these are the modes of experience most often used by psychiatric patients. The *prototaxic* mode refers to the experience of the infant. It is a discrete, momentary kind of experiencing; the infant and his world are one;

there is no before and no after, only the *now* moment. Prototaxis is also seen in panic, brain damage, and I think in sociopaths. The relevance to nursing is that the patient cannot see or make connections between the past, present, and future, implying that the only valid experience is the now moment. So for the nurse to expect the brain-damaged patient to see such relations is to pose an impossible burden upon the patient. *Parataxic* mode refers to the relation between past and present experience, to see the present in terms of the familiar elements reminiscent of the past. Here too, the relevance for the nurse is to evolve a tactic to get the patient to talk about these similarities, and then, to ask for differences. For example, if the patient says to the nurse, "You remind me of someone," there is an opportunity to get similarities and differences.

GENERAL CONSIDERATIONS IN COUNSELING

I would like to indicate some general considerations about interpersonal relations with respect to counseling. Within the characteristics of professional nursing are features that apply to all nurse-patient therapeutic interactions.

1. Structuring the situation so that the patient is clear about what the nurse intends. I think there is merit in directness, in letting the patient know exactly what is being offered. The nurse can say, "Mr. Jones, I have an hour, and I plan to give you some information about diabetes and then discuss your questions with you." If the nurse is offering a counseling relationship the patient has a right, at the outset, to know what the nurse intends. The nurse can say, "Mr. Jones, I have forty minutes, I'm offering it to you as an opportunity to talk about what happened at lunch." It seems to me that as professional nursing widens its interest in interpersonal theory, and its relevance for nursing practice, that we ought also to delete much of the so-called subtlety in nurse behavior in patient situations.

2. Behave like an expert. This requires the nurse to present herself both as a person who is not an equal of the patient but rather as one whose education and knowledge and experience in the health field are superior to that of the patient. This does not mean that the nurse knows all the answers, nor that she is required to reveal her ignorance to patients. Rather it means the nurse uses an approach that maximizes professional learning. There are two important aspects of this: asking the questions of the patient and keeping up with relevant literature. It also requires, as I said earlier, that the nurse distinguish between professional and social behavior, focusing effort on the improvement of services to patients. Personal satisfactions may coincidentally accrue from the work.

3. Showing appreciation for what the patient is up against. Patients are human and frail in many ways, but not necessarily fragile. The nurse can appreciate what the patient is up against, and show it, by genuine concern for hearing the details, aiding the patient to formulate the significance of the experience, and by helping the patient to see alternative courses of action that are open. Sympathy, reassurance—these are tactics that close off inquiry. They do not give the patient much to go on in comparison with the awareness that might otherwise develop.

4. Every human being needs to explain to the self what is happening to the self and why. In the absence of opportunity to ventilate and discuss with a professional person, patients attempt privately to make sense out of the nonsense of their predicaments. Private interpretations tend in the direction of incorrectness and distortion—and therefore in the direction of mental illness. An opportunity to check the meaning of experience with a nurse may well be the most important aspect of interpersonal relations that nurses offer patients.

CHAPTER 4

Interpersonal Constructs for Nursing Practice

INTERPERSONAL RELATIONS

There are many different theoretical frameworks which are useful in nursing practice. Interpersonal relations is one such theoretical perspective. This paper plans to provide a definition of interpersonal relations, suggest and define selected concepts which derive from this framework, and describe the relation between theory and nursing practice.

Nursing practice occurs within a relationship of nurse with

Reprinted from *Nurse Education Today,* 7(5), 201–208. Copyright 1987 by Churchill-Livingston. Reprinted by permission.

This paper was presented at a seminar on the role of psychiatric nurses in interpersonal relationships, given at Highland College of Nursing and Midwifery, Raigmore Hospital, Inverness. Selected interpersonal constructs were examined; such theoretical concepts, when applied by nurses in practice situations, provide explanations of observations nurses make and serve also to guide actions which nurses choose, to facilitate a helping nurse–client relationship. Finally, it was suggested that nurse teachers have a large responsibility in helping students to examine various theoretical constructs, learn and apply them in nursing practice, and to develop the necessary intellectual and interpersonal competencies for constructive psychiatric nursing practice.

clients. Much of the planning for, and evaluation of, practice may occur outside the relationship, but the main work goes on in an interactive process during which the participants are a nurse and patient, patients, and/or family of patient or significant others. The relationship is an unequal one, not in terms of the worth of persons, but in the sense of position within the relationship. The nurse—a professional—has specialized knowledge and competence which are translated into the services which the client or clients require. The client, within the relationship, presumably has a problem, concern, or need, related to health status, which can be defined and for which nursing interventions can be provided. Nursing services are provided in the interest of generating a beneficial effect on the client's health status. Traditionally, the definition of the health problem has been considered the task of the professional, the client providing description of the perceived difficulty and submitting to various examinations and tests. Currently, however, with an increasing number of well-educated and health-knowledgeable individuals, the client's participation is sometimes quite active in defining the problem and in monitoring treatment. This is possibly more true in nonpsychiatric clients.

Traditionally, the professional determined and carried out the required treatment. Presently, many clients present their own diagnosis, want to know the various options open to them, and make their own choices about treatment. In other words, traditions are yielding to new and more active forms of client participation in the professional relationship process. This, however, does not make the client a customer asking for and getting what he wants; it is still the professional's main work to define and to provide and recommend what the client's condition requires. The professional is the keeper of the purpose of the relationship which is to produce whatever improvements in health status possible for the client by suggesting paths toward that end.

All professional relationships, including nurse–patient interactions, encompass three overlapping phases: orientation, working and termination. The phase of orientation, a period of getting acquainted—unlike the relationship between budding friends—is primarily a one-way focused relationship. While the professional provides some personal information, such as, name and credentials,

the aim is primarily to identify the dimensions of the client's difficulty, for example by undergoing a physical examination or taking
a nursing history. Professional work requires and proceeds on the
basis of information. Information about the client and his difficulties comes from the client, observations by the nurse,
and from use of various forms of assessment, which provide the
basis for nursing diagnosis. Theories about what is already known
about phenomena, about recurring problems related to health, are
the major tools of a professional. In other words, practicing nurses
are expected to have in their heads, readily available for recall
and clinical application, a range of theories. Nurses apply such
theories as a private intellectual exercise in observing, diagnosing,
planning, and in determining treatment approaches that would
produce, in the short term or long run, the most beneficial effects
for the client. The effects are a change in the phenomena, in the
diagnosed problems of the client, produced, at least in part, as a
consequence of the nursing treatment.

Interpersonal relations is a fairly comprehensive framework which
provides many theoretical constructs of considerable use in clinical
nursing practice. The overall term, *interpersonal relations,* refers to an
array of concepts, processes, patterns, and facts. The term was first
coined by Moreno (1941), who developed psychodrama, and was
defined and elaborated by Sullivan (1953). Sullivan was a practicing
psychoanalyst but his interpersonal constructs were drawn from
both his psychiatric clinical work and from the social sciences available in the 1920s to 1950s.

The Definition of Interpersonal Relations

The definition of interpersonal relations suggests some of the
partials contained within this framework. Sullivan (1953) defined interpersonal relations as the study of what goes on between two or more people, all but one of whom may be
completely illusory. The first thing to note about this definition is
that it uses the term *relations* rather than relationships. This construct, 'relations', refers to connections, linkages, ties and bonds
between things and people. Such relations or connections are
identified in terms of their *nature* (pattern), their *origin* (history),

their *function* (intention, motive, expectations, purpose), their *mode* (form, style, method), or by *integrations* (patterns of two or more people which together, link or bind them).

In a nurse–patient relationship, and most particularly in psychiatric work, the aim of the nurse would be to study the interpersonal relations that go on (or went on) between a client and others, whether family, friends, staff, or the nurse. Such study enables identification of those human responses and patterns that are problematic in terms of health. In other words, while a client is describing an event, incident, relationship or dilemma, the nurse in that situation would be studying what was happening. Such study would include observing, noticing gestures and body movements, listening, and hearing the facts and data being presented. During this study process the nurse would also begin to notice relations and to generate inferences or to apply theory as professionally oriented intellectual operations, in order privately to interpret the data.

To put this important matter in another way, a nurse who has in his or her head a store of interpersonal constructs would most likely mentally be flipping through those constructs that at the time seem most applicable, or that best fit what has been observed, heard, or noticed. The construct in the forefront of the nurse's awareness (focal attention) would then serve the nurse as an intellectual framework, a guide. The theoretical concept would suggest further data, missing pieces, that would do two things if such data were revealed: The client would have a broader base of data for understanding his/her problem and the nurse would have a measure of confirmation or rejection of the selected construct.

The construct application suggested here is a private, mental exercise by the nurse, an intellectual operation, an empirical test of the applicability of a particular construct. Such constructs ought not to be used as labels told to the client.

Theoretical Constructs

Sullivan's (1953) definition of interpersonal relations points to many theoretical constructs. The first part of the definition: "the study of what goes on between people" suggests two questions:

1. How such study goes on—which has already been described in this paper.
2. What categories of relations—what goes on between people.

What goes on between people is transmitted through nonverbal and verbal exchanges. A major nonverbal category would be *empathic linkages*—the ability to *feel* in oneself the feelings being experienced by another person or persons in the same situation. The interpersonal transmission of anxiety or panic is perhaps the most common empathic linkage. However, various feelings such as anger, disgust and envy arising in nurse or patient can be communicated nonverbally by way of empathic transmission to the other. During psychotherapeutic sessions, in the working phase, the experienced tenderness of the therapist can be empathized by the client. In clinical work, nurses who pay attention to what they are feeling during a relationship with a client often gain invaluable empathized observations of feelings a patient is experiencing and has not yet noticed or talked about. How empathic communication occurs, and by what process, is not yet fully understood. However, Reynolds (1986) has suggested that empathic ability may be acquired by a combination of genetic factors, intelligence, and vicarious learning.

The Transmission of Gestural Messages

A second category of nonverbal relations includes the transmission of *gestural messages*. Messages conveyed by the body gesture of one person are inferred by the other, often with amazing accuracy. Such messages include forbiddance, annoyance, disgust, or approval/disapproval/indifference. Small children become sensitized very early in life, particularly to forbidding gestures; psychiatric clients tend to maintain this sensitivity more than people in the general, nonpsychiatric population.

Nurses ought to develop maximum awareness of the messages conveyed in their gestures and body posture and work for maximum verbal and minimum nonverbal exchanges in nurse–patient relationships. Birdwhistle (1971) has pioneered the development of theory in the area of body language, showing how the body can be used to say something without using words. Bateson et al.'s (1971) theory of "double blind," developed by studying schizophrenia, suggests that a message given at one level of communication can be canceled out by a contradictory message given at another level (for example, a verbal message may contradict a nonverbal message). Other researchers have studied facial expressions, which have been called the "unguarded language." Six basic expressions of emotion expressed facially are: disgust, anger, fear, sadness, happiness and surprise. The power of gesturally conveyed messages is greater in vulnerable persons—children and psychiatric patients in particular.

Patterns and Variations

A third category of relations, for instance, that goes on between people, consists of *patterns* and variations. This category of interpersonal relations is of the utmost importance for psychiatric nurses. When nurses set out to help clients change behavior which interferes with growth and healthy living, it is the problematic pattern or patterns that should become the focus for change. The psychiatric nursing literature has had little to say so far on this matter.

A pattern is a characteristic mode of behavior; it is a configuration of separate acts, variations of pattern, having similar aim or intention. The similar feature or theme, is the main indicator of pattern. Separate acts are exemplars, representatives or likeness of pattern. Pattern is the named form of behavior by which separate acts can be classified on the basis of distinctive, shared, similar features. There are few patterns and many variations of each (as with themes and variations in music). Pattern refers to the regularity, the constancy of theme, while variations are the behavioral acts (variants) of that theme. Patterns of behavior become established fairly early in life, and become familiar ways of behaving, predictable regularities in interpersonal relations. In psychiatric patients the repertoire of behavior patterns is often narrow in scope, the patterns being repetitive and quite automatic in use. Patterns can also be unique, in the sense of being temporary and situation-determined, as a response to an extreme emergency, during severe illness or panic. However, most behavior patterns are more or less enduring and persist throughout life.

Patterns can be constructive thus ensuring continued learning, growth, and perhaps health throughout life. A pattern of investigating circumstances would be one such constructive pattern. Psychiatric patients have many patterns that are destructive to their continuing development as persons. Examples would include dissociating or not noticing, intimidation, scapegoating, and "pitting one against the other." Patterns are comprised of thoughts, feelings and actions; for example, there are many behavioral acts which comprise or portray the pattern of intimidation.

The patterns (and needs) of one person are used to interact with patterns of another person (or persons); such *pattern integrations* can be complementary, mutualities, alternating or antagonistic in terms of fit, match or mismatch. Complementary pattern integrations would be like hand-and-glove or domination–submission. A message carrier (informer) seeks out a message receiver. Mutualities include, mutual dependence, in which both feel helpless and dependent on the other. Antagonistic pattern integrations occur when there is mismatch of patterns but the parties maintain a relationship anyway regardless of how stormy.

There are many patterns of patients seen in nursing situations; these include dependency, bereavement, suffering, noncompliance, self-destructiveness and hopelessness. There are also pattern integrations common to health care situations such as: subordinate–superordinate (nurse–supervisor), helper–helplessness (nurse–client), blame-blame avoidance (staff-client), guilt induction and defense, illness-maintaining and iatrogenic patterns of doctor or nurse with clients.

There are also patterns that occur in sequences, as seen in *processes.* These patterns commonly move in one direction. One fairly common patterned sequence includes: perfectionism–procrastination–paralysis of effort.

Patterns can be intrapersonal, interpersonal, and system phenomena. They occur in individuals, between two people, and among people within established institutions. In therapeutic work there are two main problems.

1. The tendency merely to diagnose, that is, to name problematic patterns.

2. The tendency to attempt behavioral change in relation to separate, random acts without considering the many other variants of persisting problematic patterns.

The aims of therapeutic intervention into psychosocial phenomena, such as problematic behavior patterns, are to:

1. Identify the problematic patterns, or diagnose them.
2. Identify some of the major variants.
3. Determine the 1 to 2 patterns most amenable to change by bringing them into the awareness of the client.
4. Focus investigation of thoughts and feelings that go with separate acts, of the 1 to 2 patterns selected, for intervention whenever these are in evidence.

In therapeutic work, particularly when it is of short duration, only a sample of patterns of a client's behavior can be investigated and worked on; but this will be sufficient in most instances. The client gains awareness of those patterns, as a basis for change, and may simultaneously gain a method for further self-study.

Processes

Interpersonal relations also has to do with *processes.* A process is a series of behaviors that occur in a definable sequence, going through identified phases and steps, each having identifiable regularities of pattern in their development and/or operation. There are theoretical definitions in the nursing literature of such processes as dying (Kübler-Ross, 1969), hallucinations (Peplau, 1963), victim response [(1) impact–disorganization; (2) recoil; (3) reorganization–integration of the event], self-system, language–thought, grieving, and others.

With the application of theory of a particular process, it becomes possible for a nurse to determine which phase of the process a patient is experiencing. Interventions, then, can be phase-specific, in accord with what is already known theoretically about that particular phase of a process.

To return now to Sullivan's definition of interpersonal relations: The study of what goes on between people, all but one of whom may be completely illusory (Sullivan, 1953). The latter half of this definition suggests another list of constructs that are useful theories when applied in nursing situations.

Autistic Invention

Autistic invention or "fantasy" refers to the tendency of people to think privately, without interaction with "real" people and therefore without external validation of private thoughts. Sullivan's definition points also to relationships that go on between one real person and illusory others. There is also a tendency of all humans to require explanations of events in which they are involved; in the absence of information, and particularly with reference to events an individual cannot control, there is a tendency to invent explanations, particularly of causation. Autistic invention, which is a human competence, is not in and of itself a problem or pathology. What is problematic is the amount of time spent in private thought as compared to public shared thought, as in talking with other real people. Long hours of private, unvalidated thought particularly by persons who are vulnerable can lead to loss of control of focal attention, invention of illusory figures and to hallucinations. Those most vulnerable are isolates who lack social skills and withdraw from people; lonely persons, and individuals having limited education or interests in the external world.

Two other forms of interpersonal relations between real and illusory figures also create vulnerability to pathology and are related to autistic invention. These are parataxic distortions and supervisory personifications.

Parataxic Distortions

Parataxic distortions are remnants of earlier, most often childhood experience. The term refers to the tendency of people to relate to new acquaintances and events in the present, as if they are known. The relationship is based upon a search for similarities or that which is familiar because it was known and experienced in the past. In this form of distortion similarities are seen but differences are not noticed. It is common for nurses to have patients say to them, "You remind me of so-and-so." This comment is the clue that the client has identified a resemblance cue between so-and-so and the nurse, and is pursuing the nurse–patient relationship on the basis of that familiar similarity. The most useful nurse intervention would be to encourage the patient to identify the similarity and then the difference. The nurse might ask: "In what way am I like so-and-so?" and then ask, "In what way am I different?" Parataxic distortions are problematic because they narrow the range of comfortable relationships to those based on similarities rooted in the past, and therefore limit the scope of a person's knowledge of people, events, and the world.

Supervisory Personifications

Supervisory personifications are the second form of relationships between real persons and illusory figures. In growing up, all children are more or less supervised by their parents, teachers, clergy, and other adult supervisors. The images and precepts of these supervisors over time are incorporated by the child and internalized during personal development. Thereafter, in certain situations, and in the absence of the real supervisors, the incorporated images and precepts are recalled and serve to guide and control the individual's behavior. In adults, however, the full responsibility for actions and their consequences ought to be taken by the individual. Actions taken are chosen by the adult. In other words, supervisory personifications in the mature adult have been largely deleted. Psychiatric clients tend to sustain relationships with persisting supervisory personifications. It is a task of psychiatric nurses to have such patients become aware of these continuing relationships with illusory figures and to assist them to generate their own beliefs to guide their own responsible actions.

Autistic invention, parataxic distortions, and supervisory personifications are three interpersonal constructs which provide explanations for experiences common to all humans and which are also inherent in such psychopathology as delusions and hallucinations, which in part are exaggerated extensions of these common human capabilities. Psychiatric clients behave as if illusory figures were real and present, making judgments of them, and influencing their choices in life. They have relationships with such illusory figures. They also selectively inattend or dissociate or ignore real people who are actually observable and in present situations with them or they minimize their significance. Therefore, psychiatric nurses having these concepts would use language with clients that encourages development of their ability to notice, to pay attention, to see, to hear, to remember and so on.

The Self System

One of the interpersonal constructs of considerable importance in all nursing practice is what Sullivan (1953) called the self-system. The self, according to Sullivan, is both an anti-anxiety system and a product of socialization. In parent–child relationships, patterns of approval, disapproval, and indifference are used along with verbal inputs which define the child and in time become incorporated self-views, particularly those that are used recurrently. Psychiatric clients have commonly had an overload of derogatory or otherwise crippling self-definitions from others which over time they have accepted as their own views of self. These recurring derogatory definitions of self by others were at first heard by the child, then incorporated, then reflected back, then acted upon, and finally serve as determinants of behavior. This theory views the self as a process, moving in a direction in the course of personal development, always open to revision—more so at the outset of entry into new situations—but tending toward a certain stability of self-views. Nurses need in-depth theoretical understanding of all of these constructs, which explain developmental and current experiences of people. Such explanations serve the nurse in determining nursing interventions that will tend toward remedial effects for patients.

Energizers of Behavior

Something needs to be said, finally, about energizers of behavior. These are useful interpersonal constructs for nurses. Sullivan suggested that there were two major categories of energizers: the tension of needs and anxiety. Needs are primarily of biological origin. Soon after birth, however, their nature (pattern), mode (form, style, method), and their function (intention, expectations, motive, purpose) begin also to serve sociocultural aims. The striving to meet needs is in part socioculturally patterned. When a biological need is operative it gives rise to tension which is reduced and relieved (satiated, abated) by behaviors used to meet that operative need. Sullivan identified biological needs as the need for food, fluids, shelter, and the "lust dynamism" (sexual physical intimacy). Nurses are not concerned about needs per se, but rather aim to recognize the patterns and style of need-meeting behavior of a client in relation to health status. Nurses are also concerned about the available resources, for instance, the quality and availability of food to meet a client's needs. The pattern interactions of others (family, nurses) with the client, during need-meeting experiences, would also be data of importance to nurses.

Sullivan referred to sociocultural needs for status and prestige as these overlie biological needs or are expressed separately as security needs. In essence, security needs have to do with "avoiding that which is not wanted." Security needs when they are operative and not met give rise to anxiety. The simplest definition of anxiety is an energy that arises when expectations that are operative are not met. Anxiety is a key concept. Professional practice is unsafe when the professional does not know this concept and, in a clinical situation with a client, fails to recognize and intervene to reduce a client's anxiety. This is particularly true when a client's anxiety rises, escalating toward panic, which neither the professional nor the client recognize. There are various degrees of anxiety—mild, moderate, severe, and panic—each having observable cues which a nurse ought to notice and recognize. These are behavioral cues, since anxiety as an energy is not directly observable. The simplest intervention is to ask, "Are you anxious?" or perhaps nervous, upset, tense, jittery. Just naming the fact of feeling anxious begins the anxiety-reduction process. To be aware of and to know what is being experienced are powerful first steps in resolution of interpersonal problems.

As pointed out earlier in this paper, the self-system is an anti-anxiety system, very much related to security needs, that is to the maintenance of status and prestige. When prevailing self-views that are operative in clients are denied by nursing personnel, negated by circumstances of hospital admission, or challenged in some way, the chances that the client will experience anxiety are increased. Since anxiety is an energy, it is then transformed into behavior which can be observed by a nurse. Such behavior, often called "defensive" is really "relief behavior"—most often behavioral acts connected to customary patterns of anxiety-relief behavior. Anger, expressed in such acts as yelling, derogating, swearing, and so forth, is one common anxiety-relief pattern. Withdrawal or becoming quiet, using private thought or leaving the situation literally or figuratively, is another such pattern. In hospitals, clients who act out anger are called "difficult patients" or "disturbed," while those who relieve anxiety by withdrawal are ignored. In both instances, the actual problem, anxiety generated by an unmet self-system security need, is totally overlooked. These, of course, are complex theoretical constructs, but they can be learned and applied by nurses toward improving nursing practice.

CONCLUSIONS

A broad range of interpersonal constructs has been suggested in this paper, briefly defined, and applications in nursing described. The scientific aspect of clinical nursing practice includes theory-guided work such as has been suggested. The nursing profession is moving in this direction. However, not all nurses appreciate or accept the substantial advantages of theory-directed nursing practice. Nurses believe that all clients are unique and that personalized nursing care is the best. That belief is only partially true. According to Sullivan, we are all more alike than not (Sullivan, 1953). Science and scientific constructs are defined in terms of universals, regularities, common elements which define phenomena.

The self-system of each person is indeed unique, in both the self-views that are held and in their arrangement, distribution in and expression of the self-system. However, the structure, general dimensions, development and function of the self-system process are composed of definable, common elements, universals and regularities which are found in the self-system of all persons. The application of theoretical constructs provides a guiding framework for understanding the dilemmas of people, uniquely expressed within a common, known structure. Interpersonal relations is not the only theoretical framework that provides useful concepts and processes for nursing practice. All of the basic and applied sciences, particularly in their published research findings, provide constructs which can be co-opted and redefined for use in nursing practice. Similarly, nursing research, when focused on the phenomena to which nursing practices are or should be directed, also provides theories applicable in practice.

In this paper only some of the constructs derived from a framework of interpersonal relations have been presented. It has been suggested that the comprehension and application of interpersonal strategies by the nurse will guide the helping process between the nurse and her client. However, the common problem shared by all nurse teachers is *how* to help their students to formulate operational nursing activity from a multiplicity of theories and psychiatric concepts.

It is suggested that those who teach nurses are often unclear about what they mean by interpersonal skills, and that where interpersonal skills have been defined there is often no clear indication of *when* or how the student is provided with an opportunity to learn and rehearse those skills (see Reynolds, 1986, Reynolds & Cormack, 1987). There is a need to examine what is meant by interpersonal skills, and to consider how teachers have attempted to teach and assess those attitudes and behaviors which are characteristic of an effective interpersonal relationship.

REFERENCES

Bateson, G., Jackson, D.D., Haley, J., & Weakland, J. (1956). Towards a theory of schizophrenia. *Behavioural Science, 1,* 251–264.
Birdwhistle, R. (1971). *Kinesics and context.* London: Lane.
Kübler-Ross, E. (1969). *On death and dying.* New York: Macmillan.
Moreno, J. (1941). Psychodrama and group psychotherapy. *Sociometry, 9,* 249–253.

Peplau, H.E. (1963). Interpersonal relations and process of adaptation. *Nursing Science, 1,* 272–279.

Reynolds, W. (1986). *A study of empathy in student nurses.* Master of philosophy thesis, Dundee College of Technology, Scotland.

Reynolds, W., & Cormack, D. (1987). Teaching psychiatric nursing: Interpersonal skills. In B. Davis (Ed.), *Nursing Education: Research and Developments* (pp. 122–150). London: Croom Helm.

Sullivan, H.S. (1953). *The interpersonal theory of psychiatry* (H.S. Perry & M.L. Gawel, Eds.). New York: Norton.

PART II Therapeutic Milieu

Introduction

Interest by psychiatric nursing in the ward atmosphere was first addressed in 1950 at a National League for Nursing, University of Minnesota conference on advanced psychiatric nursing and mental hygiene programs. This interest predated the 1953 interest expressed by the expert committee on mental health of the World Health Organization and was a forerunner of the 1956 report by the expert committee on psychiatric nursing of the World Health Organization, which indicated the nurse as the crucial representative of the therapeutic community.

In 1956, Hildegard E. Peplau, who had long been influential in this trend, held the first clinical workshop, Orientation to Modern Psychiatric Nursing, at New Jersey State Hospital at Greystone Park. This was the first of many such workshops across the country. In 1961, she presented a paper at the Illinois State Psychiatric Institute, wherein she discussed ward atmosphere as a task, a primary part of the work of nurses. She bid nurses to explore the task in detail so that "ward atmosphere" would not become simply a doctrinaire cliche, part of the large collection of unclear and undefined things nurses "should do" but never do because of lack of clarity and definition. Indeed, today this task remains in the future of psychiatric nursing. Probably it was initially derailed by the profession's excursion into the area of psychotherapy. Perhaps too, the task was so complex it required people educated in interpersonal theory and social research methods to forge ways of observing, collecting, and analyzing data on the mix of interpersonal and social system phenomena. Such people were indeed prepared by Peplau and beyond, but they joined the ranks of those leaving the shrinking public hospitals where the study of ward milieu started. So the work Peplau initiated stood still.

Peplau's focus, as part of her workshop and graduate and undergraduate teaching, was on applying interpersonal theory in diffuse clinical situations to transform brief interactions between patients or staff and patients from irritating, little-understood encounters to experiences that indeed could be clarified, explored, and understood. Furthermore, it was clear to her that there were ward social system phenomena that were part of this interpersonal system integration and these too needed to be identified and developed, a task still in its infancy today. To this end, starting in the late 1950s, Peplau encouraged clinicians and students to conduct "ward studies" to explore what she called "illness-maintaining systems." It is noteworthy that this work predated the development and interest by mental health professionals in general system theory and coincided with the work of sociologists interested in the patient and the mental hospital.

In the last several years, Peplau has been tackling the system dimension by looking closely at pattern interactions, again taking leadership in this important area as inpatients move from public facilities to general hospitals, where pathological systems are likely to emerge and become endemic and chronic unless identified, understood, and checked.

Throughout Peplau's work on ward atmosphere she has relentlessly pursued two central principles: The first is that nurses promote learning in patient situations rather than reinforce pathology and chronicity. Participating in the patients' pathology is automatic and unwitting and difficult to sort out—as the last decade of work with the borderline inpatient proves. Peplau spoke and wrote of staff participation in pathology over 20 years ago.

The second central principle regarding ward atmosphere is that, although of course one deals with pathology, in the very process, nurses promote and capitalize on competencies of patients. Again, although this sounds somewhat like a rehabilitation model of the 1980s, it was over 20 years ago that much of Peplau's work focused on capitalizing on and developing patients' competencies. Obviously, work on milieu remains ahead, as Peplau continues at the forefront of its development.

CHAPTER 5

The History of Milieu as a Treatment Modality

Asylums and psychiatric hospitals were generally considered to be dreadful environments until the middle of this century. A century ago, during the era of "moral treatment," there were a few exceptions, namely, private hospitals. Although there were a few early efforts to make hospital environments conducive to the recovery of patients, the terms *therapeutic community* and *milieu therapy* came into the language largely after the publication of a book by Jones in 1953 describing his hospital work. It was psychiatrists who first contributed to the literature on milieu as a treatment modality. Sullivan's work in the 1920s at Sheppard and Enoch Pratt; the efforts at Menninger's, beginning in 1937; Maxwell Jones' publication in 1953; the work of Stanton and Schwartz in 1954; Greenblatt, Levinson, and Williams in 1957; the innovative experiment of Caudill in 1958; and Goffman's work in 1961, all have added to an enlarging understanding of milieu phenomena.

There is the possibility that interest in the milieu during the 1950s arose as a reaction against prevailing environments, particularly in public mental hospitals. However, it is a fairly common occurrence that extravagant claims about the potential of new

Revised and edited introduction from paper originally titled *The Concept of Milieu as a Treatment Modality*, Psychiatric Nursing Symposium, College of Nursing, Rush University, Chicago, IL, April, 1985.

forms of care lead to a backlash when those claims are not realized within a reasonable period of time. Milieu, for which initially much benefit was claimed, seems now to be losing some of its popularity. Psychiatrists are turning their attention toward pharmaceuticals as a major form of treatment of mental illness, and toward biological, genetic, and brain research as more promising directions in which to search for causes and better explanations of phenomena related to mental illness.

Milieu, however, continues to be an important subject for discussion and further investigation by psychiatric nurses. While I have a publication of illness-maintenance (Peplau, 1978), I have none on psychiatric milieu. Other nurses have written on this topic, because of course the idea of nurses having a milieu function is not new. In fact, a half century ago the idea of nurses "creating and maintaining proper psychological atmosphere" was put forth (Johns & Pfefferkorn, 1934). "The manipulation of immediate environmental factors" (Render, 1947) and "the creation of a therapeutic environment" (Mereness, 1966) were considered to be nursing functions. The "nurse sets the tone" and "creates an atmosphere conducive to recovery" were popular in early psychiatric nursing literature. These vague directives, however, were not followed by specifics about how nurses might proceed in carrying out such milieu functions.

Beginning in the 1960s, writings by nurses provided somewhat clearer but still less than definitive information about nursing and milieu (Haber, Leach, Schudy, & Sidelaeau, 1978), differentiations between milieu therapy and therapeutic community, and instruments for assessing aspects of milieu (Wilson & Kneisl, 1979). In a 1975 state-of-the-art paper, Sills summarizes and analyzes nursing literature on milieu and contributes a bibliography and a sociological perspective on the subject.

There are at least three insightful journal articles written by two nurses more than two decades ago that define selected milieu phenomena. All three papers are originals, that is, they are not a rehash of previous work. Tudor (1952) described "mutual withdrawal," the way in which patients who are withdrawn evoke a similar pattern of withdrawal by nurses. Rouslin (1963) described the way in which a mental hospital system reinforced "chronic helpfulness" in patients, thereby retaining them as unpaid workers rather than promoting discharge into the community. Rouslin (1964) also presented a system concept, showing how staff participation in an individual's hostility stabilizes it and generates interpersonal hostility. These three papers still have applicability today, yet these important works have become buried, remaining largely unused for practice in the milieu.

In order to understand interactive phenomena seen in the milieu, interpersonal and systems theories are essential. Interpersonal theory, first introduced by Moreno and elaborated by Sullivan, has about a fifty-year history (Moreno, 1937; Sullivan, 1953). Systems theory, as put forth by Von Bertalanffy (1969) began to be applied during the mid-1960s, particularly in the development of family therapy. Since the late 1940s, nurses have become knowledgeable in these theoretical areas. Very few papers have appeared, however, applying these theories to the work in the milieu of staff nurses.

Nevertheless, in practice, when milieu therapy became popular, nurses took over management of such new structural or formal arrangements as ward government, "rap groups," and "token economies." What has received less attention, however, is the nature of the interactions that go on between patients, and patients and staff, and the effects these may have on patient outcomes. Nurses do interact with patients around the clock, and nursing practices in this area could be or should be their most potent contribution to psychiatric patient care. The neglected area, however, has been this unstructured, informal component of milieu, which is the most important and complex dimension of milieu.

The unstructured component of milieu consists of the people-system and its subsystems. This is a complex system of interactions among patients, professional staff, other hospital personnel, friends and family members who visit the patient. A psychotherapeutic function of nurses in relation to the inpatient people-system would not have been possible thirty years ago, when my own interest in interactions within the milieu began. At that time, the Graduate Program in Psychiatric Nursing at Rutgers employed two full-time sociologists. Part of their work was to accompany nurse faculty and graduate students to a public mental hospital to begin study of milieu interactions and of nursing's role in relation to them. Unfortunately, there were no research publications from that effort, although nurse faculty continued to explore and publish on the topic.

The idea of milieu as a therapeutic environment, as it became popular during the 1950s and 1960s, gave recognition to the idea that nurse–patient interactions within the milieu could be beneficial to patients. However, since at that time, the clinical specialist movement and graduate preparation of psychiatric nurses as psychotherapists were still in very tentative, early stages of development, consideration of the impingement of hospital systems and ward environments on patients, and the nature of interaction phenomena within the milieu, had to wait. Nurses first had to gain sophistication in theory and theory application before thinking about complex milieu phenomena. It would seem that there are many theoretically oriented psychiatric nurses who, with knowledge, skill and a computer, could now address this complex task, providing insight and direction for inpatient staff.

REFERENCES

Caudill, W. A. (1958). *The psychiatric hospital as a small society.* Cambridge, MA: Harvard University Press.

Greenblatt, M., Levinson, D. J., & Williams, R. H. (1957). *The patient and the mental hospital.* Glencoe, IL: Free Press.

Goffman, E. (1961). *Asylums.* Garden City, N.Y.: Anchor.

Haber, J., Leach, A., Schudy, S. M., & Sidelaeau, B. F. (1978). *Comprehensive psychiatric nursing.* New York: McGraw-Hill.

Johns, E., & Pfefferkorn, B. (1934). *An activity analysis of nursing.* New York: Committee on the Grading of Nursing Schools.

Jones, M. (1953). *The therapeutic community.* New York: Basic Books.

Mereness, D. (1966). *Psychiatric nursing: A book of readings,* Vol. 1. Dubuque, IA: Brown.

Moreno, J. L. (1937). Interpersonal theory. *Sociometry, 1*(3), 3–10.

Peplau, H. E. (1978). Psychiatric nursing: Role of nurses and psychiatric nurses. *International Nursing Review, 25,* 41–47.

Render, H. W. (1947). *Nurse-patient relationships in psychiatry.* New York: McGraw-Hill.

Rouslin, S. (1963). Chronic helpfulness: Maintenance or intervention? *Perspectives in Psychiatric Care, 9*(6), 257–268.

Rouslin, S. (1964). Interpersonal stabilization on an intrapersonal problem. *Nursing Forum, 3*(2), 69–78.

Sills, G. M. (1975). Use of milieu therapy. In F. L. Huey (Ed.), *Psychiatric nursing 1946 to 1974, A report on the state of the art.* New York: American Journal of Nursing.

Stanton, A. H., & Schwartz, M. S. (1954). *The mental hospital.* New York: Basic Books.

Sullivan, H. S. (1953). *Conceptions of modern psychiatry.* New York: Norton.

Tudor, G. E. (1952). Socio-psychiatric nursing approach to intervention in a problem of mutual withdrawal on a mental hospital ward. *Psychiatry, 15*(2), 193–217.

Von Bertalanffy, L. (1969). *General system theory: Essays on its foundation and development.* New York: Brazillar.

Wilson, H. S., & Kneisl, C. R. (1979). *Learning activities in psychiatric nursing.* Menlo Park, CA: Addison-Wesley.

CHAPTER 6

Psychiatric Nursing: The Nurse's Role in Preventing Chronicity

Psychiatric Nurses who hold a master's or doctoral degree are developing direct clinical practices. Such clinical work will be effective in preventing mental illness and in promoting mental health in persons who are psychiatrically disturbed. Like the other three major professional disciplines in the mental health field, psychiatry, clinical psychology, and social work, psychiatric nursing is in its infancy in evolving viable, effective clinical practice. This paper suggests one focus in the work of psychiatric nurses, namely, the prevention of chronicity in psychiatric patients.

WHAT IS CHRONICITY?

Chronicity in mental illness, like chronicity in physical illness, occurs when a pathological process cannot be eradicated, reversed,

Paper presented to hospital staff, Veterans Administration Hospital, Brecksville, Ohio and Western Reserve University, March, 1965. Schlesinger Library, Radcliffe College, Cambridge, MA. No. 84–M107, Hildegard E. Peplau Archives, carton 24, volume 838. Copyright 1986 by Schlesinger Library. Edited and reprinted by permission.

Helpful discussion with Mrs. Shirley Smoyak and Miss Sheila Rouslin in the preparation of this paper is acknowledged.

or halted. Basic sciences such as chemistry, physiology, and a host of new micromolecular sciences are providing facts and theories that may help account for irreversible physical pathological processes. These theories may have impact on the reversibility of some of these pathologies. However, closer scrutiny of all types of chronicity would probably reveal that the "top layer" is invariably "mental." In other words, all chronicity has psychological effects that burden both physical and psychiatric disorders. In unpublished research by Richard Benjamin, a clinical psychologist in New Jersey, it was found that when the real ability of aging persons was tapped, many of the observable aspects of their chronicity disappeared. Disabling effects, deadening of motivation, inability to work, hopelessness, despair, and depression vanished.

Chronicity can be defined as substitutive behavior that evolves and is utilized when use of actual capacities and abilities of a person are attenuated or rendered inoperative by illness or another reason. Forced retirement and developmental gaps, as in mental illness, force capacities and abilities to be inoperative. The main ingredient highlighted in chronicity is that the individual's abilities are no longer respected, needed, challenged, or used in rational ways. If this hypothesis is correct, then the prevention or amelioration of chronicity requires that available capacities be identified and redirected in a realistic, challenging way.

For example, a retiring high school art teacher is encouraged to take on a new and challenging experience of teaching art to senior citizens. A former professor of philosophy who developed arthritis begins moving in a chronic direction. As he leans with the distortions of his body structure, presumably caused by the illness, he begins to bend so that his chest is practically concave. Through insightful assistance he manages to become an advisor to students of philosophy; he regains status, usefulness, and self-respect. Lo and behold, the "irreversible" changes seen on x-ray disappear and the physical symptoms abate. A prominent psychiatrist upon retirement takes on the position of unofficial counselor to students in a university. He reports the work as more interesting, challenging, and worthwhile than he had ever anticipated psychiatric work could be. Biographies of famous people frequently show that those who continue to evolve as persons, who continue to refine and polish their highest human capacities—thought, reason, judgment—were less prone to chronic illness.

CHRONICITY IN MENTAL ILLNESS

Mental illness occurs in persons who have not yet developed interpersonal and intellectual competencies that would enable them to get along with people, work in the community, and evolve meaningful lives that utilize and develop further their innate human capacities. These lacks in competence are observable along four main lines: (1) disorders of the process of thought; (2) disorders of processes of perception and feeling; (3) actions that are inept, unwitting, or against the good of the social order; and (4) splitting of thought, feeling, and action in relation to particular experiences. To discuss the ramifications of all of these in detail is not within the present purview, but, in order to indicate the role of psychiatric nurses in preventing chronicity, I will indicate examples of these disorders and suggest professional interventions. (See also Chapter 21, this volume.)

Although chronicity in mental illness has its roots in development, it also results from reinforcement of the operating pathology inherent in the patient's behavior. To put it another way, chronicity in patients represents a failure of staff to force constructive change in the patient. Chronicity is not produced in patients deliberately by staff members, family, or friends. Rather, the expectations and beliefs of these significant others are conveyed unwittingly to patients who "read the message" that they are hopeless, worthless, and insignificant. Because the message confirms what the patient already believes about the self, this consensus between patient and significant others places no pressure upon the patient to change and grow; instead, it affords the patient a modicum of relief from anxiety.

Chronicity can also be seen as an outcome of serious gaps in the professional's knowledge about psychiatric problems, particularly theories about interpersonal dynamisms in relation to pathological processes. Without explanatory theory, interpersonal observations have little meaning. Such observations must be "accurately" interpreted and used as the basis for constructive nursing interventions.

Interventions are, in effect, counterpulls on pathology, pulls that slowly force behavioral changes.

A new approach to daily nursing care of patients who have mental illness could be developed along the lines of the foregoing argument that chronicity consists of substitutive behavior that evolves when capacities are not challenged, developed, and used. More specifically, it occurs when one or more of the four lacks in competence cited earlier become highly developed substitutive behaviors that are reinforced by significant others. The major questions raised by this definition would be: What are, or were, the actual capacities of this psychiatric patient? What prevented or continues to prevent release, development, and use of these capacities? What would now challenge latent capacities toward belated development in a way that takes into account the status and position the patient has actually achieved?

The linkages of integrations (patterns of relationships) that the patient has had have to be identified in a gross way and verified by continuous study of nurse–patient interactions in which attempts by the patient at replication of such patterns are made. Intensive study of each patient on first admission, specialized nursing by a psychiatric nurse for the entire first week of hospital stay, and deliberative planning by a team of all professionals involved in the psychiatric patient care plan of this patient might lead to a blueprint toward resolution of the patient's difficulties. Caudill et al. (1952) first pointed out how very important the first twenty-four hours of hospitalization are in structuring the attitudes and expectations of patients toward continuing their struggle for understanding and resolution of their problems. He has shown how patients tend to forego the struggle, hide the problem, and aim merely toward "getting out." Perhaps this helps explain the increasingly high readmission rate of psychiatric patients, for the problem remains hidden and unexplored, to surface again.

EARLY PREVENTION

The question of unused or unchallenged capacity as the main ingredient in chronicity is also related to prevention of mental illness.

For instance, with rare exception all children have the capacity to read. Yet there are many children who develop reading disabilities quite early in their educational career. What are the "causes" of those disabilities? Well, one main cause is the inability to discipline focal awareness. The question is: What aids and abets development of this ability? There is psychological literature on the theory of attention and on interferences to its development. Such theory provides a base for the development of interventions that school personnel and school nurses could use to resolve the problem of the school child. Failure to do so means continuation of "this brick in the basement" from which mental illness will later develop. Failure to correct reading disabilities may be a very early step in the long process of chronicity in mental illness.

Another preventive approach might be to scrutinize the school system, of which there are still far too many examples. When a child does something that the teacher sees as "bad," what then is the next step? In far too many schools the child is assigned to write the multiplication table 100 times or some such nonsense. To look at this "punishment" from the child's perspective, the child is required under threat of worse punishment to do extra "distasteful" intellectual work. This assignment, inevitably, forces into the awareness of the child a destructive connection between punishment and use of intelligence. This is indeed a connection that will not act as a spur to the further development of that particular capacity.

Furthermore, the assignment itself tends in the direction of automatic behavior. By the time the child has reached the fortieth time around he or she is writing "automatically," that is, without thought, and therefore is being "conditioned" rather than educated. The child is no longer learning anything, for learning requires observation, analysis, formulation, and so on. To carry this one instance a step further, the assignment omits perhaps the most important aspect. This particular punishment does not teach anything about reparative acts. The teacher has not opened up for this child the alternatives from which can be chosen the behaviors that would "fix what has been done that was bad." Instead, it breeds lack of interest in thought, for it introduces the use of intelligence in a way that is tedious and boring, demanded by irrational authorities not worth imitating.

This problem may seem a far cry from the subject at hand, namely, chronicity of mental illness, but it is damaged capacities such as in the child just described that underlie a great deal of the mental illness that now has to be dealt with in public mental hospitals. And years later it is much harder to reach latent capacities that are buried behind disuse and inept use.

The educational systems in various secondary schools must eventually be looked at with a psychological microscope to see what problems are reinforced or created by the interaction between teacher and student. For example, many teachers pick on bright girls, especially those who ask embarrassing questions or pose too many "why" questions that the teacher cannot answer. In some situations teachers use belittling tactics to deal with such students in ways that all too frequently have irreparable effects on the mental health of the student. The teacher may pick on a girl who is precocious, for behavior that would be overlooked in a boy or in a nonquestioning girl. "Stop being a leader," "Don't be a smart aleck," "Stop acting like a teenager," "Be quiet," "Fix your hair." These become the picayune responses from the teacher to the student to critical questions about something that she has noticed or about which she wants help or information. Such comments by teachers, made directly and daily to the student, in front of peers, contribute or reinforce derogation as a feature of the student's self-system. Shame and embarrassment become connected with thought. The problem is compounded if the student cannot turn to parents for help in seeing the school system for what it is. The student needs more than parental sympathy. Parental help is required to analyze what the student is really up against; in helping the student to separate her problem from the teacher's problem; in helping her to see the collision of her interests and values with those of the system and for figuring out a way not to lose her own focus, to compromise compliantly only up to a point. Real prevention of mental illness will derive from such a process.

Another way to look at the problem of chronicity is from the standpoint of what the behavior of the "chronic" patient does: what it says, asks for, and evokes in others. This of course requires the staff to be receptive in collecting data so as to infer the message, and then to check it out for accuracy. In a general way, the behavior in chronic illness says, "Take care of me, see how helpless I am." It asks for sympathy in an obligating symbiotic way. It frequently evokes anger or hostility in others because it conveys hostility, an unconscious, purposeful evening-up of some older score.

CHARACTERISTICS OF CHRONICITY

Probably, it would be possible to invent a psychological profile to predict which newly admitted patients, left largely to their own devices, will become chronic and which ones will not. The following might be some ingredients of such a profile:

> The person who tends toward chronicity lacks the ability to see constructive alternatives in the use of his or her capacities when authority figures prevent their use. As I indicated above, the schools do not teach in this manner and the more rigid the school the more the emphasis will be on instant compliance, which is an either/or situation. There are only two alternatives: Do what you are told no matter how useless, or take equally useless punishment.

> The person who tends toward chronicity cannot separate his or her problem from the problems of other persons who cannot be changed. Such a person cannot "give and take," and instead uses others and sets up situations in which he or she is used.

> The person who tends toward chronicity has an unusually strong need for approval (and was very probably a teacher's pet or "goody-goody"), and has an equally strong acquired substitute need for disapproval that has become automatic in that it operates without conscious thought.

> The person who tends toward chronicity is timid about self-expression of any kind. He or she is unable to say what is personally experienced verbally, in writing, through music, art, dance, dress, or any other means.

> The person who tends toward chronicity lacks drive in any direction, yielding to whatever brings relief rather than struggling toward solution of any kind of problem no matter how minor.

The person who tends toward chronicity lacks humor, unable to see incongruities and ambiguities in situations and make light of the more innocuous of these.

The characteristics of the person tending toward chronicity suggest where the main learning should take place. Current responses to chronic patients in mental hospitals tend more to yield to the trend rather than identify and treat the basic problems. A patient care program directed at competency building would serve as a major reeducation system.

Remotivation as a program of activity for patients is better than nothing but it is based on a "shape-up" notion not unlike that already perpetrated on the individual through a school or home situation or both. Occupational therapy frequently comes also from the same bolt of cloth. The actors (i.e., the remotivators and occupational therapists) all too often do not really believe that the patients have latent and undeveloped capacities available for use, and the patients know, empathically, by "reading" the nonverbal cues, that the program directors hold these attitudes. Schizophrenic patients particularly take cues from the nonverbal behavior of others, having learned long ago that people tend to say one thing and do the opposite, and that the latter is a more accurate index of the "true" attitude of "these people." As a result, there is a consensus that everyone goes through the motions and it keeps both staff and patients busy. One clue that staff is skeptical about patients' capacities is staff anxiety when a suggestion is made that a patient indeed has inherent capacity. That possibility collides with the more firmly held and acted upon idea that patients either lack capacity entirely or that it is completely inaccessible. This idea has requirements of its own, namely, that very elementary approaches to patients are held onto.

Chronicity in mental illness is the result of interpersonal interaction. In fact, the mental illness itself is not simply intrapersonal. In working with psychiatric patients it is clear that they use the staff to maintain their mental illness by keeping previously "sick" integrations with other persons going. They replicate in the present those relationships that in the past led to the present dilemmas of hiding capacities "under a bushel." This is understandable, for the sick behavior to the patient is the familiar behavior, the only known behavior, and it serves marvelous anti-anxiety relief functions. The patient cannot change without help.

CLINICAL CONSIDERATIONS

One characteristic of the relationship between the mother and the child who later becomes mentally ill is that there are continuing power struggles, the aim of which is to obtain an answer to who controls the child. During these struggles, which go on for quite a while before the child more or less yields and accepts "powerlessness," it is the one who becomes ill who loses the power struggle. This power struggle is replicated in the clinical situation to the extent that the nursing personnel aim at control over the patient rather than fostering learning by a variety of nonacademic means. Control involves a more or less ready-made notion of how the child (later the patient) should behave: what the child should feel, think, or do under certain circumstances. Learning involves review of experience by aiding and abetting observation, description, analysis, formulation of meaning or relations, testing such formulations in action, and the resultant foresight. On the other hand, control involves telling the patient what to do. Learning requires that the patient become involved in discovering personal wants, wishes, interests, and direction with help. The patient in a mental hospital has, with rare exception, not had that kind of help with learning from anyone; or it has occurred so infrequently, in a way so tangential to his or her experience, that it has not become internalized as a recurring useful mode of dealing with experience.

Central to the problem of irrational, recurring control-oriented situations is the problem of anxiety. Although the words *anxiety* and *tension* are increasingly common in this culture, the person who becomes mentally ill does not recognize his or her own anxiety. Sometimes when you are talking with a patient who has a great deal of anxiety, as indicated by such observable behaviors as scattering of thought or fidgeting, ask that patient right then: "Are you anxious?" or "Are you uncomfortable right now?" Most of the time you will get instant denial: "No, I am not, and I never have been anxious," or "I am anxious to get home, that's what." In a very few instances you will get doubt: "Maybe I am a little," or "Once I was anxious." Rarely will you get a direct naming of the anxiety. Naming is one of the very earliest intellectual competencies. Mothers teach their children to name an object (like a spoon), then events (like eating supper). Yet, here is an experience the patient is having, creating tremendous energy that is transformed into behavior, and for which relief in some form must be sought, and there is no awareness of the experience. The existence of anxiety is not simply the problem. Being unable to recognize and name anxiety, which is a first step in grappling with the problem, immediately implies that the patient is equally unaware of the relief behavior. Relief operations are automatic, habitual, and used without conscious thought. Because the patient uses automatic behaviors recurringly, the same thing happens to the thought process that would happen to any other body part or function that was denied usage: It withers.

Disuse is the crippling step in the development of chronicity. Disuse of the thought process by the patient, failure to seek and to acquire meaning from experience as it is lived, failure to feel it, react with, or respond to it, and plan for future experiences—all this leads to further disuse. In my experience with psychiatric patients, disuse leads to even greater anxiety. In contrast, when capacities are used, refined, polished, and respected in oneself, anxiety is not overwhelming.

The problem of anxiety in patients is not simply an intrapersonal matter. One interpersonal or interactive facet is that the anxiety of the patient is communicated interpersonally to staff. If staff anxiety is also unrecognized, if staff members are unable to say, "I am anxious" when they are, then these staff members are also vulnerable. The particular vulnerability is that staff will unwittingly participate in integrations with patients that are easiest to come by, that are automatic, and that provide staff immediate relief from their own anxiety. The aim of helping patients grow, learn, change, and regain mental health is relinquished. In other words, both patient and staff repeatedly close off learning merely to get relief from anxiety, which they do not know that they have.

The classic example follows. A patient becomes angry and begins to berate a staff member. This patient is anxious and has converted the energy of the anxiety into automatic anger, by which he mobilizes power, feeling less helpless and gaining relief from the anxiety. The staff member fails to recognize the basis for the anger but empathizes (automatically experiences as his or her own) the patient's anxiety. Now the staff member is anxious and shouts back at the patient in order to control the situation, in order to feel relief from the empathized anxiety, and to mobilize power to feel less helpless or humiliated. The patient now empathizes the staff member's anxiety and, because the automatic relief behavior did not work to reduce the anxiety, the patient's anxiety is increased. Now the patient has to redouble efforts by shouting louder and adding relief behaviors. The patient makes threats that he will break the door down. The patient's increased anxiety is now empathized by the staff member who now feels more anxiety and urgently needs relief. As the situation develops further, the staff member either uses seclusion, restraints, or medication and the patient has been shown who is in control.

Now, the situation that I have just described pinpoints the replication of the power struggle that went on previously between the parent and the child who has become the patient. The patient initiated a series of behaviors, unwittingly, but purposefully, to maintain the illness, to keep the familiar integration going. The staff person participated and has unwittingly taken that patient one step toward chronicity.

To avoid chronicity, one thing that absolutely must go on in a relationship is testing. The patient must test out changes for "new" behavior, and the staff person must survive the test if the new behavior is somehow to be included into the patient's repertoire of behavior. New behavior is tested and included; the old behavior drops out and change occurs. The patient tests a new person to see whether that person's observations of and responses to him or her are in any way different from those occurring in prior integrations. I will admit that testing behavior of patients can be trying and it accounts in large part for the reason that many private practitioners do not like to work with certain kinds of patients in office practice. Testing for embarrassment is not an easy thing to survive, for example. But it ought to be possible within the comfortable confines of the hospital, where everyone understands that the aim of the hospital is to aid and abet the patients in learning and trying out new and more constructive uses of their capacities. Furthermore, understanding the pathology at work is helpful to hospital professional staff in interpreting and dealing with the presenting behavior of patients. All will learn, rather than participate in the pathology or try to police or control it.

Each time a patient tests out a new staff person to see what works with that individual and what help obtains from that person, the patient has secured an answer about the extent to which there is hope for getting out of his or her predicament. Moreover, every test that is not survived by the staff creates in the mind of the patient the expectation that the next person will also not survive. Hopelessness that evolved in earlier situations is thus gradually reinforced, and the patient soon begins to see everyone as more or less like those awful people from earlier experience who helped produce the illness in the first place. Patients test staff members for interest, for capability in listening, for evidence of readiness to have control over the patient, for possible dependence, for honesty, for disapproval and punishment, for vulnerable areas in staff. It takes a sensitive, perceptive nurse who has theory to help interpret (privately) what she is observing, who can deal with these testing maneuvers in a direct and useful way that does not replicate previous pathological integrations the patient has had.

UNDERSTANDING INTEGRATION: NON-THERAPEUTIC AND THERAPEUTIC

Unwitting integrations between staff and patients have two purposes from the patient's standpoint: (1) They provide relief from anxiety and (2) they provide proof that what they expect of people is correct. Psychiatric patients expect to be controlled, manipulated, used, derogated or belittled, and in general seen as largely worthless. And most of their approaches to others are in the vein of confirming the expectations. Each staff member who does confirm these expectations, wittingly or unwittingly, reinforces the expectations and convinces the patient that subsequent persons will likewise reinforce them. The patient tends sooner or later to have the proof he seeks that "all people" are indeed like his or her awful parents. When the patient's expectations are more or less confirmed, he or she withdraws. When staff members make it mutual by using indifference toward the patient, the process of chronicity is speeded up. The reason this occurs is that the more the patient is cut off from verbal interchanges with real people, it becomes increasingly necessary to have relationships with illusory figures— perhaps to invent more figures for this purpose. Because the self develops in a relationship, self-definition is always in relation to others, real or illusory. Without opportunity for relationships with real people, the patient invents figures to fill the void.

I would like to point out, however, that there is a significant difference between staff indifference to patients and objective clinical detachment. Objective clinical detachment is absolutely essential if there is to be open and useful discussion with patients, and if the nurse is to be able to focus on the needs of patients. That focus requires the nurse to observe his or her own participation with patients sufficiently to separate the nurse's own needs from theirs. All too often patients are used to meet staff needs or hospital maintenance needs. Perhaps one of the most difficult clinical tasks is to focus exclusively and intensively on the needs, concerns, and learning activities of patients so that they can move in a favorable direction. This requires clinical detachment. Indifference, on the other hand, occurs when unsatisfactory integrations between staff and patients lead the staff to "give up," to move away, to leave the patient wallowing helplessly in a dilemma.

Therapeutic nursing as I have been defining it so far requires a forced change in the patient because the nurse offers a relationship focused on learning coupled with nonparticipation in the pathology of the patient. The nurse does this in millions of small ways all day long. The nurse separates herself from the patient and does not require an incorporation of nurse and patient. For instance, the nurse does not use *we*. Instead, she or he speaks for self using the personal pronoun, *I*. The nurse refers to the patient by the surname in a respectful manner. The nurse does not increase the felt inadequacy of the patient through language: She or he does not say, "Can you tell me what happened?" for this suggests doubt about the patient's ability to recall and answer; instead the nurse merely says "Tell me," assuming the patient can. The nurse that I am talking about has a sustained interest in the patient and does everything required during working hours to improve her grasp of the problem and the interventions necessary for resolution. Nursing in this sense is an active process where one is alert to what is observed, utilizing theory to explain what has been noticed, and basing nursing interventions on known theories and inferences derived from the clinical work.

One factor I have noticed in the production of chronicity is that when the patient begins to make great strides, to show improvement, the improvement at first sometimes looks like more severe illness. This is because the patient has become more open. With no need any longer to hide the illness, the patient becomes more willing to reveal it, both to himself and to others, in the hope that the meaning and purpose can be grasped. Furthermore, the patient's openness tests the staff for genuine interest. If the staff survives this test, allowing and supporting the therapeutic process to continue, the patient will then take some giant steps.

At this point, the chances are very good that the significant other, the person in the family who was the major participant in the "sick" integration that preceded the psychotic episode, will become extremely active to reinstate the illness. Generally, this is a family member, a friend, or even a physician or nurse who has some unusual need to *maintain* the patient's illness in order to *maintain* an integration based on unwitting need.

One such need is to continue the contrast that the "one" is sick and the "other" is not. This action always occurs when the patient is actively making great strides toward change. I learned this through a variety of experiences, some personal and some professional. In a hospital situation, the mechanism proceeds like this: The patient is actively trying to change his or her situation or to try out new behavior that he or she has been considering with the help of a therapist. The staff members perceive the change and become anxious because an unfamiliar element now threatens previous control that was "known" vis-a-vis the familiar, predictable behavior of the patient. The staff members use minor techniques to restore the old integration. Rouslin (1963) has described this with respect to the phenomenon of chronic helpfulness. The staff see the patient as a helpful drudge. The patient begins to see the self as exploited and expresses anger. Staff anxiety leads to such tactics as appealing to the "better nature of the patient." For example, the staff might say, "Oh, how about baking me a cake today; I'd love to have a piece of cake that you made." The detail the staff member has picked seems innocuous enough and the patient complies and may feel shame at his or her anger. The staff member, however, has not dealt with the reality of the patient's actual experience, namely anger, which is the turning point of change and accessibility in this particular patient. The patient who repeatedly experiences such events eventually gives up any hope of learning about the self, so community life outside the hospital becomes impossible. In this sense, it can be said that "chronicity creeps up on the patient." The patient, like the child in the earlier mother–child relationship, makes many tries before finally giving up when the ominous weight of staff control becomes exquisitely clear. Chronicity is a process that leads to apathetic compliance only after there have been many tries in the direction of change, tries that have been overlooked or ineptly handled by staff because they are not dramatic events. Rather, the tries were minor changes that unwittingly evoke staff anxiety.

The patients in many psychiatric hospitals, unfortunately, are dependent on their families to sign for them in order to obtain a release from the hospital. It has been my observation that on many occasions at the point that the patient is making great strides in the direction of self-change, unimpeded by staff members, a family member becomes more active in order to reintegrate the previous illness or sick relationship. Most frequently this is the parent. Not infrequently, the parent will make an appeal to see the therapist to talk about the patient's problems. The mother or father will use various rationales to make the reason for coming to talk with the therapist sound plausible and appealing.

The parental appeal includes several tactics that are worth noticing. The parent will most often use praise; the therapist is indeed trusted by the patient as no one before has been. If the therapist needs this kind of "outside evaluation" and praise, he or she is vulnerable to the drama about to unfold. The parent may say it is impossible to understand why the patient has become increasingly hostile in their relationship. Or an appeal may be made to "our common interest" in the patient. And, to be sure, there will be concealed ingratiating messages in phone conversations or letters. Many therapists will be seduced by these messages, tending to take the positive rather than the negative view, because the parent will appeal to the therapist as the "good figure" the therapist wants to be.

It is important to weigh in advance the possible real intentions of the parent's request to see the therapist. If there is the slightest inkling that it may damage the therapist–patient relationship, then a separate interview should not be held. The unspoken parental motivation is to interrupt change in the patient in order to restore the idea that no one is a better parent than the patient's parent.

A triadic parent–patient–therapist interview is much more useful. This provides the parent with an opportunity to see how the therapist and patient work together. The patient is aware of all the data conveyed to the parent and in the process can judge the reliability of the therapist. Often the therapeutic relationship is improved afterward. However, the interview may also engender envy in the parent, particularly if it is impossible for the parent to emulate the behavior of the therapist with the patient. Such envy may be the basis for appeals to higher authority to get even with or to equalize the status of parent and therapist. It may be necessary to belittle or show up the therapist—or even get the therapist into trouble of some kind with a higher authority. Most state hospitals have at least one patient whose parent has many times gone all the way to the governor's office and succeeded in destroying a therapist–patient relationship.

Parataxis goes on all over the place in this situation. The therapist becomes the patient that the parent hopes to control. On the other hand, the therapist is the parent in the patient's eyes and also becomes a competing parent in the eyes of the real parent. The therapist must be acutely aware of these phenomena. In fact, the pull on the therapist by the parent as third party in a triadic interview that has as its intention the reintegration of a sick parent–patient relationship and the destruction of the therapist–patient relationship is very strong. On the therapist's part, a deliberate effort must be made to lean with the patient and to maintain the therapeutic relationship, for if the therapist does not do this, then the parent–patient relationship is reinstated and strengthened, and a step toward chronicity has been taken by the patient with the therapist's assistance.

The patient's parent may have an uncanny way of reaching the vulnerabilities of the other person. After all, this skill worked so well with the child who has become mentally ill. In the original process the parent has used mixed messages, reading meaning into data, and other controlling operations to render the child powerless. The process is more subtle with the therapist. The parent approaches the therapist to talk about the patient, leaving the impression that the help of the parent will be useful in the therapeutic process. The therapist frequently thinks that to enlist the cooperation of the parent creates the possibility that the patient will be welcomed home and treated differently than in the past. This idea, however, represents a dissociation of what the therapist knows about the interpersonal interaction that produced the pathology, for the parent has not changed at all.

Further, therapists operate on an optimistic bias, but the net effect of a parent–therapist interview—dyadic or triadic—almost inevitably is the loss of the patient's interest in working therapeutically. Often the problem is such a ticklish one that a supervisory review prior to the interview is advisable. In this supervisory review the supervisor may well see things the therapist has optimistically overlooked; pointing these out may be tantamount to confronting the therapist with selectively inattended or dissociated areas of an immediate event. Therefore, there may be severe anxiety that has to be dealt with before the interview occurs.

If the therapist agrees to the triadic interview, it does provide an opportunity to see how the parent goes about reinforcing the pathology of the patient, thus contributing to the chronicity. For example, in one situation it was observed that both parent and patient communicated importantly only on a nonverbal level, the verbal behavior being only a reaction to the nonverbal. In one situation the patient threw her arms back and stretched. The therapist observed that the mother's anxiety increased; however, she did not respond directly to the patient. Instead, she became picky—focused on detail—and struggled with the patient on picayune items. The patient apparently perceived the "verbal disgust" indicated by the mother's forbidding gesture, but she also did not respond directly. Instead, she responded to the details that the mother was picking on. Finally, the therapist asked the mother what reaction she had when her daughter threw her arms back and stretched. Her immediate response was, "It was vulgar." This was indeed the nonverbal message and the patient understood it well. The situation was another way the patient had of acting out the mixed messages that her mother had repeatedly given in her early years: Sex was bad, but do get involved in it. By stretching, the patient could communicate half the mixed message back to the mother nonverbally.

As a result of the interview the therapist was able to see quite clearly some of the early testing maneuvers the patient had used with the therapist to evoke disgust, to gain disapproval, to eventually drive the therapist away. These included behaviors that would ordinarily call out forbidding gestures, such as picking her nose, scratching her genitals, and squeezing pimples, to which her mother, then as now, responded with derogation and forbiddance.

It is important to remember that if in a triadic interview there is a replication of the power struggle of parent and child in the parent–therapist relationship, the issue is, "Who is the better parent?" In this struggle the therapist is indeed vulnerable. In addition, because of the parent–child struggle, the therapist must lean with the patient. As the international scene demonstrates every day, a power struggle lost at one level is tried out at another level, all the way to a showdown. In most cases, the parent will appeal to the clinical director, superintendent, commissioner, and governor, in that order. Chronicity in patients will be lessened when the environment of the hospital is such that the higher authorities support the therapist—not the parent at the expense of the patient—and where therapy is also available to the parent.

SUMMING UP

My concern is that nurses participate in relationships with patients in ways that promote learning and change, rather than reinforce pathology in the direction of chronicity. For such participation, nurses need help. They need staff development programs to make theory viable for everyday observations of their interactions with patients. They need time to think about what they are doing, to talk about it with others, and the opportunity to study their relationships with at least one patient on a continuing basis. In this way their observations will be sharpened, their applications of theory will be refined, and their clinical competence will be enhanced. Nurses have what women are often credited with having: sensitivity, interest in nurturing, and intelligence. When these are brought to bear in patient care situations through direct nursing services, I am certain that patients will have enlarged opportunity to become well and get out into the community where they should be. Expert clinical nurses prepared in university graduate nursing programs can point the way, and help other nurses to improve their direct nursing practices with patients. These psychiatric nurses are trying to evolve the kind of professional nurse required to help resolve the problems of psychiatric patients.

This is to say that what is needed is a sensitive, healthy, aware person, a professional nurse who can see the dilemma of the other as it unfolds and who has tactics that can bypass the going self-system of the patient, tap healthy capacities and develop these so that the need for the pathology drops out. When the pathology works, when it goes unscrutinized, when it is merely pacified or reinforced, it becomes the habitual way of life. Pathology left to itself gets worse.

REFERENCES

Caudill, W. K., Redlich, F. C., Gilmore, H. R., & Brody, E. B. (1952). Social structure and interaction processes on a psychiatric ward. *American Journal of Orthopsychiatry, 22*(2), 314–334.
Rouslin, S. (1963). Chronic helpfulness: Maintenance or intervention? *Perspectives in Psychiatric Care, 1*(1), 25–28.

CHAPTER 7

General Application of Theory and Techniques of Psychotherapy in Nursing Situations

THE AIMS OF PSYCHOTHERAPY

Individual psychotherapy is a specific type of encapsulated experience that permits an intense relationship and focus on the life experiences of one person, so that they may be reevaluated and understood. This type of corrective experience is an important one, in which the themes and patterns of behavior of the patient are identified, placed in the perspective of his or her biography, and seen in relation to the current need of these themes and patterns. The experience is corrective mainly because it brings to the attention of the patient various dimly known aspects of his or her life, and in so doing permits a reconsideration of what was involved. This kind of a review serves as a basis for reformulation of the

Paper originally presented at Cedars of Lebanon and Mount Sinai Hospital, Los Angeles, CA., July, 1964. Schlesinger Library, Radcliffe College, Cambridge, MA. No. 84-M107, Hildegard E. Peplau Archives, carton 39, volume 1451. Copyright 1986 by Schlesinger Library. Adapted and edited by permission.

patient's views on life, and therefore as a basis for choosing and trying out new behavior patterns that generally tend to be more in line with the capacities and interpersonal interests of the patient. Individual psychotherapy is conducted by individuals who have had education that provides a theoretical framework to understand much of what goes on in the individual sessions. The education, moreover, sensitizes the therapist to personal needs and patterns of behavior so that these can to a considerable extent be under control during psychotherapeutic sessions. That is, when working with a patient the therapist tends to be less unwitting in behavior, choosing instead responses that will most likely have favorable impact upon the patient. This type of education also includes a number of tactics or strategies that can be used to more or less force the patient to take a second look at experiences, and to arrive at reformulations of the meaning of these experiences.

PSYCHOTHERAPY PRINCIPLES APPLIED

With a few exceptions, much of what goes on in individual psychotherapy has general usefulness in the nursing situation. However, it is easier to grasp the general usefulness as a result of education for individual psychotherapy than it is to start at the general end. The reason for this is that in the individual work, with a specific patient, as the novice therapist returns session after session, he or she gets a pretty good idea of the tenacity of pathology, of the need for consistency in responses over time, and enlarged awareness of the way the patient's patterns affect the therapist in off-guard moments. It is difficult to teach these concerns in a situation in which others may just as easily be responsible for unfavorable changes in a patient. The individual therapist takes large responsibility for his or her own actions and for their impact on the patient. Nevertheless, there are some general considerations, stemming from a knowledge of psychotherapy, that do apply in nursing situations.

Most psychotherapists speak of a permissive atmosphere, a climate of acceptance of the patient as he or she is. Others speak of not accepting the behavior, but of always accepting the patient. I would like to put this in still another way, namely, struggling with the problem and not with the patient. Now, how do you do this? Let me cite some aspects of this process. First of all, your response to the patient should be largely nonpersonal; that is, the behavior of the patient, whatever it is, was not perpetrated just to annoy you. If it seems so, it is quite possible that you have been set up as a "straw man" for someone else in the background of the patient; in other words, instead of annoying his father the patient annoys you. If you can use this kind of detachment, that is the first step. Secondly, the patient may indeed select one of your vulnerable areas; there is no point working for a rise out of someone who doesn't rise to the bait. So, it would be helpful to gain as much awareness as you possibly can of your touchy areas—and mostly these have to do with areas that your own parents found touchy.

Sex is a sensitive topic for some nursing personnel; they find any mention of sex distasteful. These staff members then are vulnerable to patients who use sex talk to intimidate. Another area is anger; many parents do not permit their children either to act angry, or to think about anger, or even ever to feel angry. The tendency, then, of a nurse who has had this in her own background would be for her to close off all expression of anger by patients. Yet some of them must express the "negative" feelings of anger, shame, embarrassment or hatred in order to get to the deeply buried or disassociated "positive feelings of tenderness, concern and interest."

In general, I am not saying that patients should be encouraged to have catharsis of any and all feelings at all times; in fact, I am not at all convinced that mere catharsis is useful. I am saying that the initial expression of strong feelings must be tolerated. The aim, then, is to get to the problem and to struggle with it, letting the patient's behavior go on while encouraging discussion about whatever concerns him or her at the time. This gives you an opportunity to observe the behavior, catalogue it as a pattern, and perhaps get some data that helps you to understand the pattern. Furthermore, if you work in a ward and do this regularly, you begin to see the recurring patterns of a particular patient. And once you see the pattern more or less clearly, you are then in a position to design strategies in which the whole staff can participate in the hope of producing change. Let me give you an example.

A new patient comes to the head nurse in the office and says: "That other patient in my room hit me." The nurse, of course, might give a nonsense reply like "What did he do that for?" The patient cannot answer this question; he can only speak for himself. The nurse goes after data descriptive of the situation; she asks, "When did he hit you?" The patient replies, "Oh, a while ago." The nurse privately notes the unspecific reply and says, "What were you doing at the time?" The patient says, "I was just sitting there." The nurse says, "Sitting where?" The patient says, "Oh, never mind," and walks off.

Sometime later the same patient comes up to the head nurse and says, "That other patient isn't eating his food." Again, the nurse could give a nonsense reply such as "Well, he better; he needs it." Instead, let us assume she merely says, "Oh!" The patient then baits the nurse a bit further, "He didn't eat his lunch, either." Again the nurse says, "Oh!" The patient turns away and says, "Well, I thought you wanted to know."

The next day the patient comes to the nurse and says, "Two of the patients in my room told me to get out of the room." The nurse now has three instances, all of which suggest a number of hunches about this patient's problem:

1. The patient's pattern is that of a tattle tale or teacher's pet.
2. The patient is lacking in interpersonal skills for getting along with his peers; in this instance, the patient group.

Now, with these two hypotheses in mind, the nursing staff might discuss the particular kind of interpersonal warp that leads to being a teacher's pet, and they might consider the kinds of interpersonal skills that seem to be missing, such as in this case, the ability to compete for peer attention. The staff group might want to make further observations for a day or two, to see whether these patterns do indeed seem to fit the isolated details of observed behavior of this patient. If such confirmation is secured, then the question would be: What strategies or tactics on the part of the staff would most likely aid and abet this patient in developing the needed skills? The head nurse, for example, might decide to respond to all talebearing incidents by saying: "Let me send Mrs. Jones down to the room with you to talk this over with you and the other patients concerned." That is, she would not lend a private ear to the patient, but rather would seek to arbitrate the difficulties among the several patients.

If one aspect of psychotherapy is to struggle with the problem, another is to provide a special type of experience, a type more constructive than any previously undergone by the patient. As such, the therapist attempts not to replicate the behaviors that parents used in order to produce the pathology in the patient. This would seem to suggest, for example, that staff take a look at all their behaviors that tend to cause problems for people, such as dominating the patient by telling the patient what to think, feel, or do. Problematic staff behaviors might include giving approval or praise, which foster the patient's dependence on the nurse in order to be recognized. On the other hand, members of the staff ought to take active roles with patients, not replicating indifference patients may have encountered earlier with family members.

Role reversal seems to be a characteristic of families in which mental illness is produced; that is, the growing child is placed in the position of looking after, or being a mother to, the mother or father, who tends to act helpless, or uses the children to get the work done well out of proportion to what might be expected as chores connected with normal socialization of the child. It would, then, be very important that staff take a look at the uses that are made of patients—whether these reinforce feelings of being exploited or used—in fact, denied the role of child.

Overprotection seems also to be a factor, particularly in the case of children who were born underweight or handicapped, or where the mother had a particular fear of death in general, or death of her child in particular. The crippling effect of overprotection stems from the fact that it does not allow exercise of capacities and learning by trial and error. In the clinical situation, it would be important to identify patients who had this particular kind of early childhood experience, and to develop the strategies that would reduce its replication by nursing staff.

The self or identity of the patient is often problematic. In answer to the question, "Who am I?" the patient has no confident answers, or the answers tend to be on the side of worthlessness, low self-esteem, inadequacy, and general inferiority or helplessness. The development of such a self-system started with the appraisals of parents, phrases they used very early in the life of the patient to designate him or her as an acting person. The second step in the self-system development is the hearing and interrelation of these parental appraisals. The third step is getting the actions to go with the internalized self-views. And the fourth step is seeking validation of the internalized self-views. Now, the patient in the nursing situation uses the nursing staff in subtle ways to gain validation, that is, agreement with existing views of the self. And, if the views are primarily derogatory and the nursing staff in any way agrees, then this validation has a reinforcing effect; that is, it is not corrective of the disparaging self-system.

On the other hand, to merely say the opposite to the patient does not work either. If a depressed patient says, "I'm no good," and the nurse says, "Oh, yes you are, you have three fine children," two alternative responses are then open to the patient. The patient can redouble efforts to communicate the worthlessness, such as a beautiful patient who spoke of herself as "ugly" and finally slashed her face because the nurses could not grasp the importance of her recurring statement "I am ugly" and their reassurance that she was beautiful. Or the patient can become completely dependent on the nurse, requiring an increasing number of praiseworthy statements in order to buttress the shaky self-esteem. Now what can the nurse do if a patient says, "I'm the dumb one in my family" or "I'm no good; my father always said so." Well, the nurse can attempt to open up the discussion: "When did you first notice this?" "What is the evidence for that comment?" "Who told you that?" "What did you think when you were little?" "Give me an example," and so on. The patient, of course, does not know the way in which the self-system developed; nor could the patient, in one sitting, detail all the experiences and statements by significant others that finally got indelibly structured into the current self-system. But the nursing staff can ask a question each time so that in time, the patient can begin to feel some doubt about the 100% reliability of his or her view in relation to the inherent capability or capacity, seeing the current view instead as a product of his or her past experience.

Another thing that staff can do is to assist patients to name their anxiety. It is always somewhat of a surprise to me that mentally ill patients—who suffer severe and continuing anxiety, and use rather precarious behaviors to try to reduce, relieve, or prevent more anxiety—do not know they are anxious. Helping the patient to name it is a first step. This is a very early step in child development; the child first sees objects and is assisted to name them, as for example a spoon. Then, the mother begins to help the child to name abstract aspects of events, such as "naughty." The same requirement and capacity is true of anxiety; the patient cannot get at the source of the anxiety until there is awareness of anxiety and it can be named. So, when the nurse observes that a patient is very upset, or angry, or belittling, or complaining, she can say, "Are you anxious right now?" In most instances, the first response will be denial; the patient will say no. But, as the nurse keeps asking, the patient will next show some doubt, saying, "Maybe I am." And finally a "yes" answer will occur. After the nurse has done this enough times, so that she is sure that the patient can recognize and name his or her own extreme discomfort, then she can begin to help the patient to connect the anxiety and its relief behavior. She can say: "What helps?" "What relieves it?" "What is relieving it right now?"

Patients use many relief behaviors such as anger, rage, rocking, sleep, and hallucinations. When the patient has been able to make connections between anxiety and relief behavior a sufficient number of times so the nurse is fairly confident of the ability, then the nurse can get at what went before the anxiety. It is helpful not to ask, "What caused it?" It is more useful, and easier for the patient to answer, if the nurse says: "What were you thinking or doing just before you got anxious?" This maneuver should yield the expectations of the patient, which can then be compared to what happened instead of what was expected. In general, this is what causes anxiety—when expectations, prestige, or status needs that are operative are not met. In most instances, the best way to reduce chronic anxiety is to change the expectations that are held.

For example, a patient believes that her stepmother should love her. She rushes home from work each day, confident that when she telephones her stepmother that a loving response will occur. Each time, however, the stepmother comes through with a comment like, "What did you call me now for? You know I am having my supper and anything you have to say to me can wait." But she goes on hoping, reinforcing a noble but worthless "should" system, and being recurringly anxious and increasingly unable to cope with its deleterious effects upon her thought and relationships with other people. Lastly, I think it would be helpful if nursing staff put their emphasis on helping patients to learn from experience rather than emphasizing arbitrary controls over behavior. Much of the behavior of the patient is rather automatic anyway. It is an immediate response that has as its aim the relief of anxiety or the prevention of more anxiety. Control of behavior is not possible unless you are able to observe, describe, and analyze the situation, then formulate what is going on (which is the learning product), validate, test, and use new behavior based upon the formulation. This concept of learning (as contrasted to the ones that have more to do with stimulus–response conditioning, adaptation, or brainwashing) suggests that the patient can put up with the anxiety while he is helped to observe and describe what is going on. So, in all instances that come to the attention of the nursing staff, it would be helpful if nurses aided and abetted description of experience. First you get the structural elements in the experience; this tactic reduces some of the anxiety. "Who was there?" "Where did it happen?" "What time was it?" "How old were you?" Then: "What happened?" The aim is to be a blow-by-blow description of the experience rather than classifications or generalizations from the experience. The nurse, then, must know the difference between description and generalization, between detail and classification.

One aspect of mental illness is disorder of the thought process, and one variant of this disorder is the tendency to lose the detail and become vague, general, overabstracted. The corrective experience is to ask for the opposite—instances of experience given in verbatim fashion. It would help if all nursing staff made a conscious effort to give less opinion, advice, or conclusion, and sought instead some further description from every patient, regarding every statement or complaint of the patient. In the first place, it would convey to the patient that the nurse was interested, concerned, and listening; if the nurse handled the questions comfortably and capably, it would help develop trust and respect between nurse and patient. Many patients who become mentally ill are persons who have been unable to evoke tender concern and interest of others in hearing about their experiences. It would be most useful if nursing personnel would develop this kind of interest in patients, to listen, to ask simple questions such as "Tell me more about that," "What does this have to do with you?" or "What was your part in that situation?" Patients who have been in psychiatric hospitals repeatedly or long show that the next layer of illness is the institutional overlay pathology. Such patients often give up expectation that anyone will ever be interested in them. In fact, in working psychotherapeutically with chronic patients, it takes the most painstaking effort and sustained interest to get the patient to talk about the self at all. Instead the patient is all too willing to tell in great detail about the lives of others because his or her own seems to have shriveled down to almost nonexistence.

I think you would find it useful, also, to study a particular patient and to pursue through direct transactions with that patient the nature of his or her pathology. You need to do this for purposes of refining your understanding of the difficulties of patients. You can learn much more by studying patients than by studying textbooks in psychiatric nursing. By studying, however, I mean collecting notes, reviewing them, trying to figure out what is going on. And one important aspect of what is going on is the way in which the patient is using you to maintain his or her pathology, to keep the illness going. This is understandable; it is familiar behavior; it has served the patient well in reducing and preventing more anxiety; and so the patient is loath to yield familiar behavior for new behavior. But you need to determine your participation with patients on the basis of the possibility that changes in your behavior will be influential in altering their views and behavior in a favorable direction. And this requires you to study what goes on, to take a second look—at least in your relationships with one patient on a regular basis—so as to improve your own techniques and enlarge self-awareness.

CHAPTER 8

Pattern Interactions

Pattern interaction is a phenomenon rarely researched, infrequently written about in psychiatric literature, and mostly overlooked as a topic for discussion. Pattern interactions that occur at the unit level, between patients, and patients and staff, surely are an important area for study and for therapeutic intervention.

In psychiatric units where staff nurses are not engaged in scheduled psychotherapeutic work with patients, their interactions with patients—which constitute a large part of their work role—ought to be viewed as a significant contribution to the outcome of hospitalization.

In this chapter I will define pattern interaction, tell you some illustrative stories, and then discuss significant dimensions of this subject.

PATTERN DEFINED

A pattern is a characteristic mode of behavior. It is a configuration comprised of separate acts, each having a similar aim, intention, or theme, the similar feature or features serving as cues or indicators of the pattern. The regularity or constancy of theme in pattern is exemplified or represented in variations or separate acts, which are exam-

Originally titled *Pattern Interactions at the Unit Level*. Paper presented at the Menninger Foundation, Topeka, Kansas, November, 1985.

ples of the pattern. A pattern is an abstraction, a named form of behavior by which separate acts can be classified. Pattern is the genre, or category, or style of a group of separate acts having distinctive, similar features, including thoughts, feelings, and actions. The name of a pattern pinpoints the regularity, the feature that separate acts share. That characteristic feature is observable or can easily be inferred from observations. The construct (theoretical concept or process) defines what is known about a particular pattern from observation, interview data, experience, or research. In terms of usefulness and ease of applicability for nursing practice, such constructs ought to be defined in two ways: (1) by identifying the essence of the phenomenon in a serial order of its defining aspects; and (2) by elaborating in a detailed, descriptive, and general form, including facts about the dimensions of the phenomenon and its variants. The construct provides explanation and guidance for intervention.

Patterns are intrapersonal, interpersonal, and system phenomena. A spectator observer can notice and infer patterns of a single person or pattern interactions and integrations occurring in relationships between two people. On psychiatric units, in families, and in other established social situations, pattern integrations are system phenomena. Patterns can be unique, temporary, and situation-determined, as for example during a disaster or acute illness; or patterns can be recurring, stable, and repetitive, enduring throughout life.

PATTERN INTEGRATIONS

The term *pattern integration* refers to the fitting together, or merging, or the patterning of need of one person with that of another or others so that there is a match, a fit, compatibility, union, or bond—a linkage between them that unites the two into a whole. Each becomes a part essential to the functioning of the whole. The incorporation of a part of each, as being necessary to the functioning of the whole, is required for relative completeness of the unit.

Need-pattern integrations go on between real people, such as spouses, parents and children, friends, employer and employees.

They also occur between a real person and an illusory figure such as supervisory personifications, incorporated significant others, or hallucinatory figures and other autistic inventions. Many of the expectations and functions associated with problematic need-pattern integrations tend to become automatic, that is, they transpire without thought. Certain pattern disintegrations such as the sudden disappearance of a kidnapped child, or death or divorce, and various forms of "hostile disintegration" such as the suicide of one partner, are always stressful and anxiety provoking for at least one partner. Panic may be evoked and even personality change in the extreme. Because there is a human tendency toward pattern maintenance and pattern perpetuation, persons often seek reinstatement of pattern integration with a new partner to "complete the unit." And there is the expectation that those strategies that have worked in the past to maintain the pattern will continue to do so in the future. Anxiety occurs when those familiar strategies fail to work. There are at least four overall categories of need-pattern integrations:

1. Mutualities such as mutual withdrawal, mutual dependence, or mutual hostility. In this type, both parties use the same behavioral pattern although there may be differences in the variants, the behavioral acts.
2. Complementarities like "hand-in-glove," that is, two patterns with complementary fit such as domination-submission. You cannot have an informer pattern operative unless another person fits in by using a pattern of information receiver.
3. Reciprocal or alternating, when, for instance, partners in a pattern integration of dependent person and helper reverse roles.
4. Antagonistic, whereby two persons use patterns that do not fit, but the relationship is kept going anyway, as for example one person using a general pattern of domination and the other one a pattern of independence. Another example would be a boss whose pattern is mainly approval seeking, that is, showing an inordinate need for approval, praise, or "strokes." An employee of the boss who says, "She's a grown-up; I'm not going to butter her up" has an antagonistic pattern. Needless to say, this pattern integration will

give rise to much distress for the boss, and therefore much trouble for the employee.

Observing Pattern

One aspect of therapeutic work is to identify recurring and newly emerging patterns, those that tend to preclude further personal development and those that tend to favor it. Aims of therapeutic intervention include bringing into awareness and fostering a patient's efforts toward constructive change in recurring problematic patterns and processes. Another therapeutic aim is to stop the professional—the staff nurse in the psychiatric unit—from reinforcing a patient's pathological patterns, thereby halting further stabilization of the patterns. At the same time, staff need to recognize and reinforce newly appearing constructive behavioral patterns. In therapeutic work, especially in the milieu, not all behavioral patterns are addressed; a sample of the more obvious problematic ones will suffice to help the patient to gain methods for observing, considering, and changing behavior.

The process by which nurses perceive patterns from observed behavior of their own and of patients is not clear. Patterns are abstractions. They are inferences drawn from observed data. Sensitivity to patterns derives from many sources: social experience, self-knowledge, competence as an observer, or detached analysis of collected data. For example, knowledge held in the mind of the nurse and readily available for recall and application during clinical work is of the greatest value. Theoretical constructs descriptive of particular patterns and their variants, such as have been carefully drawn from empirical clinical research, serve as cognitive structures that sensitize a nurse to known patterns. When observing a patient in interaction, the nurse simultaneously notices and privately interprets what is seen or experienced. The advantage of the nurse's having and using conceptual knowledge lies in the stability of the concept's definitional structure. The essence of particular patterns (the regularities, universals) remains the same across variants and cases. The pattern is seen as a gestalt, a set of essences of behavior experienced as a whole, the set being more than the separate acts that are observable and illustrative of the pattern to be inferred. This theory, known by the nurse in advance of observation and interaction with patients, serves to sensitize to theoretically defined patterns.

Psychiatric patients tend not to recognize the patterns inherent in their separate acts of behavior. Most often they do not recognize the meaning, that is, the intention or theme of similar acts. Frequency and duration of one action, although observable, seems to be less significant than variation in repertoire with persistence of theme in each variant. The variability is in the behavior; the relation occurs by way of the theme, which is an observer inference about the pattern.

Patients, especially chronic schizophrenics, seem to have a hierarchical ordering of acts in a series related to any one presenting pattern. Failure to achieve integration of that pattern with the expected or desired pattern of another person tends to call out, one by one, acts related to the whole series. This illustrates the immense richness and great variety of imagination in the cognitive capability of these patients to defend and assure continuance and survival of their existing self-system.

Behavior expressed in patterns has utility in the psychological economy of the individual, and the tendency is not to change but rather both to maintain familiar behavior and to integrate relationships so as to achieve a fit that assures pattern perpetuation. In chronic schizophrenics, where those tendencies are portrayed in the extreme, pathological patterns are quite automatic, and therefore unwitting, rooted in long-standing unmet needs, and operate as relief behaviors when anxiety is experienced. Moreover, most of these patients have enduring, built-in anxiety systems, in that they hold and operate on expectations that are least likely to be or cannot be met.

I believe that the interactions of staff nurses in psychiatric units can be guided to become more scientific, systematic, specific, and definitive and less a matter of addressing whatever is presented as random data. This would require ordering the randomness by addressing a few problematic patterns and processes of each patient. Progress for the patient then becomes in part an effect of the nurse's scientific competence in theory application, investigative interviewing competencies, and ability to analyze observational data as gathered. Progress is a matter of chance or serendipity when random acts are not ordered and analyzed, the patient struggling to order his or her own disconnectedness and that of the milieu interactions. Determining and planning to deal with recurring problematic patterns of a patient in milieu nurse–patient interactions ought, at least tentatively, to occur as part of the admission process. What is needed is a new kind of nursing history, one that obtains from the patient and other informants critical incidents that occurred in various phases of life, in which the patient's interactions with others are described in sufficient detail to infer problematic patterns. That would enable staff nurses to avoid pulls from the patient toward participation of the nurse in problematic patterns of the patient at the outset of care, and would also enable early planning related to a few problematic patterns of each patient.

PROBLEMATIC PATTERNS

Now I will mention some nonuseful patterns of patients that prevent further personal development in the direction of constructive social living. Therapeutically, a beginning point would be staff discussions of each of these patterns, raising such questions as: What acts are observable? What do you as nurse say and do when you notice that? And what, then, does the patient say and do?

Some illustrative stories prove interesting. Some years ago, when I was still giving clinical workshops in public mental hospitals, one of the exercises for the nurse participants was to make ward observations, analyze the data collected, and make suggestions for improving these situations. On one ward there was a beautifully embroidered pillow placed high on a mantel. One day when patients and staff were at lunch, the workshop nurses moved the pillow from the mantel to a chair. Later observations, on the return of staff and patients to the ward, showed that the head nurse immediately noticed that the pillow was out of its place. She grabbed it, dusted it off, and quickly returned it to the mantel. The other staff and patients exhibited effects of high anxiety and then great relief once the system was restored to its familiar arrangement. Similarly, in another hospital and another ward, all chairs were lined up in rows in front of the television and along the walls. In the absence of patients and staff, the workshop nurses rearranged the chairs in functional, small circles and semicircles, such as would promote social conversation. When staff and patients returned, it took them exactly three minutes of cooperative activity to restore the previous dysfunctional arrangement of chairs. Patterns of control of patients by nurses integrate with obedience patterns of patients in both of these situations—to the detriment of progress for patients.

In another state hospital, on the first morning of a workshop, I was having breakfast with a group of staff nurses in the dining room around a large table. As a patient entered the room and approached our table one of the nurses said, "Put your hand up," which I did, as did everyone at the table. The patient then circled the table and tapped the fingers of each nurse's hand. I said, "What was that all about?" and one of the nurses said, "Oh, that's his way of saying good morning; he's mute." So the next morning, when the scene was replayed, instead of putting up my hand I said, "Good morning" and the patient replied, "Good morning." The staff nurses said it was the first time the patient had talked in years. They were unaware of their well-intentioned participation in the patient's nonverbal communication by their expectation that he would not or could not talk. There was mutual agreement of nurses and patient that talking was not necessary, a pathological integration.

Some years ago I was consulting with a staff group. One of the staff nurses reported that a medical resident, for whom she had previously had the highest regard, was now someone whom she thoroughly disliked. Puzzled by this shift in their relationship, she realized after lengthy and probing discussion that a patient had used her daily medication as the focus for bringing about a marked dislike between these two fine professionals; it was a pattern of dislike that gradually became mutual. The patient would ask the nurse, "Should I take my medication?" "Is it good for me?" "Do I need it?" or "Is he a good doctor?" Then the patient would take whatever the nurse said and add a twist of her own when she spoke to the resident. She would ask the resident, "Should I take the medicine exactly every four hours?" "Should I take it with a little or a lot of water?" and otherwise hinting at the nurse's ineptness. The pattern the patient was using was "pitting-one-against-the-other," and it worked! The resolution was simple: Resident and nurse had a joint session with the patient and thereafter they separated the physician and nurse content to which they would respond. The nurse referred all medical questions of the patient saying, "Take that up with the doctor," and the resident did likewise with nursing-related questions of the patient. But well-established behavioral patterns do not disappear. The patient finds new targets in the interest of maintenance of familiar patterns. The scene shifted to two patients whose budding friendship became the target, with the other patient trying to separate them. Nurse conferences with the three patients and stepped-up efforts of the patient's individual psychotherapist to seek awareness and the long history of the pattern became the new intervention strategies.

In the 1960s, I gave a clinical practice workshop for nurses in a public mental hospital. While there, I visited a long-term inpatient whom I had known in childhood. I knew, for example, that as a child she had been the family favorite and pet, a position she defended at the great cost of making friends and participating in peer groups. She also was a talebearer—first to her parents about siblings, then to her teachers regarding classmates. These adults accepted the information and in some instances encouraged her to bring more. The several long evenings I spent on the ward visiting this woman provided considerable observational data about the patient and particularly regarding her interactions with staff members (in this instance, mostly licensed practical nurses). Inferences drawn from these data were inescapable.

The patient had managed to involve staff and patients in an almost identical replication of pattern integrations, carried forward from earlier family and school and later work situations. She was the favorite and pet of staff on all shifts. She was the ward informer, carrying tales about patients to staff who accepted them and often protected her from the wrath of other patients. Her bed was next to the nursing office; she was the only patient permitted to enter and stay in the nursing office whenever she wanted. Her strategies for accomplishing this pattern perpetuation were also very similar to those that had worked in earlier situations. She used a pattern of ingratiation represented in such acts as diligent work for the staff, passive obedience to their requests, and of course talebearing. At home she had offered to do housecleaning, scrub floors, and do the dishes; at school she was the pupil who always volunteered to clean blackboards, clap the erasers, and pick up debris in the classroom. In the hospital, she scrubbed the nursing office and, among other ingratiating work, was taken to the homes of nursing personnel to do their housecleaning. The patient's chart showed that over a 30-year period she had virtually every known (up to 1960) form of treatment, but the patterns of behavior that for life had precluded social acceptance by her agemates remained intact and in fact were reinforced daily by staff.

It is nursing interventions into the ordinary patterns of behavior—ones that portray the social ineptness, that preclude growth-enhancing relationships, that are demonstrated in interactions with patients and staff within the psychiatric unit—that are the main work of staff nurses.

In the 1970s, after I "retired," I had a two-year visiting professorship in Belgium. While there, I visited Gheel, a community in which for centuries foster families provided a residential program for psychiatric patients. A group of nurses, including me, and a physician and social worker were permitted to visit one of the families that had taken in two psychiatric patients. The assumption was that these were "normal" families and that living with them would have a beneficial effect for patients. The family we visited consisted of a husband and wife and two patients, all of whom were present during our stay. One of the patients sat silently at the dining room table eating large slices of jelly bread; the husband, equally noncommunicative, sat next to her. The other patient was an attractive, middle-aged woman, physically active, socially graceful, and seemingly very intelligent. She had travelled around the world and was fluent in several languages, including Flemish, French, German, and English. She spoke knowledgeably to the nurses about places she had visited and about current events. She asked relevant questions of the nurses and easily shifted to the native language of each visitor. All of that seemed to be quite an accomplishment and certainly a clue that there were large capacities in this woman that could be tapped for personal improvement if not for recovery.

However, during conversations with the nurses, the patient would suddenly, abruptly, cut off the communication, dash to the other side of the room, and stand, meekly, with bowed head, beside the wife. Standing there, she looked like a very frightened little girl. Then, in due time, the patient would return and resume conversation with the nurse group. After this happened twice, suggesting a recurring pattern integration of patient and wife, I decided to investigate. I asked one of the nurses to observe, so that perhaps we could determine the signal used by the wife to call out such instant obedience in the patient. After two more almost identical occurrences, the nature of the patient–wife interaction became clearer. The illness-maintaining system went like this: As the patient became more pleasantly engrossed in social relationships with the visiting group, and began to show enthusiasm and enjoyment, and at the point when she glanced toward the wife, the wife issued a minute facial gesture of forbiddance. Later on, the wife's pattern of forbiddance was also noted in other body gestures, such as frowning and hands on her hips. The gestural pattern of forbiddance, shown in separate acts, was the powerful signal, quickly obeyed by the patient, that very probably coexisted with and supported a pattern of dependence in the patient. In this family's milieu the wife obviously was the central figure. She stood up, talked the most and loudest, at times almost drowning out the conversations of others. Obviously, she exemplified a major pattern of domination; her husband and the other patient, to whom she issued "do this, do that" directives, clearly showed a pattern of passive-submissiveness. The one patient who made an effort to get out of a domination-submission pattern integration with the wife was nevertheless controlled by a pattern of forbiddance used by the wife.

This, of course, was a very brief observational visit. In the group there was a governmental supervisor of foster care. It is of interest that even under conditions of knowing that he was an "inspector," the wife could not audit and control her own behavior in order to edit out this pattern, if only for a short time, suggesting that her patterns were automatic. Interestingly, neither the inspector, physician, nor social worker noticed; they thought the wife was wonderfully kind. The nurses had been sensitized to a theory of patterns and pattern integrations, a theory that served as their observational framework.

In another workshop, in a public mental hospital in the southern United States, the participants were learning to do group work. The patients were a captive group, brought to the group session by attendants who then sat at the door to "protect" the nurses. The anxiety of the patients was exceptionally high in the first session. The inference was drawn that their expectations related to the presence of the attendants may have accounted for their high anxiety. The attendants were removed for the second session, but the anxiety of patients was again high, if not higher. No clear explanatory inferences could be drawn from the data presented by the nurses in a review session held afterward. So I paired the nurses and asked each to observe the other, instead of the patients, in the third session. On review of these data, what seemed a very clear inference emerged: Several of the nurses were unwittingly using a pattern of seduction that these southern men recognized as a come-on technique clearly forbidden under the circumstances. One nurse even used a periodic wink while another batted her eyelashes. Once the nurses gained control and edited out their own behavioral acts—variants of a seduction pattern—the anxiety of the patients decreased and group work got started. In the last session, one of the patients who spoke for the group said, "At first we didn't know what you wanted, and then that stopped," some sort of validation that the seduction inference was correct.

DISCUSSION

Patterns of behavior are inferences drawn from data of observed behavioral acts and interactions. The methods of observation—spectator and participant observation—and theory application are the scientific tools the professional uses in the process of inferencing. Discussions with another observer, with the possibility of validation of inferences, help to reduce if not obviate errors. Inferences in clinical work ought to be viewed as hypotheses, tested against further observational data and revised as the data suggest. However, with psychiatric patients it is quite a good bet that each one has, and uses, more or less automatically, one or more patterns of behavior that prevent personal growth, development, social relationships, and productive living in the community. In this chapter it is suggested that these patterns are carried forward from the home and community situations and into the psychiatric unit by patients. There patients once again use those patterns and integrate relationships with other patients and staff in ways that tend to perpetuate the patterns. The work of staff nurses in the unit, in cooperation with other professional treating personnel, ought to be directed toward corrective interventions into problematic patterns.

Patterns of behavior are learned responses. They become familiar, known parts of the self-system of the patient. Such patterns are triggered by need, anxiety, and by self-system maintenance. Without awareness of these connections such patterns are repeated, become habitual, and in the case of chronic patients become almost totally automatic. One patient called them her "trap-adaption." On the other hand, learned behavior can be unlearned, but that is no easy task. However, a first step, after nurse identification of problematic patterns, is to generate a patient's awareness of behavioral acts and the pattern they represent. Awareness provides the basis for change, for trying out other, new alternative patterns.

There are, of course, many issues. I have not said that nursing intervention into problematic patterns at the unit level is the only work of unit staff nurses; I have said that it is an important, often-overlooked part of their work. The focus on a few problematic patterns would fit into a planned nursing approach and reduce a common tendency in some units, particularly in public mental hospitals, to intervene in random acts in random fashion.

Rules of organization of units can be seen as aspects of institutional patterns against which, in a testing pattern, most patients will play out their own problematic patterns, once again checking for limits, boundaries, fairness, and trust. Similarly, unit privileges— whatever they are—call out patient patterns. Some patients will try for the most—a pattern of exploitation; withdrawn patients expect failure and often do not try at all. The expectations of staff and of patients, often privately held and unverbalized one to the other, also at some level interact. Often, psychiatric patients are sensitive to the expectations and vulnerabilities of others, reading staff well while being unaware of their own expectations and how they govern their behavior. The clearer that a nurse is of his or her expectations of patients, and their relation to the nurse's behavior, the better.

CHAPTER 9

Psychiatric Nursing: Role of Nurses and Psychiatric Nurses

The psychiatric nurse's role is today in an "identity crisis" (DeShouwer & Buerl, 1975). The crisis is being resolved, in different ways and at different speeds, in various countries. The emerging role of psychiatric nurses in the various countries is in relation to the developments in mental health as a field and to the social sciences as another source of explanatory theory relevant to mental health.

It may be most useful to think of *nurses* who practice in psychiatric settings and *psychiatric nurses*, who also work in such facilities. Nurses have only *basic* nursing education, of which a part includes knowledge and supervised practice related to psychiatric work. Psychiatric nurses have specialized *post-basic* nursing education and therefore have more knowledge and competence for their work.

The *role of nurses* in psychiatric settings of all types is the same generalized one as in other types of health care institutions, but adapted to the special considerations of psychiatric patients. This role includes assessment of nursing needs of patients, developing nursing care plans, implementing such plans through direct nursing

---

Reprinted from *International Nursing Review*, 25, 41–47, March/April, 1978. Copyright 1978 by *International Nursing Review*. Reprinted by permission.

care or through other nursing personnel, evaluating the results of nursing care and coordinating the care of other health professionals. The nurse also helps to create and maintain an environment in the service unit that is beneficial for patients. Through visitors and other program plans the nurse stimulates continuing relationships between patients and their family members and community contacts. In addition, of course, nurses carry out medical orders. The knowledge base which the nurse uses to guide these nursing practices is whatever is included in the basic nursing curriculum. Additionally, inservice and continuing education opportunities should be available so that the knowledge base will be gradually updated and expanded.

The *role of psychiatric nurses* also depends upon the length of post-basic nursing education, the scope and depth of knowledge included in it and the clinical modalities for which supervised clinical practice is provided. There is great variation in what psychiatric nurses are able to do, for their competence is largely dependent on the foregoing factors. It is not a matter of intelligence. There are just as many intelligent nurses as there are intelligent persons in all other health professions. It is a matter of educational opportunity to develop that intelligence into competence for practice in psychiatric nursing.

What nurses or psychiatric nurses do—or learn to do—in any given country has much to do with prevailing definitions of the phenomena called "mental illness" and of definitions of the nature of the corrective professional work that is needed to put patients in the direction of "mental health." It is a characteristic of all professional work—that of physicians, nurses, lawyers, dentists, and the like—that the starting point for deciding the practices, and therefore the role, must be an understanding of the problems, difficulties, needs, or phenomena, which the practices or role to be used are intended to fix, correct, change, or improve in some way. As shown in Table 9.1, the conceptions and theoretical explanations of "mental illness" are changing. Only three major trends are shown. There are, of course, many "schools of thought" about what is mental illness. Some of them are blends of these three trends; others are elaborations of one piece of one trend. In any given hospital or mental health center it is possible to find most, if not all,

TABLE 9.1 Changing Conceptions and Theories Explanatory of Mental Illness

Intrapersonal	Interpersonal	Systems
Within-person phenomena	Between-persons phenomena	Within social systems phenomena
Medical model: – Psychoanalysis—intrapsychic: – Biochemical—disturbed body function: – Genetic—inherited traits: – Behavior modification—extinguish problem behavior by rewarding acceptable behavior.	Dyadic interaction model: – Psychotherapy—therapist a model for changing client's problematic pattern integrations with sick-making and sick-maintaining others: – Therapeutic modalities: individual and group: – Dyadic therapy: patient and significant other person.	Social interaction model: – Family therapy—therapist promotes change in family network of patterns, linkages, and strategies of family: – Milieu therapy—an environment that provides various mechanisms for change of behavior in groups.
Mental illness is a disease of a person; the "patient" is "sick."	"Mental illness" is a disturbance in a relationship with two or more people: the relationship is problematic.	The "identified patient" is merely the signaler of a disturbed system in a "closed family"; the family is disturbed.
The "cause" of mental illness lies in the patient's past, in his genetic inheritance, and/or in bodily dysfunction—neurological, biochemical, etc.	The "generic roots" of mental illness lie in past relationships but the "purpose" of present behavior, which replicates and perpetuates past relationships, determines the continuation of the behavior.	One member of a family is assigned or takes (for some purpose) the role of signaler of ongoing family system disturbance; that member is "labeled" mentally ill.
Spectator observation is used: – The patient's symptoms are studied. – A diagnosis of the type of "mental illness" is made. – Treatment is ordered for the patient: – Drugs, EST, behavior modification, activity schedules, etc.; – Acute disturbance and acting-out are	Participant observation is used: – Interactions between patient, patients, patient/staff member and patient visitor are studied so all become aware of them. – Diagnosis of problematic pattern-integrations of patient with others is studied. – Diagnosis of "type" of "mental illness" is done	Sociological observation is used: – The entire family and its networks of patterns and strategies are studied so all family members become aware of them. – Options for revised or new patterns or strategies are openly considered. – No diagnosis is indicated.

TABLE 9.1 Changing Conceptions and Theories Explanatory of Mental Illness (Continued)

Intrapersonal	Interpersonal	Systems
Within-person phenomena	Between-persons phenomena	Within social systems phenomena
seen as signs of illness and are often "treated" with drugs, restraint, seclusion, etc.	when required for official records. – Drugs are used to reduce severe anxiety. – Acute disturbance is treated as panic and acting out is a basis for discussion of purpose and pattern integration.	– Separate sessions with parents, children, or one member may be held but not to discuss absent members.
– The professionals *do not* observe or study their behavior in interaction with the patient's behavior. – Family are "informants." – Care: Doing things *to* or *for* the patient.	– Professionals observe and study their participation in interaction with patients. – Family data are taken in front of patient. – Care: doing things *with* the patient.	– The "treatment" experience is open and aims to open up a closed family. – The professional is an educative agent for system change and detached from the family system.
The concern is about symptoms, entities and their amelioration. The sick person is seen as "different" from others.	The concern is for processes, mainly interpersonal and intellectual processes. The person's behavior is seen as different in degree not in kind—an exaggerated expression of ordinary human processes.	The concern is about systems, networks and ways in which they are maintained. The patterns of behavior of family members are seen as needful and purposeful, based on past experience often being replicated, but open to awareness and change.
The tendency is to hospitalize the "mentally ill," to remove from family (often to exclude family) and to protect the community. – The family tends to "close ranks" and enlarge distance from the "sick" person.	The tendency is to maintain in the community, using outpatient care and short-term hospitalization when absolutely necessary. – Family members may be invited to dyadic or individual therapy. They are participants in care of patient.	The work with families is done on an out-patient basis—in the home when possible; the tendency is *not* to hospitalize or treat individually the "identified patient."

TABLE 9.1 Changing Conceptions and Theories Explanatory of Mental Illness *(Continued)*

Intrapersonal	Interpersonal	Systems
Within-person phenomena	Between-persons phenomena	Within social systems phenomena
"Chronicity" in patients is explained as evidence of genetic defect, failure of the organism to respond to drugs, EST, etc., or failure of the patient as a person.	Chronicity in hospitalized patients is explained as "institutional pathology," failure of the therapist to infer patterns and apply successful interventions, lack of explanatory theory, or insufficient time.	
– The institutional tendency is toward routines and custody and occurs as a consequence of staff failure to observe staff participation in evoking patient disturbances and in perpetuating psychopathology unwittingly. – Institutions tend to become "closed systems."	Out-patient care prevents institutionalization and its effects and allows the patient opportunities for contacts in which to try out new behaviors that may result from therapy.	
Theories used:	Theories used:	Theories used:
Descriptive psychiatry, genetics, biochemistry, biology, psychoanalysis, conditioning theories (behavior modification), psychology.	Interpersonal psychiatry, social science—especially sociopsychological interaction theories, communication theory, behavioral theory.	General systems theory, social science—especially sociopsychological interaction theories, family theory, communication theory, matrix theory, behavioral science theory.

of the prevailing schools of psychiatric thought. Each physician on a hospital staff may represent and adhere to a different psychiatric theory to explain the phenomena called "mental illness."

The dilemma of nurses and psychiatric nurses is clear. No basic or post-basic nursing program can teach all possible theories used by psychiatrists in their work. There isn't that much time! Should one theoretical framework be taught to nurses? If so, which one and on the basis of what criteria should it be selected? Or, should nurses take an eclectic approach—learning a little bit about as many different theoretical orientations as possible but not gaining any depth in one of them. In the latter case, what would be the nursing practices, for these, like medical practices flow from the theories that are used. A consideration of some characteristics of patients' living in hospitals is in order. Some of the usual things that nurses do in general hospitals are bathing, feeding, toileting patients, attending to mouth and skin care or positioning or changing dressings or other kinds of bodily care. In psychiatric hospitals patients do these activities for themselves and only a minimal surveillance of them by nurses may be needed. Patients' beds need to be made, but patients also do this. Furthermore, if a patient has had a mother who was compulsively orderly and demanded precision in bedmaking, any rebellion of that patient about bedmaking in the hospital may be a healthy, independent stance, in which event the nurse would be well advised not to make an issue of bedmaking. But that would, of course, depend on whether refusal of the bedmaking was taken as a sign of health or of illness, which would depend upon the theoretical framework being used, by physician and nurse, to explain the patient's behavior.

Nurses pass out medications. It is common in psychiatric hospitals to medicate patients, often quite heavily. Nurses can, of course, observe and report drug effects. But the effects to be observed are also related to the theoretical aim in giving them. The aim may be to take the edge off severe and recurring anxiety of the patient, thereby enabling nurse/patient talks of a substantial, beneficial kind, or the aim of the medication may be to "tranquilize," to produce in the patient the effect of quiet that may stimulate thought, undisturbed by talk.

Nurses also often schedule patients for activities, on and off a hospital unit, providing surveillance of adherence to such schedules. Nurses may also arrange and participate in ward activities: ward government meetings, birthday parties for patients, coffee-break sessions when patients have completed "cleaning duties," if these are required of them in a unit. The "activities of daily living" in a hospital unit are often considered to be the nurses' concern. These include such activities as hours of arising in the morning, nap times if permitted, sleep hours–deciding these matters and providing surveillance of these activities.

The critical question is whether the nurse is to carry out these activities within an intrapersonal framework—being a detached observer and mother-surrogate; or whether an interpersonal framework will guide the nurse, as a participant observer, alert to verbal tactics and considering them from a standpoint of nonreplication of "sick-making others" in the previous interpersonal environment of the patient. No one can monitor or direct the nurse/patient verbal exchanges at all times. Only the nurse who has a theoretical knowledge of communication theory, and who can recall and use it during nurse–patient verbal exchanges, can be held responsible for the short and long-term effects of such exchanges.

The work of nurses in psychiatric settings can be defined in different ways: (1) as manager of the routines of life on a unit with kindness, but only a modicum of unselected theory; or (2) as a change agent who uses substantial theory to guide nurse interactions with patients with the aim of evoking substantial change in patient behavior. Two generalizations in psychiatric literature are instructive (Stanton & Schwartz, 1954). One is the generalization that panic in patients is staff-induced, most specifically when there are covert, undiscussed, staff disagreements as to what care should be or how it is to be carried out. The other is the idea of illness-maintenance by staff, which is, of course, unwitting. The latter idea generated from study of "the other twenty-three hours"; that is after a patient's fifty-minute hour of therapy with a physician. If these two generalizations are taken seriously, as they should be, then nurses, in order to be more fully knowledgeable and responsible in their work, need substantial postbasic nursing education in theories that aid them to see qualities of illness-maintenance in their daily work, and aid them to change their own participant behavior so as to become agents for new and more self-evolving behavior in patients (Table 9.2).

The definition of the nature of "mental illness" is in effect the definition of the work which the patient is to do in order to change himself into a more fully functioning person. The role of physician and nurse and other mental health workers flows out of the definition of the patient's work (Table 9.3). The question of who will define the patient's work is another matter: whether it be defined in very general terms, as in Table 9.3, or in terms more specifically related to the particular patient.

TABLE 9.2 Some Illness-Maintaining Behaviors of Nurses with Inpatients.

1. The nurse using a patient (who was similarly exploited at home) to do errands for her (bring coffee, clean office, carry messages).
2. The nurse burdening the patient with tales of her exciting social life—putting the patient in the position of "audience" and at the same time having little interest, if any, in his concerns; to cheer him up by "one-upping" him!
3. The nurse making "pets" of a few patients and thereby reinforcing previous "pet" status for those patients and reinforcing "unfavorable comparison" for other patients. Giving gifts to some but not all patients.
4. Arbitrating sibling-like disputes among two patients so that one loses and one wins, as in sibling disputes at home.
5. Responding to dependency bids in ways that confirm and re-confirm the patient's self-view: "I am helpless, dependent," etc.
6. Responding to patient bids for derogation or punishment by giving in, thereby confirming and reconfirming these patient self-views.
7. Permitting, inviting and responding to "tale bearing" in which one patient "tattles" on another, thereby reinforcing the patient's "informer role" which further isolates the patient from constructive interaction with other patients as peers.
8. Allowing or permitting "coalitions across generations"; i.e., participating in nurse–patient discussion to the detriment of some other staff member. This replicates the patient's previous pattern of "pitting one against another" which may have effectively disunited mother and father, who are then reunited in concern for the now "identified patient."
9. Entering into pseudo-chum relationships with patients.
10. Nonuseful channeling of anxiety into overmedication, seclusion, EST, or work rather than into investigation of circumstances that evoked the anxiety in a given situation.
11. Using various problematic verbal inputs such as "mixed messages," "double-binds," etc.

In some community mental health centers in the United States the professional staff is organized into "focus teams." Each team includes physicians, nurses, social workers and psychologists but not according to a particular ratio. Each team serves a defined population in a geographical area of the region served by the mental health center as a whole. Initially, each team spends some

TABLE 9.3 Different Definitions of Mental Illness and Therefore of the Work of the Patient and the Role of the Nurse.

Definition	Work of the patient	Role of the nurse
Socially inacceptable behavior of the patient has previously been "rewarded": he has unfortunately been "conditioned" to behave in these ways.	Submit to treatment using behavior modification (reconditioning) techniques.	Surveillance of patient following treatment plan. Pass out rewards. General nursing routine care.
Inacceptable behavior is the result of genetic inheritance.	Submit to whatever ameliorative treatment of symptoms is ordered.	Surveillance and custody. Reporting. General nursing routine care.
Inacceptable behavior is due to a biochemical imbalance.	Submit to tests and prescribed treatment drugs to rectify the imbalance.	Surveillance, reporting. Pass medications: tranquilizers, stimulants, lithium, hormones, etc. Observe effects. General nursing routine care.
Inacceptable behavior is due to some unknown but adverse brain activity.	Submit to prescribed treatment (electrostimulation, electroshock, lobotomy, etc.).	Surveillance, reporting. Pre- and posttreatment "preparation." General nursing (and surgical nursing) care.
Inacceptable behavior reflects problems in living with people and lack in intellectual and interpersonal competencies to understand and solve those problems.	Participate in psychotherapy sessions and in ad hoc talking sessions with the available professionals, so as to investigate, understand and resolve those problems and in the process gain new intellectual and interpersonal competencies on an experiential/educative basis.	Use all "activities of daily living" as a basis for observation, discussion and intervention in ways that enhance the patient's intellectual and interpersonal competencies to change his own behavior. Also general nursing care. Using "situational counseling" to aid patients involved in disputes, violence, other grossly inacceptable

TABLE 9.3 Different Definitions of Mental Illness and Therefore of the Work of the Patient and the Role of the Nurse. *(Continued)*

Definition	Work of the patient	Role of the nurse
		behavior, to investigate the problem inherent in the acting-out situation. Referral for other professional services, (e.g., clergy) and coordination and follow-up on discharge.
The inacceptable behavior is due to "lack of insight" into intrapsychic causes.	Seek psychoanalysis for those who can afford it.	

time seeking a consensus on its views of mental illness. When a patient first comes to the center the receptionist calls whichever team member who has that hour free to do the "intake," the initial history. At its next "team meeting," usually held every other day, the team reviews the intake, decides more specifically what work of the patient may be required, and assigns one team member to arrange appointments through the receptionist and to proceed with the work. The criteria for assignment include who has the necessary competence and who has time free to take on another patient. The work might be brief counseling, individual psychotherapy of somewhat longer duration, participation in group therapy, family therapy, referral to a "sheltered workshop" and the like. Very nearly all team members are competent to do the various forms of therapy including the psychiatric nurses and general nurses who are members of the team. The work of each team member is subject to periodic data review by one other team member: When a case is to be closed a team review and decision is made.

It is easy to see that there is a great deal of planned role overlap. All professionals provide psychotherapy although some may prefer group therapy, some individual therapy, and some prefer family therapy. Some teams also include graduate students in nursing (master's program in psychiatric nursing) as well as psychiatric residents and psychology and social work students. They are supervised in their clinical work by faculty in their respective programs but the final team review before discharge also occurs.

There are also some separate roles. Diagnosis and prescription of medication is a physician role. Study of a home is a social work or psychiatric nurse function. Follow-up care after discharge is most often a nursing function due to medication that may be involved. Psychological testing is a psychology role. Fees that are charged to patients are the same for all psychotherapists but are adjusted according to the economic status of the patient.

The aim of the mental health centers is to provide "talking" therapy for all patients, to do that early and only for as long as needed.

The concern in the development of community mental health centers has been with early and effective treatment to prevent hospital admissions and to stop the continuing backlog of patients in public mental hospitals. Another aim has been to keep families and communities involved—to see "mental illness" as a problem of a family which it must help to solve. The family is a part of the problem and of its solution.

There are similar developments with respect to mental retardation and psychogeriatrics. Special homes are of course available for patients who have for years been in such institutions, but the trend is toward home-care and community-based supportive services. Nurses are often the primary care persons who visit homes, arrange for services needed, and contact physicians when there is a medical problem. In institutional care, nurses, of course, are needed for direct, bedside care of the severely handicapped (idiots, hydrocephalics, etc.) and for the medically ill psychogeriatric patient: cerebral vascular accident, Parkinson's, etc.). With regard to the less severely retarded who are institutionalized, the "training" is seen as the function of special teachers, while nurses use "activities of daily living" and group modalities other than therapy (behavior modification, remotivation groups) to stimulate the human development and social behavior of the retardate. Similarly, in psychogeriatrics, nurses are studying the aging process and developing nursing interventions which prevent or slow up institutionalization and which tend to ensure human functioning at the highest level possible for each patient.

In public mental hospitals the tendency is to place the most competent psychiatric nurses in admission wards or with newly admitted patients. Such nurses provide counseling, individual and group psychotherapy, and "specialing" for patients in panic. In "chronic wards" the effort is toward resocialization with nurses most often being the program planners.

An attempt has been made in Table 9.4 to show an array of possible activities connected with the role of the nurse and psychiatric nurse in various kinds of psychiatric/mental health settings. What nurses and psychiatric nurses will actually do in any given setting depends upon:

1. The competence brought to the work as a consequence of basic or post-basic nursing education.
2. The definition of mental illness and therefore of the work of "mentally ill" patients that prevails in a given setting.
3. The extent of consensus around the question of whether each profession should or should not have only discrete, unique, circumscribed roles or whether there can be overlap (as, for example, in

TABLE 9.4 Summary: Role of Nurses and Psychiatric Nurses

Nurses (basic nursing education only)	Psychiatric Nurses (post-basic nursing education)
Assess patient needs	*All activities listed under "nurse", plus:*
Develop nursing care plans	Intake (history taking)
Implement nursing care plan:	Sociological observation of homes
Carry out direct care	Member of mental health team:
Assign and supervise nursing personnel	Counseling
Evaluate effects of nursing care	Individual psychotherapy
Create and maintain an environment in service unit of benefit to patients	Group psychotherapy
Stimulate patient relationships with family:	Family therapy
Dyadic patient/visitor conferences with nurse	Supervisory review of clinical data (own and other)
	Discharge planning with team
	Follow-up and evaluation of patient outcomes
	File case reports

TABLE 9.4 Summary: Role of Nurses and Psychiatric Nurses *Continued)*

Nurses (basic nursing education only)	Psychiatric Nurses (post-basic nursing education)
Carry out medical orders:	"Special" patients in panic.
Pass prescribed medications	Model for constructive interven-
Monitor medication effects	tion in "ward disturbances".
Carry out physical procedures	Experiential teaching of nurses.
Surveillance of bathing, mouth care, toileting, bedmaking, food intake, sleep.	Writing professional nursing papers.
General nursing routines, especially for severely retarded and medically ill psychogeriatric patients.	*In hospital* Work with newly admitted patients as above.
Prepare for and/or participate in special treatments: behavior modification, electroshock, lobotomy.	Work with acutely disturbed patients, especially regarding panic. Work with autistic and otherwise acutely disturbed children.
Referrals to other professions—clergy, social work, etc.	Work with acting out and otherwise acutely disturbed adolescents.
Coordination of patient care of other professionals.	Serve as a resource and consultant to nurses.
Schedule patient activities (off the unit):	Present patient data at staff meetings.
Surveillance of adherence to schedule.	Arrange supervisory review of clinical data with equally or more experienced professional colleague.
Arrange and participate in unit "activities of daily living":	
Ward government	
Various modalities of group activity	
Remotivation and resocialization groups	
Work groups	
Patient parties	
Make follow-up home visits after discharge.	
Talking with patients:	
Situational counseling	
Disrupt illness maintenance.	
Attend in-service education sessions and ward staff meetings.	
Attend outside continuing education meetings.	

talking with patients which all professionals do) and if so, to what extent (i.e., only counseling, counseling and the various psychotherapies).

4. The cost of certain kinds of care (e.g., psychotherapy) the difference in status and salary levels (e.g., physicians, nurses, etc.) and the numbers of persons needed and available to provide certain kinds of care may also be countervailing or influential factors.

REFERENCES

De Shouwer, P., & Buerl, A. (1975, March 10–13). *The role of nursing personnel within the psychiatric and mental health team — As seen by a medical administrator* (mimeograph). World Health Organization Working Group. Saarbrücken.

Stanton, A., & Schwartz, M. (1954). *Mental hospitals.* New York: Basic Books.

PART III The Teaching of Psychiatric Nursing

Introduction

On March 1, 1956, the Elizabeth, NJ *Daily Journal* reported that at Rutgers, Hildegard E. Peplau was developing a graduate psychiatric nursing program, the first program in the country devoted exclusively to preparation of clinical specialists in psychiatric nursing, under a grant from the U.S. Department of Health, Education, and Welfare. The only two-year clinical program of what were then 28 graduate programs, students would work with psychiatric inpatients and would also have a "mental health in public health" clinical experience. The public health dimension was not only a foray into work with disturbed families, it also represented an emphasis not suggested formally until the 1960 report of the Joint Commission on Mental Illness and Health, Action for Mental Health.

In 1958, *Psychiatric Nursing: Nurse-Patient Relationships,* an educational film made at New Jersey State Hospital at Greystone Park, was released. Peplau had been a major force in creating the film. Within 18 weeks of its release, over 800 showings were arranged by producers Smith, Kline, & French alone, not counting those handled by coproducers American Nurses' Association and National League for Nursing. One hundred sixty prints were made, making it one of the most widely used films in nursing education. At the time, Peplau suggested a companion film depicting the psychiatric nurse and patient at the community level, comparing similarities and differences in hospital and home care. The community mental health movement was not yet with us, but obviously it was on Peplau's horizon. Problems with deinstitutionalization have only in recent years been noted, yet 30 years ago Peplau saw the need to closely scrutinize a phenomenon then not commonly observed or even named. If there was ever a master teacher, it is Peplau. In education and practice she gave new meaning to the notion of learning through experience. Every clinical observation is worthy of description and review. Clinical observations are to be collected and analyzed, and neither ignored nor read into with meaning beyond the data. As a teacher Peplau has always been singleminded and straightforward in her task of encouraging learning. The roles of teacher and supervisor are as objective as is humanly possible, the teacher/supervisor critically auditing clinical data and facilitating the learning of the student. Constructive use of capacities is as much a focus of the nurse's learning as it is of the development of the patient. Know-how is encouraged by providing clinician-students with ways of understanding and interpreting raw clinical data—tools of the trade that have become Peplau hallmarks—providing clinicians with ways to communicate with patients, to understand interpersonal and intrapersonal processes, and to intervene into pathological modes of thinking, feeling, and action.

Peplau's systematic review of verbatim data (handwritten in the days before tape recorders were used routinely) began when she first taught at Teachers College, Columbia University, in 1948. Surely this was the beginning of qualitative research in psychiatric nursing. Her systematic collection and interpretation of data in a manner reminiscent of anthropological research has influenced the thinking and approaches of nurses she has taught. In this way she has stimulated curiosity and serious scholarship in nurses and has influenced the development and refinement of logical thinking—often different in content from her own.

As a teacher, then, Peplau is a sensitive guide and facilitator of inherent capacities of the learner rather than a disciple-maker. Thus she has influenced average nurses and superior nurses, all pressed to their limit, even to diverge from her views and to surpass her if that is where they are headed.

CHAPTER 10

What Is Experiential Teaching?

"Learning by experience" is a phrase that is widely used. It suggests that a person's experience can be used to promote his learning. To understand the phrase, therefore, it is necessary to grasp and use the concept of *learning* and the concept of *experience,* and to know the teaching method that can be used to promote learning by experience.

The purpose of this paper is to propose definitions for these two concepts and to describe the form of teaching, in a way that clarifies the meaning of the phrase and distinguishes the method from more traditional or didactic forms of instruction. Experiential teaching is an important function performed by nurses in their work with patients. An understanding of this method of teaching should facilitate health teaching in all types of nursing situations.

WHAT IS EXPERIENCE?

Experience is anything lived or undergone. It is the inner perception that a person has of events in which he participates. It consists of the "felt relations"—the connections which a person feels concerning an event—or the inferences he draws. It is, for example, the inferences which occur to nurses in a relationship with a patient. These "felt relations" or inferences can be identified. Descriptions of responses of the separate senses, reports of the total organism, and observations which the nurse makes of others are the major components of the raw data from which nurses formulate what they experience in a work situation. Thus, when experiential teaching is the method used in nursing education, the nurses identify and describe what has been seen, felt, thought, or done in a situation with a patient, and what has been noticed concerning the patient.

Experiential teaching aids students (or staff nurses in an inservice program) to organize the meaning of experiences in clinical situations, and has three principal components: (1) what the nurses or students have *experienced,* as just described; (2) what is *learned,* or the meaning of that experience; (3) the *instructional process* or the interacting roles of teacher and students in discussion of clinical experiences. The nurses or students bring the content to the classroom with them and the teacher functions as a critical auditor and facilitator in formulating meanings.

In traditional education the content is usually decided upon, prepared in advance, and introduced by the teacher, possibly from a course outline or teaching files, and the students are expected to absorb what is said and later recall and use it in their work. So this is one difference. In experiential situations, reports of events are presented by students, usually verbally, sometimes from notes. In the discussion of these, data are analyzed and the meaning abstracted. A blackboard helps to keep formulations before the students as they are made and revised. These may be statements of problems encountered, as they emerge from discussion. They may be generalizations to explain what went on in the clinical situations. They may be hypotheses or clinical hunches, which serve as guides for future observations. Discussion often reveals biases and misconceptions, particularly those of very young student nurses. In these situations, individuals can learn something useful when they become involved as participants, and what has actually been experienced is organized, and its meaning to the observer checked against experiences of others in the peer group.

In undergraduate and graduate training programs, formal and

informal events (called "learning experiences") are usually arranged or occur so that students have a series of varied experiences which permit them to see relations between different kinds of experience. In inservice programs, the everyday work situation provides many experiences which ought to be analyzed and organized in their meaning to nurses. This can be crucial to the recovery of patients. What nurses actually experience when patients are anxious, self-derogating, express feelings of worthlessness, resentment, hatefulness, and the like, influences these situations.

Knowingly or unknowingly, nurses make inferences—assign meanings to what is experienced—and these are part and parcel of the meaning to which they respond. Some awareness of this is needed and effort at such awareness is the nurse's obligation. Otherwise, the nurse and patient act in juxtaposition, each observing the other's behavior, without seeing her own participation. And, short of mechanical restraints, the nurse cannot really control the behavior of patients. She can only be aware of, and in some degree control, what goes on in her responses.

This kind of awareness, or understanding of her own participation when patients express various kinds of behavior, cannot be taught. It can only be *learned* by examining and slowly getting clear about what is felt, thought, and done by each nurse.

WHAT IS LEARNING?

Learning is a concept that is often used very loosely in the literature. It is used to indicate formation of automatic or habitual responses, as a result of trial and error, reward and punishment, and the like. Other concepts, such as conditioning, adaptation, integration, and so forth, are often defined as though they were synonymous with learning. It is uncommon to find in the literature the opinion that pathological patterns, such as those in patients diagnosed schizophrenic, are learned. From the standpoint of this chapter, these patterns would be called adaptations.

A workable definition of learning, which educators and therapists alike would find useful, ought to help make the use of this concept, especially in the field of education, more precise.

Learning can be defined in terms of the behavior of the person who is in the process of learning. Such behavior can be observed or inferred from behavior that is observed. The process involves a series of operations, each one reached by the learner at a given time. The operations, in the order of their appearance, are as follows:

1. A person who is in the process of learning *observes what goes on* in the course of an experience, event, or situation in which he is participating, actively or passively, overtly or covertly. A person who is reading a book, hearing a lecture, watching a patient, listening to a colleague, is observing. To observe means to use the five senses to notice the details of an event as it is happening. One of the most important interferences with noticing the details of what goes on is anxiety (Sullivan, 1957).

2. As the next step in the process of learning, the person *describes what went on and what was noticed* during the experience. Anxiety can also interfere with this step. Perception and attention are selective—to maintain comfort, one might see the familiar rather than the new, or hear only those ideas that are in agreement with one's personal views on a subject. The tendency of all people to avoid anxiety is supported by patterns of selective perception and selective inattention. Severe anxiety, therefore, may automatically rule out description of some facet of experience that was not noticed enough to be described. To describe what was observed means to tell it to somebody else, or to be able to write down a verbatim account of what transpired during an event or after it has occurred. In this way, using observation and then description, the learner *collects the data of an experience* from which something will be learned.

3. A person who is learning then *analyzes the data collected* so that the possible and significant meanings can be determined. Identifying the significance or abstracting the essence from the variety of details in an experience is a principal task of the learner. Here, too, anxiety and parataxic distortion (the tendency to see present events only in terms of past experiences) often operate to hinder learning. Data are analyzed by sorting out the common and the unique elements, by comparing one aspect with another, by applying known concepts to explain the data, and by drawing inferences as to the connections among the various occurrences that were observed and described. Analysis should lead to fresh, new inferences from the data of an experience, or should suggest other data which may be required before conclusions can be drawn.

4. The learner then *formulates the significance* of an experience by making statements which reflect precisely the gist of what went on. These formulations are the learning products; they are the conclusions drawn from data secured while undergoing experience. The most common interference with this step is the tendency in our society to assign clichés to denote the meaning of experience. It is common to have students conclude, "I liked her," "it's terrific," "she didn't cooperate," and to offer other such noncommunicative phrases as the significance of their richly varied observations. In formulating the significance of an experience, various standpoints must be considered—the significance to the learner, to the teacher, to the author of a book or to its reader, for example.

5. A person in the process of learning *validates* the learning product. Validation, as it is used here, refers to checking the meanings, the inferences drawn, for their correctness in the light of data collected. The nurse who is using experiential teaching with a patient helps the patient to formulate the meaning of his experience and then checks that meaning with him to see whether they both agree on it.

6. Finally, the learner *tests a learning product through usage* and, with this step, the learning process—with reference to the particular experience—is brought to a close. Through such testing, learning products are evaluated as one step in the development of foresight which will be useful in later experiences.

COMPARING LEARNING AND ADAPTATION

Both learning and adaptation are influenced by the tensions of need, by anxiety, and by conflict in which there are opposing goals. Both learning and adaptation go on during, and as a result of, experiences but they lead to different products. We have already shown that a learning product is developed by sustaining anxiety, tension, or conflict while collecting and analyzing data in order to determine the meaning of an experience. Adaptation indicates more static patterning.

The steps in adaptation include: (1) observing a difficulty that is felt, or experiencing vague discomfort, or feeling an unexplained and immediate need for comfort or relief in the form of approval or disapproval (as relief from indifference, for instance); and (2) using familiar patterns which in earlier situations reduced tension automatically—that is, without critical examination of the meaning of what is experienced. It would clarify thinking in the field of education if the formation of patterns that work automatically merely to relieve tension were classified as adaptations, or as products of conditioning. The term *learning* could then be used in a more precise way, indicating use of critical facilities, such as the capacity for conceptualizing experience, for generalizing, for abstracting the meaning of events in original patterns—that is, responses that are new, spontaneous, and significantly specific to a current situation.

The operating difference, then, in these two concepts lies in the recognition and handling of anxiety, and the use of available skill in sustaining doubt, delay, and uncertainty until an experience has been understood. In this concept of learning, anxiety would be recognized as an aspect of the data collected, analyzed as a relevant part of the experience, and would provide the energy for use during a stage of inquiry. Anxiety-relieving phenomena offer security by restricting awareness; the relief is a sort of payoff for not noticing, not profiting from experience, not grasping the meaning of what has been observed. Everyone has seen phenomena such as transferring blame from the nurse-as-observer to patients or other personnel, operating on the basis of wishes rather than what is experienced or observed, shifting a discussion from the point of focus, or being otherwise distracted from a task at hand. These are examples of automatic actions used to relieve tension.

In this sense, then, "learning by experience" (which the psychiatry textbooks say "psychopaths" do not do) implies generalizing from what is felt, thought, or done as a participant in an event. It implies development and refinement of the human capacities—to conceptualize, to comprehend, to formulate significant relations as they are experienced in a situation, and to use and refine this ability in personal and work situations. This, then, is one component of preventive psychiatry in education. Experiential teaching in nursing education offers nurses a way of using and refining their capacities as persons and as nurses.

THE TEACHER'S ROLE

When experiential teaching is used as a method, the role of the teacher is rich and varied and is limited only by the boundaries of endowment, training, and the policies of an educational institution. The teacher has two principal functions—as a *critical auditor* and as *facilitator.* She listens intelligently to students' descriptions of experience, and uses her own capacities and skills to encourage learning, that is, the recognition of what can be generalized from these descriptions.

She might act in the following ways: ask for further description of the situation in which a student participated; frame simple but provocative questions which challenge the student to clarify an experience or to notice other possible meanings; suggest gaps in data which require delay in making inferences; pose likely alternatives to generalizations made by students; call attention to sources for further exploration of relevant information; restate what has been presented to suggest a new relation, theme, or variation; and the like. These actions stimulate constructive use of capacities to clarify what has been experienced in a clinical situation.

The teacher must be sensitive to latent, or partially recognized, creative capacities in others and be able to observe and to relate herself to these constructive aspects. An optimistic bias—an expectation that the student can and will learn—is particularly helpful when coupled with sensitive observations of the interaction of teacher and students.

The intention of the student to learn becomes a central feature of the kind of educational situations described. Knowledge that is useful and practical, relevant to the work situation, is an inevitable outcome. Helping students to find out what they know intuitively, or what they can know more fully, of their experience and participation with patients is at first the aim of the teacher, but the students soon recognize this and make it their aim, too.

Nurses want to be as helpful as possible, to intervene constructively in the nursing problems of patients. To function in this way, expertness of a particular kind is required of them. The kind of expertness needed is determined by the nature of problems, and by the kind of intervention likely to reduce the strength of, or solve, those problems with patients. I think this kind of expertness can, in some degree, be described, and that there is a relationship between it and the outcomes of experiential teaching situations.

USING EXPERIENTIAL TEACHING

Health teaching is a part of the work role of the staff nurse in all situations. In psychiatric nursing, however, experiential teaching may, at this time, have wider applicability.

Technical or mechanical expertness is not the major requirement of psychiatric nurses. The problems of patients in psychiatric situations are problems of living—unawareness, disorders of feelings, thinking disorders—problems which have to do with communication, symbolization, perception and the like. Professional nurses, who get into more or less immediate touch with the patient undergoing stress in the ward situation, need particularly to observe, conceptualize, and comprehend how the situation looks to the patient. They ought to be able to observe changes in situations and the concomitant shifts in the behavior of participants. This requires rather expert use of their conceptualizing capacities. It requires development and continuing refinement of the abilities to observe, to recall vividly, to describe and record significant details, to analyze situations and determine the nursing problems, to generalize and infer meaning from observational data, to formulate and state problems and generalizations, and to validate with other nurses and patients the meanings inferred. These abilities are needed by nurses in their everyday work role, and for improving the collaborative relations with other professional workers, particularly in hospital situations. Research which involves nurses can hardly proceed without these important abilities and opportunities for refining them.

OBSERVATION, PARTICIPATION, AND INTERVENTION

To summarize another way, the predominant features of the work role of nurses in psychiatry are observation, participation, and intervention in social interactions within the hospital ward or the professional work situation. In this work situation, day in and day out, both nurses and patients experience something. There is, therefore, always the possibility of learning something useful to living, here and later, through the nurse–patient relationship. If nurses focus on the learning possibilities and view psychiatric hospitals as special educational institutions in which neglected learnings—gaps in learning by experience in the past—can be rectified, this can be an important element in the patient's recovery.

Instead of this view of psychiatric hospitals (where patients learn about living by learning from experience in the ward situation) there are various current views and misconceptions. One particularly important here is the idea that if you work in psychiatric hospitals long enough, you will become "crazy" too. Perhaps under present conditions, and in some situations, there may be a kernel of truth in this. Given a ward situation in which the pathology of perhaps thirty patients operates all day, every day, and the nurse is more or less unaware of the possible meanings of that pathology and of her own participation in relation to it, she may be affected by it.

There is a vast difference, however, between that kind of situation with its long-range effects on patients and personnel, and a nursing situation in which the nurse is competent. And by competent I mean that she has become fairly adept and is interested, in a continuing way, in identifying and using what she experiences. This kind of participation—conceptualizing that "inner component" of ward events and situations while participating with patients—is guided by awareness, intention, purpose, and foresight as well as some inferences concerning the consequences of her actions.

Nurses can only communicate and interact in terms of what they actually know, or are aware of—by way of their feelings, thoughts, and immediate actions. Experiential teaching offers a way of both clarifying and expanding that awareness and self-knowledge.

In the nursing profession, and particularly among psychiatric nurses, there are many who are expecting fruitful outcomes of the research projects now being conducted. What is available in textbooks gives us some plausible explanations of what is observed in nurse–patient situations in psychiatry, and there are some useful guides to action. But there are carefully selected and able nurses, participating in research activities, whose observations should prove valuable in enlarging and clarifying the principles of psychiatric nursing practice. To get these observations formulated for review, and to give these nurses full opportunity for refining their skills, I suggest inservice educational programs, using experiential teaching as a method for finding out what does go on in nursing situations. This would seem more useful than relying on textbooks, which can only tell us about what others believe does, or should, go on.

The informal review of day-to-day experiences may well provide a fresh view of psychiatric nursing practices. It may indicate the points at which nurses tend to reinforce or go along with the pathology of patients, instead of helping them to learn something new about living among people. It may clarify this method of "learning by experience" as a preventive-psychiatry aspect of education, as a way of identifying roles and activities of nurses which are most useful to patients, and as an aid to nurses themselves in learning healthy ways of living with people.

REFERENCES

Sullivan, H.S. (1953). *The interpersonal theory of psychiatry* (H. S. Perry & M. L. Gawel, Eds.). New York: Norton.

CHAPTER 11

Interpretation of Clinical Observations

An interpretation is an explanation, a construction, representation, or conception of the meaning or sense of a subject or event. In other words, interpretation is a process by which raw data secured by clinical observation are worked over and translated so that the various meanings of the data can be formulated. The process is one of rendering significance (intention, purpose, sense) from the raw data. For purposes of this chapter I use the term *interpretation* in two ways: to refer to the form or structure of a situation; and to refer to the intention, purpose, or function of a situation. Bergman (1951) distinguishes between what he calls Meaning I, the formal, operational meaning, and Meaning II, the significance, usefulness, or fruitfulness. In a general way, my use of the term is similar.

Perhaps I can clarify these terms by using them in relation to a brief clinical example. A young girl has a problem that centers around food rejection and overeating. These recurrent patterns of behavior are described by the girl in a way that suggests among other interpretations that her not eating is related to a wish to have

Paper presented for the Class of Interdisciplinary Communication in Psychiatry of the Nebraska Psychiatric Institute, The University of Nebraska College of Medicine, Omaha, Nebraska, January, 1958. Schlesinger Library, Radcliffe College, Cambridge, MA. No. 84-M107 Hildegard E. Peplau Archives, carton 39, volume 1441. Copyright 1986 by Schlesinger Library. Edited and reprinted by permission.

full self-control in the area of food taking. In this interpretation, the wish is a part of the structure of the meaning; the nature of the wish, to have self-control, reveals something of the intention or purpose of the pattern of not eating. Both of these formulations derive from analysis of what the girl has described as she talks about or uses these recurrent patterns of behavior.

I find it very useful to point out when students have *only* the structural meaning of what is going on, that is, they know that there is some kind of goal, pattern, force, theme at work in the situation but they do not yet know the nature (that is, the significance or function of this goal or pattern) to determine intentions and purposes of behavior takes more time and effort. The clinical instance I have given was meant to be illustrative of both structural and functional aspects of meaning; it is certainly not a comprehensive presentation of either the raw data or of the various interpretations that could be made.

In any clinical situation there are at least three sources of raw data to be interpreted: (1) the context, which is those conditions or circumstances that precede, surround, and give rise to current clinical observations; (2) the process, which comprises the structural operations of individuals in a context; and (3) the meaning, which incorporates the functions, purposes, and significance of the behavior toward which individuals move within a context. Full interpretation requires collection of data with regard to all of these sources, analysis of these data, and information about the various meanings. When these three aspects are considered, it is obvious that both observation and interpretation are complex tasks. In this chapter I do not go into detail about various patterns of observation that can be used to secure these data, but rather confine my remarks to some of the ways professional people unscramble clinical observations in order to derive the meaning.

WAYS TO INTERPRET CLINICAL DATA

Interpreting clinical data has become something of a parlor game—indeed, television has long taken to presentations with a psychiatric bent. The kind of interpretation that I discuss is at first a difficult and exhausting task; in the course of educating for these tasks some of my students fall by the wayside and all of them suffer fatigue. This, I suspect, is due to a conflict between customary or social modes of interpreting data and the ways that I describe here.

There are a number of different ways to interpret data; each parallels a level of development of ability to reason. The more complicated the method, the more highly developed the process and capacity for reason. In order to illustrate this, I discuss various ways to interpret in a sequence that parallels somewhat the development of a person.

Autistic Invention

The very young child interprets his experience by what Sullivan (1953) calls *autistic invention*. The child has no other way to interpret experience until language, a considerable vocabulary, and some patterns of relating to others have been learned. By autistic invention is meant the ability to invent and assign meanings to events in a highly personal way. Using this method, both the very young child and the schizophrenic patient have in common a tendency to interpret events in light of what they wish or expect will happen, rather than in terms of observation of what is actually happening. At first, students frequently use autistic invention to explain clinical observations; that is, they frequently draw conclusions from sources other than the clinical data, more often than not from their own wishes or personal experience. I use a very simple device to rule out autistic invention as the primary way to interpret data, even though I recognize that personally based speculations may give clues that are of value. I ask the students to interpret the statement "When the cat's away the mice will play," or some other proverb. I point out to the students their tendencies to add to the given data. I also ask them to identify the cues in the raw data that led to their interpretation.

Decoding

Another way to interpret is to *locate the key symbols in any set of given data and decode them*—that is, transpose them into other words that reveal the meanings. Then *restate* the original data in terms of the decoded meaning. In the proverb just cited, the key symbols are *cat*, *away, mice,* and *play.* When these are decoded, keeping the given data within its context and without additions by autistic means, they can be transposed as follows: *cat* stands for authority, *away* represents gone or absent, *mice* indicates subordinates, and *play* refers to fun. The restatement of the decoded meaning would be, "When the authority is absent the subordinates have fun." This type of interpretation is of some value in working with dreams or highly resymbolized statements of schizophrenic patients.

I use proverbs in teaching to help locate a tendency toward autistic elaboration of given data as a way of interpreting it; it is also a way to begin to teach decoding as a method of interpretation. There are a number of other errors that occur and can be pointed out in reviewing students' work on the simple exercise of interpreting a given proverb. Students often interpret feelings (of the cat or the mouse), largely because this is an area currently emphasized in psychiatric work. Students often prophesy what will happen if the circumstances are changed, as for example, "when the cat comes back," or if the "mice run away." Instead of decoding a key symbol, students often will interpret what the key symbol *is not,* as for example, "the mice are not the masters of their own lives." Or the students will use imprecise decoding, as for example, when cat is said to refer to "danger," or when play is said to refer to "doing what you want." Sometimes students will alter the key symbol, removing it from the class of objects to which it belongs—as for example, when the cat is seen as the "supervisor of nurses" or the "mice" are seen as children. Some students will decode several key symbols without showing significant differences in the meaning of each, as for example, when the cat is said to refer to "no one is present" and mice are decoded as "a person's behavior."

Other problems are located through the proverb exercise. Partial interpretation of the given data occurs when one of the key symbols is omitted in the decoding process. Piecemeal interpretation of aspects of the proverb—without restatement of the phrase subsequent to decoding—is a very common problem. Circumstantiality and "making sure you guess correctly" are two glaring errors. It is not uncommon for students to insert phrases that have no relation to the given data (for example, "the peer group will respond to their absence") or to give long unnecessary preliminary statements about the use and value of proverbs, or to give four or five different interpretations in the hope of hitting the one that the teacher deems correct. These failures to come to the task directly sometimes signify major difficulties in the thought process of the student; to pick them up early gives the teacher an opportunity to work with the student in correcting the situation, if this is possible through academic means.

There are also other problems, which might be classified as a tendency toward concreteness or toward overabstractness. When concreteness is used, the student might say, "The cat is the cat who is away but the mice aren't." As you can see, this is a simple reshuffling of the given data without any attempt at decoding. Or, the student's response might be too overabstract to see the relations to the given data, as for example when the response is as follows: "When the danger restraints are loosened, freedom results."

I have spent a good deal of time on this particular method, decoding the key symbols and restating the data in transposed form, because it is one that reveals much about the interpreter; it is not, however, the most important type of interpretive method. One danger in teaching decoding is that it may encourage students to use a one-to-one equational type of thinking in making interpretations. This danger decreases when students acquire additional interpretive methods.

Subdividing and Categorizing

Hardin (1957) refers to two other methods by which data may be analyzed and interpreted: (1) Data may be subdivided, as for example when a child asks, "Is all fruit, fruit or are there apples and oranges?" (2) Data may be categorized, as for example when a child asks, "Is it an apple or a bird?" (p. 395). Both of these methods are useful in psychiatric work; we subdivide when we ask, "Is what is observed to be classified as behavior or further subdivided into independent or isolated behavior?" We are categorizing when we ask, "Are we dealing with an emotional factor or a biochemical factor?" These methods have a place in interpretation especially when effort is directed toward finding out a dominant pattern of behavior; in order to do so, it is necessary to transpose various acts of behavior into larger categories that indicate the same dimension. In other words, you cannot add apples and bananas unless both are "reduced" to fruit, that is, to the same dimension. The game called "twenty questions" in which children ask, "Is it animal, vegetable, or mineral?" helps them to learn these two methods.

To this point I have discussed four methods of interpretation—autistic invention, decoding, subdividing, and categorizing; there are still other, more complicated ways to interpret clinical observations.

Conceptual Interpretation with Operational Definitions

It can be assumed that professional education supplies knowledge the professional worker applies in his work. This knowledge consists of concepts that help explain observations, principles that guide the observer in his or her work, general facts and information used in the reasoning process, and techniques for securing data and for intervening in ways that are favorable in relation to the work situation. Of these various forms of knowledge, concepts, principles, information, and techniques, I now discuss only the application and use of concepts in the interpretation of clinical data.

A concept is a standardized interpretation developed as a result of the experience of many workers in the same field. A *concept*, as I am using this word, is a term that is defined by stating the operations usually associated with it in their serial order of emergence. In psychiatric work we have very few objectively verifiable, operationally defined concepts; this is a serious limitation that handicaps interpretation of clinical observations. There are also many quarrels about whether operationalism is possible or useful.

An *operationally defined concept* is a term that is defined by stating all of the behaviors usually associated with it. These behaviors, however, are not itemized as separate acts of individual behavior, but such separate acts are reduced to a dimension that generally refers to all of the individual acts that classify under that dimension. In other words, whatever term is being operationally defined, the person making the definition is required to ask and answer such questions as: What are the different dimensions of behavior associated with this term? What are the operations of each dimension? In what serial order do they appear in the sequence of behavior as it can be observed? What instances or acts of behavior can be classified under the heading of each dimension? For example, I will give an oversimplified operational definition of *conflict*. A person can be said to be in conflict when: (1) Two incompatible goals are held; (2) there is avoidance of one or both of these goals; (3) there is movement toward both goals; and, as the conflict becomes more emergent, (4) there is hesitation, vacillation, blocking, and/or exhausting fatigue not due to physical causes. You will notice that each operation is stated in general terms and that separate acts of behavior of the person in conflict must be classified as properly falling under each of the stated operations. Perhaps I can illustrate how this works by specifying first how a concept is applied in clinical observation and then how the concept is used to get at the structural and functional meaning of what goes on.

In order to apply a concept one must, (1) first know that the concept exists and be aware of its definition, that is, its operations; (2) some, one or all of the operations must be observed, or inferred from separate acts of behavior that are observed in the clinical situation; (3) the observer selects from memory the concept that includes the observed or inferred behavior; then (4) the observer uses the remaining operations of the concept to secure more data. For example, an observer notices that a patient is unable to make a decision. The patient hesitates, walks back and forth vacillating as to whether to participate in a ward activity or to avoid the work or the contacts or something related to participation in that activity, or whether to speak or not to speak. The observer may notice this for several days before deciding that this is behavior that can be classified as hesitation and vacillation. In the definition of *conflict* that I have just given, this was the fourth operation indicated in the serial order statement. Having observed and decided that this patient is hesitating and vacillating, the observer would now apply the concept further. The observer would identify the two goals either by observing the patient directly or by talking with the patient. Which goal is being avoided, or are both being avoided? What steps toward these goals have been taken? Which goal is the strongest? I am not suggesting that the interview situation be structured to include the questions as I have stated them; I am suggesting that these are the

questions for which the observer needs answers. In the interview
situation the observer might say: "I noticed that you are reluctant to
join the group, could we talk about that?" The data relevant to the
foregoing questions would unfold. The interviewer, therefore, has
to keep track of the direction of the inquiry and of the relation of
this direction to the questions that need answering in order to determine whether conflict is present and to determine the nature of that
conflict. It takes time to secure sufficient data for full application
of a concept; in many instances, many hours of interviewing are
required.

An operationally defined concept works, then, to explain behavior that is observed. But it explains it largely by giving the form or
structure of meaning for use in the subsequent inquiry; it does not
give the reasons for that form or structure. For example, the concept
of conflict, the way I have defined it, will not help explain why a
person holds two incompatible goals. It merely suggests that hesitation, vacillation, blocking and/or fatigue, which are directly observable, are related to conflict—and it suggests what else the observer
needs to know in order fully to identify the nature of the conflict.
The hesitation, vacillation, and fatigue abate as the patient begins to
recognize and to deal with the nature of the incompatible goals. This
recognition, however, is not a simple matter either, as the various
layers of meaning of the goals have to be dealt with in turn until the
central conflict is revealed. It is these different levels or layers of
meaning that make the difference in what a staff nurse might do and
what a psychoanalytically oriented psychotherapist might do in relation to a presenting conflict. For example, the staff nurse is presented with and has to deal with patients who express conflict about
going home *or* staying in the hospital. The psychoanalytically oriented psychiatrist would work toward dealing with the conflict in
terms of dependence and independence. These, however, are different levels of expression of the same conflict.

Generalization

Generalization is the ability to move from details to general meaning, and from literal or concrete to figurative meaning. Considerable skill in generalization is needed by all professional workers.

Generalizing is used in the application of concepts, but it is also used to derive the problem, pattern, theme, relation, or connection inherent in descriptions of experiences, as well as direct observation of behavior. Generalizations serve the professional worker as structured standpoints for further observations or they may serve as conclusions that indicate closure of a problem situation. In nursing, the observer must notice and then evaluate the demands of the patient so that these can in part be met through nursing services.

In the education of nurses, I have used several different approaches to the development of ability to generalize. For example, initially, I give the students copies of fairy stories, such as "Henny Penny," "The Emperor's New Clothes," and the like. I ask the students to derive several general ideas from the given data that best express the patterns, themes, or hidden meanings—meanings that are not *directly* stated in the story. I frequently locate errors in thinking that are similar to those described earlier. I ask the students to show me where in the given data are the cues, the hints, to the generalizations they have drawn. Once this has been tried using several myths, stories, or song hits, I may give the students a dream, and then an extensive report of statements by a schizophrenic patient in which the language is highly resymbolized so that the meaning is hidden or very nearly lost. Here again, one problem of students is that of going beyond the given data, of adding data either by autistic invention or from private and personal experience and then interpreting this, rather than the given data. The teacher's task is one of helping students to recognize differences between generalizing by abstracting from given data and reading meaning into data.

Generalizing is one of the principal methods for getting at the functional meaning of the difficulties of a patient in a nurse–patient relationship or in the patient's relationships with a group of patients in the ward setting. This method can be classified into two aspects: (1) overall impressions and (2) more precise classification of details of clinical observations. Overall impressions are really sweeping speculations that apply in situations in which many of the same details are similar to those observed in previous situations and therefore call out the same impression. For example, a student may tell me: "I don't really know on what basis, but I have the feeling that this patient is very envious of the other patient." A review of the observations made by this nurse may reveal certain details that point to operations of the concept of envy. Some students, of course, have quite standardized impressions, like stereotypes, of particular forms of behavior, and these must be ruled out to produce a really useful clinical observer. But there are also gifted students who do have sweeping first impressions, of an intuitive kind, that are often later revealed to be empathic observation. Speculations of this kind are very useful, so long as the observer knows that they are mere speculations and serve as hypotheses for further structured observation.

More precise classification of the data of clinical observation requires that data be sorted and analyzed in order to locate connections, or relations, such as the problem, trend, pattern, theme, need, and the like. I teach students, for example, to review and analyze all of the data they have on their relationship with a particular patient in terms of the patient's view of self, as the patient has stated its variations directly and indirectly. This is painstaking work and often requires an hour or two of review of the data, but it yields not only patterns and themes of the self view but also variations in the expression of these patterns and themes. More often than not, the patient is unaware of the overall pattern and theme, but may recognize an individual expression of self and lay claim to it. The patient's patterns of relating to people, including nursing personnel, are something that nurses need to know about, especially if they intend to be helpful. For example, one patient that I am concerned with has a stereotyped pattern of giving. He gives compliments, all of his food and gifts, and at Christmas time tried to give a gift to the student, as he was able to do with other nursing personnel. The student recognized this as a recurrent pattern and from a review of her data knew something of the variations and of some of the stated reasons for giving things. She therefore, steadfastly turned down the gift with a very brief statement to the patient—each time that she did not wish to take the present. This intervention by the nurse in this pattern of behavior began to spread to relationships with other people and eventually to beginning inquiry on the part of the patient about why he needed to relate himself to others in this way. If this student had merely taken the gift without recognizing either the pattern or any of its significance, the patient's pattern of giving would merely have been reinforced; nothing favorable or new would have happened. It was not the refusal of the gift alone that brought about change, but understanding of the patient's use of this pattern of behavior.

Generalizations that are made about clinical observations refer to connections or relations between objects, classes of objects, events, or acts of behavior. In order to formulate a generalization from data, the observer ought to be able to return to the raw data and identify the connections.

For example, on one ward in which I was teaching a group of basic students, we made observations of all patients in order to determine certain characteristics of the ward society. We were interested in securing answers to the following questions: Who was the central figure? Who carried the messages to and from the central figure? What devices did they use to include others from the in-group? What were the linkages that bound this in-group together? What were the characteristics and themes of the patients on the periphery? The students took each of these questions and phrased other questions they could casually ask patients in order to secure the data needed for this study of the ward society. For example, they wanted to know: Where were the favorite beds for that season of the year? What did the patients consider important privileges on the ward? and so forth.

A great deal of information was collected by this study group in a very short time. The analysis of these data yielded some very interesting patterns and themes, but the central theme in the in-group was, "It's hopeless; we will never get out." This was the tie that held the group together, and it seemed that all else revolved around this theme. The history of this theme was then sought in the case histories of the individual patients in the in-group, and there was good reason for each of these patients to feel their situation was hopeless. For example, the central figure had been admitted as a "mental defective" at the age 14 and had been committed for life because of her behavior in other institutions and because she was the last remaining member of her family. The students were indeed interested that it was not a member of the nursing personnel but a patient who was the central figure around whom the life on the ward turned. Knowing this information, and having generalized not only the themes but answers as well to the questions posed at the beginning, the nurses could then determine what to do about it. This, then, is an instance in which a more specific structured type of generalizing was used for purposes of locating the meaning of what goes on in a ward as a society of people.

Developmental Framework

A developmental frame of reference may be used to interpret clinical data. This method requires the observer to have in mind definite information about each era of development, which can then be compared with what is observed in a particular era and in this way determine what lies ahead as the patient moves forward.

There are, of course, many different frames of references about human development. Some years ago, a group of graduate students in nursing prepared an outline they entitled "Tools and Tasks of Personality Development" (Peplau, 1969). In preparing this outline, these nurses surveyed some fifty-two different points of view about development of personality; their outline represents areas of agreement among the works surveyed. The outline placed various "tools" in the serial order in which they become available for use to the human organism. Moreover, they have defined each era by marking off the beginning and ending of the period by the emergence or ripening of another tool. I find this outline most helpful because the definition of each tool facilitates translation of clinical observation and, as I said earlier, the whole outline suggests successive steps in forward movement as a person develops and uses more mature capacities. (See Chapter 2, pp. 31–41.)

For example, one tool that emerges in infancy is the tool of *autistic invention,* the ability to interpret experience in a highly personal way. Between ages 6 and 9, or the juvenile era, the tools of *competition, compromise,* and *cooperation* ripen in that order. In preadolescence, ages 9 to 12, the tools of *consensual validation* (reaching agreements about the meaning of experience and ways of action) and *collaboration* (deriving satisfaction by participating in group accomplishment) develop. These tools illustrate parts of a developmental frame of reference. Observing these separate patterns in an individual places him at a given moment in an era of development; recurrent usage of earlier patterns in the absence of later ones suggests that the person has been stalemated at that point and that movement ahead will require development of subsequent tools. With adults, however, we rarely see complete absence of later tools but rather dominance in the use of earlier ones. The use of autistic invention by the schizophrenic patient, for example, meets a need to avoid loneliness, for instance, but it also prevents refinement of such other tools as cooperation and consensual validation on the simple basis that these later patterns are not used enough to gain comfort and skill in so doing. This tells the observers something of the nature of the helping task.

There is of course always the need for a word of caution in the use of established knowledge, concepts, and frames of reference—although no one individual can build up all of the knowledge he needs by making all of his own generalizations and testing them as he goes along. There is also the need to maintain awareness of the role assumptions play and of the difficulties in interpreting freshly, with and without the use of established knowledge. Yet Sigmund Freud developed psychoanalytic theory and method because his clinical observations did not meet the prevailing cultural explanations nor his own earlier ideas of the meaning of what he observed; as a result, a major change or shift in his thinking was required, which led to a new formulation. But it is the pressing obligation of each professional worker to *determine* whether this now-established formulation helps or hinders interpretation; whether the data observed corroborate a favored theory, or whether the theory really explains or points toward the meaning of what is observed.

The purpose of interpretation, from the standpoint of the observer, is to secure the meaning of what is noticed, to revise this meaning with further observation, and to base actions on established formulations of meaning. This purpose requires professional workers to go beyond mere naming or labeling of behavior and to reach the point where there is precision in the knowledge used and in the pattern of using it. It is toward this effort that I have concerned myself with interpretation and with the ways of doing it, to the end that I will be more aware of what I teach and how my students are using this important process in psychiatric nursing practice.

I have not considered, in this chapter, the question of how interpretations are developed or used in clinical work: I have only described some of the methods that are used by the observer. How these are woven into the interview situation is another matter. Whether the interviewer gives interpretations to the patients, or under what conditions it is safe to do so, is still another important question. These, however, are questions beyond the scope of this chapter. One thing is certain, however: the mode of thinking and interpreting of the interviewer serves as a model, one that the patient notices and may copy.

INTERPRETATION BY NURSES

There is, however, one pressing question I do want to discuss: the question of whether nurses should interpret clinical data or whether they should merely report it for the use of other professional workers. In my opinion, a work situation that forbids the nurse to make interpretations is one that places obstacles in the way of the development of nursing as a profession. More than this, such a situation also restricts the growth of nurses as persons—of the use of their capacities for reason. Moreover, nurses who are forbidden to use interpretations are not fully free to develop their own clinical abilities. Everyone, layman and professional alike, interpret what is observed. Unless all professional workers are aided to refine the knowledge and methods of interpretation that they use in clinical work, they will use their own autistic inventions and parataxic distortions of the meaning of what goes on around them. Nurses do interpret and should be assisted to develop the ability to interpret.

SUMMARY

This chapter deals with seven different ways of interpreting clinical observations. These are: (1) by autistic invention, making up the meaning in a highly personal way; (2) by decoding and translating the key symbols in given data; (3) by subdividing data; (4) by categorizing data according to general classes; (5) by the application of concepts that explain the structure of meaning and suggest sources for getting at the functional meaning; (6) by generalizing from given data through the use of overall impressions or specifically structured patterns for analysis of data; and (7) by application of a developmental frame of reference. Each of these methods is defined and to a limited extent illustrated.

Interpretation is a way of making sense out of what is noticed; it is one important step in the total process of working with people in difficulty. Equally important are the other functions of the professional worker in the psychiatric field. These include observing so that there are sufficient data with reference to the context, the process, and the content of a situation. Once interpreted, meanings need to be validated; that is, the meaning needs to be checked in various ways. There is always the possibility that the meaning to an observer and the meaning to the person observed will differ. Checking the meaning with a patient is not always possible, so the professional worker often checks with other observers in the situation, with other colleagues, or one can check with similar cases reported in the literature. Once the meaning of a situation is formulated, the next step is the problem of intervention—what to do to change the situation in a way favorable for the patient. Intervention is followed by further observation and reporting of the results of such effort.

It seems to me, from the standpoint of a nurse educator, that teaching how to interpret is the more complicated. We need to have some more careful ways to estimate development of the abilities represented in the methods I have described, and we need to know more about the reasons for the absence of these abilities in students who come from particular contexts.

Interpretation will be improved when we have more precise concepts. The social sciences are sources to which the professions turn for new knowledge, for more careful definition of concepts, and for objective verification of what we now know and use.

REFERENCES

Bergman, G. (1951). The logic of psychological concepts. *Philosophy of Science, 18,* 93–110.
Hardin, G. (1957). The threat of clarity. *American Journal of Psychiatry,* 114(5), 392–396.
Peplau, H. E. (1969). Theory: The professional dimension. In C. Norris (Ed.), *Proceedings of the first nursing theory conference*, pp. 33–46. Kansas City, MO: Kansas University Medical Center.
Sullivan, H. S. (1953). In H. S. Perry & M. L. Gawel (Eds.), *The interpersonal theory of psychiatry.* New York: Norton.

CHAPTER 12

Clinical Supervision of Staff Nurses

In nursing there is considerable discussion, mostly in the back rooms, that administrative supervision should be replaced by clinical supervision. I have suggested that each clinical supervisor should have an administrative assistant to take care of management details, thereby freeing the supervisor to do clinical supervision. What would it be like? What kind of regular sessions should be set up for orderly and continuing review of the work of the staff nurse with a clinical expert who is the clinical supervisor? With what frequency should these conferences occur? What would be a useful duration, one hour, two hours, or an indeterminate period? What kind of preparation for the conference should be expected of the supervisor and the staff nurse? Does the work situation allow this kind of time and effort? These and many other questions about the best form of clinical supervision are being raised by nurses. I address these questions from an interpersonal standpoint.

From *Further Aspects of Nurse-Patient Interaction.* Paper presented at the Institute on New Dimensions in Nursing, Pennsylvania League for Nursing, Altoona, Pennsylvania, October, 1964. Schlesinger Library, Radcliffe College, Cambridge, MA. No. 84-M107 Hildegard E. Peplau Archives, carton 39, volume 1451.

THE SUPERVISORY CONFERENCE

The supervisory conference should occur at least once each week, preferably twice, and last at least one hour at the beginning. The conference may be shortened after approximately two years of supervision. A definite time should be scheduled; the hour should begin and end on time. Regular conferences are necessary and desirable if the supervisor is to gain a picture of the major and dominant patterns of thought and action of each staff nurse.

Initially the focus of the supervisory conference is upon the staff nurse's interactions with patients. Eventually the supervisor may wish to concentrate on patterns of behavior between the staff nurse and the supervisor. It is important to avoid discussing the nurse's private biography and interactions in social situations because the supervisory conference is work oriented. The aim is to review observations and explanations of the nurse's patterns of practice with patients under different conditions and circumstances; these same interpersonal patterns will tend to be used in the relationship with the supervisor. If the patterns indicate disturbed relationships that go beyond the help of the supervision, the nurse should be referred for therapy.

The staff nurse should come prepared with notes, verbatim data, or tape recordings. As the supervisory conferences progress the staff nurse should begin to organize the material for discussion of a particular clinical problem: for example, some systematic study of instances of clinical data in one case or in several similar cases; relevant literature; and a beginning formulation of an explanation of the data. In order to keep pace with the developing competence of staff nurses under supervision, the supervisor must have time to keep up with review of the literature.

The procedure of the review will vary with the nature of the concerns and data presented. The staff nurse should take the lead in talking about the nurse–patient interactions while the supervisor listens, and ask questions when clarification is required. Theories that explain the data are suggested, and the nurse should be referred to literature in order to enlarge her understanding of the clinical issues. The staff nurse does most of the talking and discussing. The aim of the supervisor is to try to perceive the interaction the way it appears to the staff nurse in the context of the situation, and to suggest alternative modes of responding.

Both staff nurse and supervisor should keep some kind of record of these conferences. Periodic evaluation of the records should show evidence of variation or change in behavior and development of new competencies.

DIRECT OBSERVATION

The supervisor may directly observe the practice of the staff nurse, providing another dimension of data for review. The supervisor may notice something in the practice of the staff nurse that has been overlooked through review of data in the supervisory conference. The aim of direct observation, however, is to enlarge the staff nurse's self-awareness, individual responsibility, and capability for making sound judgments so that on-the-spot supervision will become less needed as conferences go on.

The supervisor should share openly her views regarding the quality of work, the competencies that still need to be developed, and should provide direction for such development. The staff nurse should know—every step of the way—where she stands and where she needs to increase effort to develop. Termination of work may result as a final step in the supervisory process, but it should never come as a surprise if the supervisor has been open and direct with the staff nurse.

SUMMARY

In summary, the supervisory conference is an interview mechanism through which staff nurses can become expert in interpersonal relations. The supervisor must be a person who has high tolerance for ambiguity, who can allow human error, who can think clearly, and who has no covert need to dominate and destroy. A concern for the slow but sure growth of the staff nurse nurtures and stimulates development of competencies in work with patients. The supervisor must be a nurse who can tolerate disorder in the presentation of data, and who knows something about the procedures by which data can be ordered into theories toward a science of nursing practice. It will take nurses who really have a passion for details and for seeing relations among facts, but who are largely uninterested in the power of administrative tasks as compared to the fascination of inquiry into clinical problems. These nurses will want power to do something, not power over people or their lives; this is a limited, rational power, based upon knowledge and the eagerness that others also become more knowing and capable.

The service-based clinical supervisor in the year 2000 will be an expert clinician in one area of nursing practice, will be an authority on methods of studying interpersonal situations within a particular clinical service, and will be eager to communicate her knowledge to the young so they can grow and change and enlarge their clinical learning. The clinical supervisor in the year 2000 will publish literature on various interpersonal aspects of clinical problems; she will become as much of a theoretician as will the university-based faculty member.

The opportunity to observe and understand clinical data in service settings is immense. In this chapter, I have briefly outlined some dimensions of the work of clinical supervision of staff nurses so that they may increase their competence in work with patients by using the results of analysis of this gold mine of data.

PART IV Psychotherapy

Introduction

In 1952, when Hildegard E. Peplau first wrote about psychotherapy, she distinguished it from counseling. Therapy, she said, took place at a certain time in a certain place, the therapist devoting the full therapeutic hour to the patient to focus on a central interpersonal difficulty that affects the patient's life. Counseling, on the other hand, was but one role in a combination of nursing roles. It often used the more immediate interpersonal events in the current context of round-the-clock contacts with patients in order to facilitate learning. Even in her early work, however, the main intent, ideas, and principles of psychotherapy and counseling sound identical. Ironically, however, Peplau's counseling as originally intended—that is, the application of matters psychological and interpersonal to immediate clinical situations, as one among other nursing roles—is surely part of milieu practice and is more difficult than formal psychotherapy.

In any event, over the years, as Peplau developed the clinical specialist position where the counseling role became the prominent nursing role and interpersonal techniques the crux of psychiatric nursing, the term *psychotherapy* slowly started to replace *counseling* in her work. At the same time, a focus on the application of psychotherapy knowledge, skills, and principles to the more diffuse, unplanned clinical encounters (as part of the milieu in psychiatric facilities) refined the original counseling role.

Interestingly, this latter refinement still seeks a name, for although the intervention is psychotherapeutic in intent and benefit, it is not psychotherapy itself in relationship, process, and structure—though some might call it "brief encounter therapy" of sorts or "situational interviewing" or "consciously executed experiential relationships." Too, this on-the-spot therapy is equally useful, productive, and necessary with physically ill patients. However, physically ill but emotionally distressed patients, unaccustomed to interpersonally focused and skilled nurses, would be surprised to learn they had received psychotherapy as part of their treatment.

Starting in the 1960s, Peplau was also pressured to start using the term *therapy* by graduate students who soon recognized there was perhaps another level operating in the use of the term counseling for what they were being taught. In addition, in the early 1960s, at an American Psychiatric Association meeting where Peplau was presenting, Dr. Henry Davidson (well-known forensic psychiatrist, long-time friend of psychiatric nursing through Peplau, superintendent of Essex County Overbrook Hospital in New Jersey, and the Dr. Whatsisname of the publication *Mental Hospitals*) urged Peplau to tell the M.D. audience what psychiatric nurses where actually doing. Prior to that time, in the late 1950s and very early 1960s, it would have been impossible to gain access to patients if the term psychotherapy had been used. Agency doors would have slammed shut to these avant garde nurses doing "psychotherapy," even though nobody else was doing it with these public hospital inpatients. Counseling, as part of the nurse–patient relationship, sounded benign and unthreatening to the turf of the more established psychiatric hierarchy.

Peplau's psychotherapy is characterized by its organization, by distinct psychotherapeutic strategies that are designed and always related to the pathology involved and the outcome desired. Both structure and content of the nurse–patient interview is analyzed for themes, patterns, and integrations. In distinguishing psychotherapeutic closeness from other kinds of closeness, Peplau, in the 1960s, was the first and only psychiatric nurse to clarify the similarities and differences between professional closeness and interpersonal intimacy at a time when it was popular for psychiatric nurses and other professionals to blur the two boundaries, thereby courting trouble in their work with patients.

Peplau the supervisor was always intrigued with the psychotherapeutic process, with the way the mind worked and people behaved. That intellectual curiosity has spawned the interest and scholarship in human behavior that is her legacy.

CHAPTER 13

Interpersonal Techniques: The Crux of Psychiatric Nursing

The time is past when a nurse could become, in one lifetime, an expert in all clinical areas. Advances in all fields of knowledge and within nursing science itself point to the inevitability of clinical specialization.

When you begin to think about specialization, however, you think not only of a focus in a particular area but of considerable depth. As the scope of the specialists' work narrows, the depth intensifies at, I submit, the point of the uniqueness of the clinical area. The unique aspect of a clinical area is twofold: It is that which occurs in other clinical fields but is not emphasized to the same extent and it is that which is almost entirely new—the uncommon, promising developments which result from thinking deeply about a particular facet of work in just one area.

Each of the areas of nursing practice has a particular clinical emphasis. This emphasis does not preclude attention to all the other aspects of the workrole of the nurse practitioner, but more time, effort, and thought are given to this particular facet. For example, nurses in public health programs emphasize health teaching, not to the exclusion of the technical aspects of nursing practice nor of the supportive, reassuring, mother-surrogate type of nurse activities. But, by and large, nurses who visit patients in their homes spend a proportionately larger part of their time teaching. Medical-surgical nursing emphasizes technical care; pediatric nursing emphasizes the mother-surrogate role; in this chapter I want to consider the particular emphasis of psychiatric nursing.

I have indicated various subroles of the workrole of nurses. Briefly, these include mother-surrogate, technician, manager, socializing agent, health teacher, and counselor or psychotherapist.[1]

Psychiatric nursing emphasizes the role of counselor or psychotherapist. It is true that this idea is not a universally accepted one in all psychiatric facilities. But note that I say "psychiatric nursing," not "nursing in psychiatric units."

There are two levels of professional nurse personnel practicing in psychiatric units—general practitioners (general duty nurses) and specialists (psychiatric nurses). Let me clarify the difference. A general practitioner is a nurse who has completed only her basic professional preparation. From my viewpoint, a "psychiatric nurse" is a specialist and at this time specialist status can be achieved by two routes—experience and education.

Before the passage of the Mental Health Act in 1946, experience was the route by which a nurse earned the title "psychiatric nurse"; since 1946, however, some 25 graduate-level, university-based programs in advanced psychiatric nursing have been established. There are stipends available for study in these programs. Any nurse who can qualify—because she has completed her full basic professional preparation and has the intellectual and personal qualifications for graduate study—can secure a stipend for graduate study toward becoming a clinical specialist in psychiatric nursing, that is, a "psychiatric nurse." From my point of view, then, the route of clinical specialization for any nurse who was

[1] For a more complete discussion of subroles see Peplau's "Therapeutic Concepts" in *The League Exchange*, No. 26, pp. 1–30, published by the National League for Nursing, New York, 1957.

graduated since 1946 is through a university-based graduate level program.

I realize this is a status problem, but the profession of nursing will strengthen its position in relation to all other professional disciplines when it recognizes the culturally accepted fact that university education is the route for clinical specialization. There is good reason for this. Theoretically the university is free of the service commitment of the hospital—it can take objective distance, look dispassionately at the work of nurses, and dare to consider gross changes in the workrole.

When you are employed in a service agency, on the other hand, you become a participating member in its social system, ties of friendship and loyalty become binding as well as blinding, and dispassionate inquiry is greatly lessened. There is another reason why universities have culturally been charged with graduate education: The scope of established and newly formulated knowledge represented in a university faculty is ever so much wider than that represented in a professional staff group. It is access to this knowledge and its application to clinical observations that transform the student into an expert clinician.

There is clear distinction then between nursing in a psychiatric unit (what a general duty nurse does), and psychiatric nursing (what an expert clinical practitioner does). This distinction should be kept in the foreground for in this chapter I will refer to nurses and nursing, when speaking of the common and basic elements, and to psychiatric nurses and psychiatric nursing when speaking of the more specialized clinical functions.

A psychiatric nurse is first of all an expert clinician. She may also be a teacher, supervisor, administrator, consultant, or researcher, but underlying all these functional positions there should be advanced clinical training. Such clinical expertness revolves around the field's unique aspect or emphasis, in this case, the role of counselor or psychotherapist. I want to develop the importance of this idea for the general practice of nursing in a psychiatric setting, but, first, I wish to pinpoint why other aspects of the work in a psychiatric unit are not the central focus of psychiatric nursing.

The emphasis in psychiatric nursing is *not* on the mother-surrogate role. Some nurses believe that the unmet needs of a patient's infancy and early childhood can be met by the nurse's taking on various mothering activities. This belief assumes that the corrective experience is largely an emotional one resulting from a relationship in which the nurse complements a need for mothering of the patient, by supplying its counterpart—need-reducing mother-surrogate activities. This is analogous to the notion that when calcium deficiency produces tooth decay, supplying the calcium will fill up the cavities! A patient needs love, warmth, acceptance, support, and reassurance—not to supply the unmet needs of the past but for current reasons; having these emotional experiences makes it possible for the patient to come to grips with the earlier unmet needs on intellectual rather than on experiential grounds.

The notion that a made-up "good mother" experience will correct the patient's pathology is based on the assumption that the patient has not moved ahead in other areas compatible with chronological development—for example, language, vocabulary, and thought develop despite emotional deprivations.

To give mother-surrogate activities the central emphasis would be to deemphasize these tools which have developed and can be utilized.

There is another inescapable fact: The small number of professional nurses in psychiatric facilities has for a long time required that the necessary mother-surrogate activities—the bathing, feeding, dressing, toileting, warning, disciplining, and approving the patient—be taken over largely by nonprofessional nursing personnel. I do not foresee that any great benefit would accrue even if the supply was such that professional nurses could take on fully these mothering activities. Note that I have not said that a nurse never bathes or feeds or dresses or warns a patient in a psychiatric unit; what I have said is that these mothering activities are not the central focus.

The emphasis in psychiatric nursing is *not* on the technical subrole. Some nurses believe that the cause of mental illness will ultimately prove to be some biochemical or otherwise organic problem, identifiable by the results of various laboratory test procedures and correctable by some technical manipulations analogous to the injection of insulin in the therapeutic management of a person diagnosed as diabetic. Other nurses in the past and present have believed that technical expertness in giving tubs, packs, coma insulin and care in the pre- and postphases of electroconvulsive therapy or lobotomy would lead to solutions to mental illness. Technical expertness in giving medication or carrying out procedures associated with nursing is, in my opinion, not the desirable emphasis in psychiatric nursing.

CUSTODIAL ACTIVITIES

The emphasis in psychiatric nursing is *not* on managerial activities. Historically, these have been aspects of custodial care with restraint, protection, cleanliness, and order the dominant themes. Many of the housekeeping activities associated with these themes have been shifted not only to nonprofessional personnel but to work details made up of working patients as well. The housekeeping activities have given way to a host of clerical and receptionist activities, which nurses have taken on, and which presumably have to do with the management of the patient's environment in the interest of his care. I submit that the time is near at hand when administrators will recognize that these clerical and receptionist activities can be performed far better and more cheaply by a high school graduate; that these are not "professional" activities but instead are largely busywork which keeps the nurse away from direct contact with patients.

The emphasis in psychiatric nursing is *not* on socializing-agent activities, such as playing cards and games with patients, taking walks and watching TV with them and the like. In some basic schools of nursing, students are taught that these activities are central in the work of the nurse; I submit that the preparation of a nurse is not required for such activities; that the use of a nurse's social experience as an interesting diversionary activity in the patient's daily life is not the best use of the time of a professional nurse. Nonprofessional nursing personnel, volunteers, and visitors can do this game playing just as well as a nurse can. The professional education of the nurse is wasted; it is not needed to perform these activities which most laymen learn some time during their teens.

Group activities along these lines might better be planned and carried out by the recreational department or some department other than nursing service (or nursing education since students are largely "used" for this purpose). I have not said that a professional nurse *never* plays cards with patients; however, these activities are not the central emphasis in psychiatric nursing and at most should take a bare minimum of the day's time of a professional nurse. The emphasis in psychiatric nursing is *not* on health teaching although this subrole, in the workrole of the nurse, is an important one which needs to be developed further. I have pointed out that this is an important part of the work of nurses in public health. But the patients in the case load of these nurses are more often immediately able to use information than are patients in the psychiatric setting. Even so, teaching psychiatric patients about diet, nutrition, grooming, sex, and the like, may be very helpful. There has also been one promising study reported in which psychiatric patients were taught a concept of anxiety to apply to their own experiences; several similar studies are now under way (Hays, 1961).

The emphasis in psychiatric nursing is on the counseling or psychotherapeutic subrole. This generalization is based upon the assumption that the difficulties in living which lead up to mental illness in a particular patient are subject to investigation and control by the patient—with professional counseling assistance. It is also based on a second assumption: That formal knowledge of counseling procedure is absolutely essential for the more general type of approach which may be useful in very brief relationships with patients. Further, these general approaches are in the nature of "interpersonal techniques" useful in relation to specific problems—such as withdrawal, aggression, hallucinations, delusions, and the like—and these are the crux of psychiatric nursing.

There is being developed in psychiatric nursing a theory and procedure of nurse counseling. This development is proceeding along two lines:

1. A "surface type" of formal counseling procedure, such as a general nurse practitioner might use with patients in all clinical areas, is being described. Many schools of nursing already are beginning to teach interviewing—of a therapeutic in contrast to a biographical type—as a basis for counseling. A companion result of this development will surely be the identification and description of a variety of general approaches to specific problems—

interpersonal techniques—which nurses can use in everyday brief contacts with all types of patients.

2. Depth counseling, such as might be employed by a psychiatric nurse specialist who had completed two years of master's level clinical training, is also being described. Several nurses are now employed in situations in which they are doing long-term counseling of patients, utilizing the competencies secured through such clinical training. It is conceivable that in another decade or two nurses will share offices with psychiatrists and psychologists and social workers for the private practice of psychiatric nurse counseling, although now there are no publishable instances of such practices.

TEACHING STUDENTS

In many basic schools of nursing, students are being taught counseling technique in connection with nurse–patient care studies, particularly in the psychiatric setting. I have talked with a number of teachers in these schools and their general conclusion seems to be that when the student has an opportunity to work directly with one patient—say in one-hour sessions twice a week over a period of ten weeks—a great deal of learning takes place.

The student gets more than a textbook picture of pathology; she gets a full view of the complexity of the difficulties of a psychiatric patient, of the variations which occur in particular patterns of behavior. Many students find out, for example, that there are infinite variations of the pattern of withdrawal and that observed changes in the behavior of a patient are more likely to be changes from one variant to another of a central pattern that persists. Thus, a patient who uses gross withdrawal—by muteness, for example—can, as a result of a nurse–patient relationship, eventually, begin to speak; the verbalizations, however, are also classifiable as a variant of withdrawal, particularly when the patient talks but doesn't communicate anything descriptive of his difficulties.

In a carefully guided nurse–patient relationship, the nurse learns the art and science of counseling technique. She discovers that the art part of it is intuitively based—it is a clinical judgment which she herself makes, minute by minute, that this maneuver or that maneuver might conceivably be useful to the investigative effort. The student also learns the value of knowledge and procedures for their application to explain observations; this is the scientific part. The student gradually ceases to use such terms as anxiety, conflict, dissociation, and the like, as mere labels for behavior; she begins to use these concepts as scientific tools to guide her in assessing the investigative effort under way and in getting more information. Both the nurse and patient need as much descriptive information about the patient's life experiences as can be obtained without making the patient too uncomfortable. It is this information which will be worked over by the nurse and patient together so that the patient can understand and benefit from his previous experiences in living.

ANOTHER BENEFIT

Another important learning accrues from teaching counseling in the nurse–patient relationship. The student learns detachment; she learns—with the help of her teachers—how not to usurp the counseling time to meet her own needs; how to use the time instead, to help the patient formulate and meet his needs. She learns to make clearer distinction between techniques that are useful to her socially, outside the professional work situation, and those specifically useful in a clinical situation.

Moreover, the student learns a lot about herself as she begins to understand her reactions to the patients' behavior and verbal content, her own need for approval, the points at which she is particularly vulnerable. Patients have a way of unwittingly locating the vulnerabilities of students—be it their need for approval, their sensitivity to their appearance, their embarrassment in discussion about sex, or any one of a host of similar problem areas.

Once a student nurse has had successive counseling interviews with a particular patient, and has responsibly reviewed her nurse–patient data with an expert psychiatric nurse teacher, she is able to transfer—or generalize—the learning products to much briefer relationships with patients. Students invariably report that learning about counseling of one patient helps them to use to better advantage the two-to-three minute contacts they have with patients in the ward setting. Nor do I know of any other way for a student to achieve these understandings except as a result of talking with one patient about the patient's difficulties, in designated, time-limited sessions occurring over a period of time, and following each session by a substantial review of what went on with an expert psychiatric nurse. You cannot tell students what to do along these lines and then expect them, magically, to be able to do it. The student must not only experience this day-to-day process but she must have interested and active help in examining, bit by bit, the interview data which she thus collects.

One result, then, of the nurse–patient inquiry is the ability to transfer a substantial amount of learning toward more generalized interpersonal techniques. I believe that such techniques are the crux of psychiatric nursing and it seems to me that it ought to be possible for psychiatric nurses to develop specific interpersonal techniques useful in intervening in specific patterns of pathological behavior of patients. And it is possible; several nurses I know are currently involved in developing and testing such techniques.

It is my premise that interpersonal techniques can be devised and utilized by nursing personnel in relation to problematic behavior patterns of psychiatric patients. I believe that these interpersonal techniques, rather than modifications of medical-surgical nursing techniques, are the crux of the practice of nursing in a psychiatric setting.

REFERENCES

Hays, D. (1961). Teaching a concept of anxiety. *Nursing Research, 10,* 108–113.
Peplau, H.E. (1957). Therapeutic concepts. *The League Exchange, 26,* 1–30.

CHAPTER 14

Psychotherapeutic Strategies

The aim of nursing care of psychiatric patients is to assist the patient to struggle toward full development of his potential for productive living in the community. This aim requires nursing strategies which will aid the patient to resolve obstacles that stand in the way of full development. These obstacles are primarily of two kinds: (1) disturbances in thought, feeling, and action, which might be called the pathological use of one's potential; and (2) lacks and gaps in the development of intellectual and interpersonal competencies which are absolutely essential for healthy social interaction in the community.

It is not easy to design nursing tactics that will bring about realization of this aim of nursing care, for most, if not all, psychiatric patients. Theoretical knowledge concerning the observable pathology and hidden assets of persons diagnosed as mentally ill is still quite limited in quality and quantity. The social sciences and the applied psychiatric disciplines are still in very early stages of theory development. Nevertheless, it is possible to suggest some feasible dimensions of such nursing care which merit clinical trial as well as further careful study.

Reprinted from *Perspectives in Psychiatric Care, 6,* 264–270. Copyright 1969 by Nursing Publications, Inc. Used with permission.

For a tactic used in nursing care to be considered psychotherapeutic, the strategy or approach must have demonstrable impact on the item of behavior which is representative of an aspect of the pathology or an asset of the patient. Furthermore, the tactic for which there is anticipated a beneficial effect on the patient or a coercive pull in the direction of mental health must be sustained over time; there are no "magical" tactics which, if used once or twice, will produce substantial, constructive, and lasting effects observable in the behavior of a patient. Nursing strategies which are considered to be psychotherapeutic must be used persistently, many times, in situations in which a specific pathological item is presented by a patient and observed by the nurse. Therefore the alertness of the nurse in immediately noticing, assigning meaning to, and then responding specifically to the item of behavior presented by a patient is crucial to psychotherapeutic outcome.

One facet of mental illness is the tendency toward replication of inept behavior and, frequently, of the earlier social interactions from which it derived. For example, it is not uncommon for a firstborn child to attempt to retain his initial status as an only child by reporting to his parents the "bad" behavior of his siblings. If the parents accept the messages and court further "informer" behavior in this child, his relationships with his siblings will deteriorate. Since his focus is upon getting more rewards than the siblings get from the mother, the child will not particularly notice the reasons the other siblings manage to enjoy each other and to exclude him from their play.

On entrance to school, this child will attempt to use the same talebearing tactic to enhance his powers with the teacher. Again, if the teacher listens and courts further messages from this child, one major consequence will be isolation from his peers. Six-to-nine-year-olds particularly do not like teacher's pets, informers, tattletales. They tend to exclude them from the informal peer groups in which the major focus is learning interpersonal competencies essential for group living. The child who does not get into the peer group feels less human—an isolate set apart from others substantially like himself. To assuage this very lonely feeling he may increase his obsequiousness with authority figures, thereby becoming a more perfect, though exceedingly lonely, "apple polisher." Later on, through high school, sometimes in schools of nursing, and in the employment situation this behavior is used, exploited, and held in contempt by others. The informer perceives these responses to himself but is disoriented by them because he cannot, without help, see what is problematic about his behavior, and he has not to date experienced the acceptable behavior of a person valued by a peer group.

This item of pathological behavior, coupled with other kinds of slowly evolving pathology and interpersonal incompetence, is seen in some patients diagnosed as schizophrenic. In the ward situation the patient will use the only behaviors he knows to negotiate interpersonal relationships. He will work to become a ward pet—and in most hospitals, I regret to say, he will succeed—by bringing messages to the nurse about the misbehaving patients. This behavior is a perpetuation and replication of the initial sibling rivalry. If the nurse responds in the same manner as the mother, school teacher, employer, and so on (that is, if she merely accepts the "messages"), the patient's expertness as a talebearer is further developed. However, if the nurse wants to carry out the aim of nursing care, she will use repeatedly a psychotherapeutic strategy which, in time, will require the patient to stop being an informer. This response by the patient is a first step in developing social competencies which, when achieved, will make him acceptable to a group of peers. Patients in group psychotherapy are quick to spot the patient who informs outside the group and not infrequently they find many ways to evoke such discomfort in him that he will withdraw himself from the group. This situation repeats the isolation from his peers that went on in the school situation.

The psychotherapeutic strategies of the nurse, when a patient brings her tales about another patient, are verbal tactics. The nurse can say, "What are you telling me for?" or, "You have something to say about Joe Smith? Very well. You and I will go and talk with him directly." The aim of the nurse tactic is not merely to receive the patient's message—as did his mother, school teachers, and employer—but rather to introduce into the situation a new stimulus which will force the patient to evolve new behaviors in response to it.

The dependency of psychiatric patients is another area of concern to psychiatric nurses. In dealing with this area, the psychotherapeutic strategy of the nurse is not used in relation to the whole problem of dependency but rather is directed toward the item—the particular variant of dependency that the patient presents at a particular moment. In interview situations, for example, it is not uncommon for the patient to test the nurse to see whether she will dominate, take over, and run his entire life—that is, whether she will replicate the previous known mother domination. The bids are subtle, varied, and innumerable, but the nurse can choose not to reinforce dependence by acting as if the patient were helpless and unable to make these simple decisions for himself. The patient may ask, "May I smoke?" "May I go to the bathroom?" or "May I lie on the bed?" These bids for permission sound innocuous, but if to each one of them the nurse responds yes, she has not only given permission but also has communicated that she is the one who decides these matters. The patient will then make bids for disapproval by remaining silent, by leaving the interview without saying anything, or by coming later than expected. If the patient is dependent on an authority figure for disapproval—which is also quite characteristic of schizophrenic patients—and if the nurse comments about the foregoing bids, the dependency need is reinforced.

There are also more subtle approaches, as when the patient says, "What time is it?" "Did I tell you yesterday what the doctor said?" or, "Did I tell you my brother's name?" In these instances the patient is acting out his dependency by requiring someone else to be his timekeeper or to function as his memory. The more the nurse functions as the memory of the patient, the less he develops his memory, because potential is developed through use—more through use than through models. It is not the nurse's direct response to any one of these items that reinforces the dependence; it is the pattern of the recurring response to most of them which sums up in the mind of the patient that the nurse takes charge and that he need not think or act in his own behalf.

Sometimes there is evidence of improvement in the patient when the nurse responds by encouraging dependency. What actually happens is that the nurse replaces some previously incorporated figure, and in the early phase is seen as a "better" person than that wicked old disapproving autocrat, or mother. Later, when the patient feels fully the fact that he is tied, dependent, incorporated with this new person—and he feels helpless to extricate himself and act with freedom and independence—the situation becomes problematic. It is much more useful not to court such dependence in patients, but rather to aid them to recognize their own abilities to decide whether to smoke or not, to remember what has been said, or to find out the time by referring to the clock.

This is what milieu therapy is all about: recognizing recurring problematic behavior patterns which had their beginnings in early childhood situations in which the child rearing tactics of the mother or of the other significant adults were not equal to the power maneuvers of the child; recognizing the replications of these patterns in subsequent school, peer group, community, and employment situations; and disrupting such replication within the day-to-day nurse–patient interactions in the ward setting. It can be added that such disruptions increase the anxiety of the patient, at least initially. Anybody's anxiety is increased when his familiar behavior is not participated in, when somebody else does not participate in the same pattern integrations that he has been accustomed to. So the dispensing of comfort in the psychiatric setting—that is, decreasing the anxiety of patients—is largely a matter of reinforcing the pathology of the patient and abetting the development of chronicity.

You always have to think of the strategy in relation to the pathology. The more the staff in the unit participate in the replication in an attempt to disrupt the pathology, the more chronicity is developed. I recently had occasion to talk with the physicians and residents in a psychiatric unit in a hospital in the West. They said, "We have a patient who's constantly pitting one person against another. She comes to the doctor and says, 'You know, the nurses don't like you. You know they think you're a fink. You know they think you don't know what you're doing.' Then she goes to the nurse and says, 'You know the doctors around here think you're a slave. They just see you as a handmaiden. They think you're dirt!' What do you do about this patient?" The pitting of one person against another was not a new behavior in this particular patient; she had used it to sow discord between her girlfriend and her friend's mother, between the high school teacher and the principal, between her mother and father. So the more the nurse and doctor played this game with her, the more they were reinforcing that piece of pathological behavior. They said to me, "What do you do? We've tried everything. We've talked to her and we've lectured her. We've had her in group and individual therapy." I said, "Try dyadic therapy. Put your unit in front of her. Take your nurse and doctor together and present a front that she cannot disunite."

Psychiatric nurses are only now beginning to develop psychotherapeutic strategies having to do with recurring replications of problematic behavior such as playing the informer role, pitting one person against another, initiating and perpetuating power struggles with authority figures, and the like. The interaction of a particular patient with all other patients and with all staff members is the unit for study to locate the difficulties for which nursing strategies are needed at the ward level for milieu therapy. Needless to say, this is a complex, difficult task—perhaps an impossible one in ninety-bed wards having one nurse who has limited education in the nursing of psychiatric patients. However, if we are going to talk about milieu therapy with any kind of sense, then we must look at the replications that do go on, and we must develop the strategies to help disrupt them, to help the patients develop the patterns they need for getting along with other people by dealing with the obstacles that get in the way.

A second and equally complicated area under development in psychiatric nursing has to do with recognizing the thought pathology inherent in a patient's language behavior. Benjamin Whorf's (1956) great contribution to psycholinquistics is that first you get the language, which then helps you to assign meaning, and you get the thought secondarily. You know this from your own grade school education where you get spelling lists first; then you looked up the words and got the meaning; then you used the words to assign meaning, that is, to think with the words. There is need to develop psychotherapeutic strategies that will have impact upon the problematic language item of the patient and to study the effect which the persistent use of these strategies has on patients. You need to listen to the language of the patient and then get the strategy to link in with that language item as soon as it is presented.

For example, the patient diagnosed as schizophrenic usually has a marked disorder of the thought process manifested in a wide variety of language behaviors. He uses language to conceal rather than to reveal information, to increase rather than to decrease the work of the hearer, to allude to ideas rather than to state them directly—I might add here, to test the competence of the therapist. For instance, the statement of a patient, "I have two hearts. I have one and you have one," was not literally true. She did not have two hearts, one of which she could assign to the nurse. She was using this language behavior to say something else; she was not talking directly, but rather indirectly.

At first the language of the patient and the tactics that later reveal a thought disorder are probably used consciously—possibly on retaliation to the maneuvers of a dominating mother or a dominating teacher or a sibling or someone. However, as these tactics become habits—habits of language usage which then become habits of thought—the patient loses control over them. Subsequently, the language behavior makes constructive interpersonal relationships in the community more, rather than less, difficult, because language is the main medium of exchange in social relationships.

One variant of language difficulty that reflects thought disorder is the inept use of pronouns. Healthy people use *he, she, it, we,* and *they* as shortcuts in communication. However, if the hearer does not know the person or persons referred to by the pronoun and asks who *he* is or *they* are the healthy person can immediately respond by giving the name of the individual or individuals. Schizophrenic patients, however, lose the referents to the pronouns. Their original use of pronouns was purposive—to hide the information being conveyed—but because the use of *they* has become a habit, the actual identity of the people to whom this pronoun refers has been lost. You might say that they are experts in concealment and get trapped in their own language habits.

Patients diagnosed as paranoid use the pronoun *they* recurringly. If the nurse and the other staff members persist in asking "Who are *they*?" the patient will follow distinct steps in finally achieving the names of the persons so referred to. This is one of the observable regularities in the behavior of paranoids, if you work with them long enough. At first the patient will say something like, "I'm not going to reveal anything," or use some such avoidance response. In the case of a very sick paranoid, a very chronic paranoid, the avoidance response will always come first. But if you do not go away and if you use the psychotherapeutic strategy over time, persistently, by continuing to say "Who are they?" eventually the patient will respond with "the people" or "everyone" or some other global term. This response is the second step. Then, if you persist further in asking "Who are *they*?" the patient will finally respond by saying "the nurses" or "the doctors" or "my family" or "my friends"—in other words, he will name a class of people. Finally, weeks or months later, the patient will produce the names of the people he is referring to when he uses the pronoun *they* in talking with staff members—that is, he will have recovered the names or the referents to the pronoun.

This result involves hard work; it is not achieved overnight. You might have to ask some paranoid patients, "Who are *they*?" two hundred times over two hundred days before you get names. But you will get them. Newly admitted and chronic patients use the pronoun *they* predominantly in their language. What the nurse's response is to this pronoun usage can make a difference in the perpetuation of this faulty language habit. If you are going to help a patient, you have to correct his language, which corrects his thought. You do not work on the thought disorder; you work on the language item with which the patient does his thinking.

The nurse can ignore the pronoun and she can ask about something else; or the nurse can assume that she knows who is being talked about, which is the most common response; or the nurse can ask, repeatedly, "Who are *they*?" "Whom did you have in mind?" "Whom were you referring to?" "Whom do you mean by *they*?" on and on, varying the language of her question, but not the message. The message is the stimulus.

Similarly, a patient may say, "It bothers me," or some equivalent covert use of the pronoun *it* may be employed. If the nurse fails to ask, recurringly, "What is *it*?" "What do you have in mind by *it*?" "When you say *it*, what are you talking about?" the patient will not recognize that he has failed to be direct in giving the necessary information. If the habit of language is of long standing, he will not be aided to recapture such referents to this pronoun, and he will get sicker.

Many patients who have the problem of nonseparation from some incorporated authority figure use the pronoun *we* to speak for the unit (me and the incorporated figure). Here too, if the nurse fails to ask, "Who is represented by 'we' as you are using it?" the patient perpetuates this language behavior. He also perpetuates his tendency to think of himself as an extension of or as incorporated with some other person. What frequently happens in nursing situations is that the nurse assumes that she grasps the referents to the patient's use of *we*. In the community, you do not have to ask everytime somebody says *we*; you can guess to whom the pronoun refers. With a schizophrenic patient you cannot rely on your ability to guess because he has a private way of using all language, including pronouns. The nurse may also unwittingly use the pronoun *we* to refer to herself and some incorporated others—in which case she helps to perpetuate the patient's difficulty as well as her own. There are many greeting cards about nurses that say, "Have we had our enema today?" or "Have we had our bath?" Get rid of this language behavior for other good reasons.

In one of our workshops the clinical director had found a pair of twins for two of the nurses to work with. One of the nurses heard me when I said "Don't use *we*. When the patient says *we*, ask her 'Whom do you mean?' 'Who's *we*?' 'Whom are you referring to?' 'Whom do you have in mind?'" The other nurse never heard me say this. When her patient would say, "Well, we went out and did thus and so," this second nurse would say, "Well, where did we go?" At the end of the week the patient of the nurse who did not use *we* showed a substantial change; she no longer wanted to dress like her sister and she named all of her relatives by name (and she had the biggest extended family I've ever heard of, and *we* meant all of them). The other twin did not show this progress because the nurse was incorporating herself into the we-unit.

Another language pattern of patients which represents a problematic aspect of the thought process is inherent in the use of "you know" or "everybody knows" or some other clause suggestive of mind reading. If the nurse acts as if she does know without asking for details or otherwise receiving adequate information from the patient, she compounds the patient's language difficulty, which in turn reinforces his mindreading tendencies and ideas of reference, and, finally, at the end of the line, delusional thinking.

The psychotherapeutic tactic that in time will have impact on this language usage, and then upon the thought process of the patient, is to ask, "What is it I am supposed to know?" or, "What are you suggesting I ought to know?" or to say, "No, I don't know. Tell me." The idea to convey is that the nurse needs information from the patient and that she can neither assume knowledge with any accuracy nor read the patient's mind. If the nurse persists in this tactic, eventually the patient will say, "You know—no, you don't know; let me tell you." Thus, pathologic and healthy behavior will be exhibited side by side. (A similar juxtaposition will occur with the pronouns: "They—I mean my wife and children.") When this language behavior is observable in the patient the nurse has evidence that the psychotherapeutic verbal tactic is beginning to have impact upon the patient's language and thought. Finally the "you know" piece will drop out. But it will never drop out if no one provides a new stimulus so that some doubt is thrown into the language system.

There are, of course, many other variations of language and thought difficulty, each of which, when studied carefully, can lead to a design of verbal tactics which nurses can use to undermine the presenting pathology of patients.

I have very briefly discussed two areas in which psychotherapeutic strategies are being developed: (1) behavioral interactions within the ward milieu in which patients and staff have encounters which ought not to replicate pathology-producing situations, but which instead should provide stimuli to the development of new behaviors; and (2) verbal tactics used by nurses to force change in the use of language and thought in the patient. It should not be assumed that these tactics encompass all there is to psychiatric nursing—a very complex field which at present is beginning to develop psychotherapeutic strategies that may be quite useful in helping patients to get on with the business of living in the community with a modicum of comfort and success.

REFERENCES

Whorf, B. (1956). *Language, thought, and reality.* New York: Wiley.

CHAPTER 15

Therapeutic Nurse–Patient Interaction

Virtually all of the practice of nursing with psychiatric patients takes place within a nurse–patient relationship. Unlike other specialized areas of nursing, there is very little hands-on practice. There are, of course, medical orders, medications, and treatments with which nurses help or carry out; but only the nurse–patient relationship, within which such prescriptions are carried out, can properly be called nursing. Quality nursing in psychiatric work requires very little technical skill and is very much a matter of competence exercised within the relationship of nurse with patient. The nature of such competence is often greatly misunderstood. Nurses and other professionals often erroneously advise nurses that their work is simply a matter of being pleasant, friendly, obliging, accessible, unconditional, and completely open in revealing oneself to patients. Friend, companion, chum, mother, or parent substitute are all suggested as nurse roles. Competence in nurse–patient relationships is a much more complicated expertise.

In a distinguished lecture, Sills (1983) takes the stance that it is "in the process of relationships with individuals, groups, families, and communities that nursing helps (assists, facilitates, enables) to

Therapeutic nurse–patient interaction. Paper presented at Hamilton Psychiatric Hospital, Hamilton, Ontario, April, 1984. Schlesinger Library, Radcliffe College, Cambridge, MA. No. 84-M107 Hildegard E. Peplau Archives, carton 32, volume 1181. Copyright 1986 by Schlesinger Library. Edited and reprinted by permission.

promote, maintain, and restore health." Sill's position derives from the idea of Hughes (1963), who said: ". . . . professionals profess. They profess to know better than others the nature of certain matters and to know better than their clients what ails them or their affairs" (pp. 655–665). As to the "certain matters," about which nurses claim expertise greater than their clients, Sills asserts that "nurses profess relationships." The definition of nursing according to *Nursing: A Social Policy Statement* (American Nurses' Association, 1980) sharpens the focus proposed by Sills. This definition states that "nursing is the diagnosis and treatment of human responses to actual and potential health problems" (p. 9).

DEFINITION OF PSYCHIATRIC NURSING

Psychiatric nursing is the diagnosis of those human responses of clients, in relation to psychosocial or psychiatric problems, that detract from and prevent healthy living in the community, which nurses treat during the course of nurse–patient relationships. It follows, then, that nurses and clinical specialists who provide nursing services for psychiatric patients are experts, to an extent consonant with their education, in the nature of psychosocial, human responses presented in nurse–patient relationships.

The "certain matters" about which nurses who work in psychiatric services should be expert include those human responses of patients related to mental illness and those that are not. As professionals, nurses would be expected to provide corrective services in relation to the former, and to enhance use of the latter human responses. Expertise, of course, is related to education. Therefore, a clinical specialist in psychiatric nursing who holds a graduate degree would be expected to know more and have more competence than would a staff nurse. Nurses in both groups, however, have a professional responsibility to keep up with new knowledge and to continue to learn more and improve their competence through retrospective analysis of daily experience in their work with patients and by keeping up with new knowledge.

The corrective work that nurses do, occurs within a nurse–patient relationship. Clinical specialists in psychiatric nursing use

specialized modalities, such as individual, group, and family psychotherapy. Staff nurses, however, can also aim for therapeutic
benefit by making the best possible use of every nurse–patient
contact they have within the psychiatric unit. In comparison with
psychotherapeutic modalities, staff nurse contacts with patients
tend to be random, discontinuous, and of variable duration. Nevertheless, these contacts are opportunities for initiating, establishing, and reinforcing a therapeutic direction for patients. In this
chapter some ideas on the nature of mental illness are presented
and discussed in terms of constructive, corrective efforts of nurses
that can occur during nurse–patient relationships.

NATURE OF MENTAL ILLNESS

There are some important ideas about mental illness that have been
learned in the last few decades. Views about mental illness shape
attitudes and treatment of patients who are so diagnosed. The history of psychiatric care clearly shows this relation. When mental
illness was thought to be caused by demons, theological exhortation
was a treatment. More recently, when mothers were blamed for
faulty child rearing, the patient was hospitalized and mothers were
not allowed to visit. When destructive behavior of patients was
thought to be "badness" within the person, such disturbed patients
were put into seclusion rooms so that, somehow, from within themselves, they would learn to shape up. Now it is recognized that panic
is often the energizer of disturbed behavior and that its cause may be
found in whatever sets off the panic.

A great deal is being learned about mental illness from family
therapy, particularly about the dysfunctional communication and
pattern integration that tend to go on in sick-making families.
Individuals do not get sick alone. Mental illness is a product of
relationships that go on in systems such as families, military units,
occupational units, and even psychiatric units. The patient is often
the signaler of a disturbed system; within that system other members may be more disturbed than the patient. The one who is
diagnosed mentally ill may be serving a system function, such as
reuniting members about to leave what had been a close family

system. In other words, the mentally ill use patterns of behavior to maintain family systems, and therefore disturbed patterns tend to be perpetuated.

Withdrawal

For example, withdrawal is a behavior pattern used by many psychiatric patients. This pattern, when first used by the individual, had great utility. It makes sense to pull away or retreat from a fear-evoking situation, or to use this means to escape from a domineering father. Withdrawal, however, does not make sense once situational circumstances have changed. When patients come into a psychiatric hospital where there are helping professionals, the pattern of withdrawal continues to be used when it may be dysfunctional.

Nurses need to gain understanding of complex behavior such as withdrawal. They need to learn when it was initiated, the basis on which it was purposive, and what prevents a patient from giving up the pattern in later situations. One patient put it this way: Her mother preferred her older sister. The patient gave many descriptive examples suggesting such preference and also pointing to the mother's use of "unfavorable comparison" of patient to sister. In order to gain a modicum of approval from her mother the patient used ingratiation as a pattern having many variations. For example, one Saturday, the patient and her mother spent the whole day cleaning the house. In late afternoon the sister came home from a football game and showered confetti all through the house. The patient said, "Look what you are doing—getting confetti all over. We just cleaned the house." The mother immediately said to the patient, "That is a despicable thing to say to your sister." The patient ran to her room; she used a pattern of withdrawal.

There are several points in this vignette. The withdrawal was purposive. So was the ingratiation pattern but it did not work to reduce the patient's anxiety. The patient's self-views were affected by the mother's patterns of behavior: "unfavorable comparison" and "sibling preference." The mother's behavior failed to confirm or enhance the patient's feelings of self-worth or introduce useful views of self into the patient's self-system. The clincher, the exit signal that set off the withdrawal pattern, however, was the mother's distorted communication. The patient had merely cited facts; the mother transformed what the patient said into further onslaught of the patient's self-system.

This problematic event does not end there. For full understanding, it is necessary to pursue what went on during the withdrawal. In this instance, when the patient got to her room, feeling totally helpless, she cried. What did she think about? One thing is certain, rumination goes on during withdrawal. Moreover, the interaction between patient and mother-as-illusory-figure went on. The patient asked herself, "What did I say?" Then she recalled her comment to her sister. Then she thought, "But if I said that, my mother wouldn't have called me despicable." After further rumination along these lines, by autistic invention, and in a predictable self-derogatory direction already laid down in interactions with her mother, the patient concluded, "But I must have said something else, something awful. My mother is a good person. She wouldn't have said that unless. . . ." It is during the withdrawal that the patient initiates a self-fulfilling prophecy, saying, "I can't remember. I'm losing my mind." She is indeed on the way toward mental illness. It is no accident that, shortly thereafter, as this outpatient examined many such events, she became less withdrawn and more assertive of her own position. At that point her mother committed her to a mental hospital. It is also not surprising that the admitting physician sided with the mother. His theoretical framework was that mental illness is a one-sided affair, and he took the mother's words for facts without talking with the previous therapist or the patient. Nor was the mother to blame. She was acting on her own self-system and needs, whatever they were.

In this vignette, some facets of interaction within family and hospital systems have been used to show complexity of pathology, to illustrate points about mental illness given earlier, and to prepare for a discussion of therapeutic nurse–patient relationships. The event presented already suggests that the way to mental health for patients is to talk about their experiences, to understand what went on and their part in it, and to strengthen their intellectual and interpersonal competencies in that process. The data presented took about thirty minutes of nurse–patient discussion and occurred in the seventh session, previous contacts being less productive warm-up.

THERAPEUTIC NURSE–PATIENT RELATIONSHIPS

Nurses who work in psychiatric units have endless opportunities to initiate relationships with patients, use them to help move the patient in a direction favoring productive social living outside of the hospital, and incidentally to learn a great deal about psychotherapy first hand. Nurses will find such opportunities every time a patient approaches them, in every ward "incident," and also by seeking out the more passive patients. Nurses say, "But we don't have time for that." In that case, one should review current uses of time and make time for patients. Moreover, no one can say how long it takes to set a new direction in motion for patients.

During nurse–patient relationships, what is being suggested here is an investigative approach. Such an approach has the following major characteristics: It is primarily *verbal*. The general principle is that anything patients act out with nurses, will most probably not be talked about, and that which is not discussed cannot be understood. Understanding, for both patient and nurse, of troublesome events or behavior patterns of a patient, flows from analysis of data. That data is produced verbally, the patient talking, describing, and the nurse listening, thinking about what is heard and providing prompters for the patient to do his or her work.

The language and thought of the nurse are crucial to any investigative effort with patients, however brief. It is well to keep in mind that social conversation is not what is being suggested. Patients do not come to hospitals to find friends among staff. Patients can socialize with other patients. Staff are employed to help patients see the need for and to do the work required for their recovery. The language of the nurse conveys this message. The nurse might respond, for example, to a patient's bid for social data about the nurse by saying, "Use this time to talk about you" (or some variant of that message). Patients do not need and most often cannot wisely use personal data about the nurse. Many patients use bids for social data about the nurse so as not to take a look at themselves; nurse participation in such bids tends to reinforce such patterns of concealment.

Some years ago, in a workshop, nurses were seeking advice on what to say to alcoholic patients. When asked to tell what the nurses had said previously, they recalled telling patients about bad effects of alcohol on themselves, parents, and friends. Now patients were saying to the nurses, "How can you help us when you couldn't help your own father?" What does the patient need the personal information for, and in the short- and long-run how might he or she use it?

The general idea in an investigative approach is that anything that has happened or is happening now, in the experience of the patient, can be talked about, looked at, made sense of, and put into a useful perspective. This includes what goes on in a nurse–patient relationship but not that which occurs in the life of the nurse outside of the hospital, or in nurse–staff relationships. In other words, the focus of the investigative effort is largely one way, on the experience of the patient.

This approach is often difficult at the outset for nurses (and for other professionals too). The tendency is to talk with patients in pretty much the same way as one talks with family and friends. The manner and sometimes much of the language has become automatic, so it is necessary to shift gears, to stop and listen to one's own word usage and to think about its usefulness in a nurse–patient relationship intended to be therapeutic. To be therapeutic means to have the intent that the effects for the patient will, at least in the long run, be beneficial.

Consider this instance. A nurse talking to her friend about the nurse's family says, "We would like it if you came to dinner." The friend assumes that by *we* the nurse means her husband and children and that by *you* she is referring to her friend and husband. At work, a psychiatric patient comes to the nurse and says, "We would like permission to go shopping." The nurse responds by saying, "We will let you know." Who are they talking about? If this patient has an identity problem (and most psychiatric patients do) and is so incorporated with his mother that he is unsure where his self begins and his mother's ends, the nurse has helped to perpetuate that problematic pattern of incorporation. She has done so by not asking, "Who wants permission, you and who else?" and by her use of the "nursery" *we*. To some nurses this sounds like hair-splitting. The fact is that many patients who use *we*, when asked for the referents, cannot specify them—and they do not use the personal pronoun *I* in talking about themselves. However, as the nurse keeps asking, each time a particular patient uses *we* in the nurse's presence, the patient will change. He begins to think. Soon the patient will say "We—I mean Joe and me," and eventually he will use *I* and begin to speak for himself. Separate identity has been set in motion.

There are many such problems of patients that are implied in language usage that if used in social situations might not have the same connotation of difficulty. Examples are: the use of *you* or *one* in speaking about oneself; the clichés *you see* or *you know*, which in mental patients imply mind reading; or the paranoid *they* when the referents are lost. In regaining adequate use of the pronoun *they*, patients work their way back through this sequence: *They* refers to "the people"; *they* refers to a class of people (e.g., the bankers); and finally, *they* refers to named real people. Pronouns are used to designate people and objects, and in healthy people these referents will be named directly or can be if asked about. As for *you know*, nurses ought to ask, "What is it I'm supposed to know," or some variation on this inquiring message. Otherwise there is tacit agreement that both know something without asking or telling.

Psychiatric patients have difficulty focusing their attention. The jargon of psychiatry labels this "scattered thinking." So nurses who intend to be therapeutic with patients who have this problem can, during a nurse–patient relationship, either test the patient for this ability and/or assist the patient with this attention problem. The way to do that is to structure what the nurse says to the patient in such a way that the ability to attend is brought into play and exercised. This is best done by attempting, not once but in many successive contacts, to get the patient to describe one experience as a whole, in all of its dimensions. Patients have difficulty not only in describing, but in recalling details of events. The effort to do so, after long disuse of this ability, is likely to give rise to anxiety and to make use of such automatic relief-giving patterns as changing the subject, asking about the nurse, withdrawal, and the like. So the greater effort in this endeavor occurs on the part of the nurse. Attention is focused when one event is the content of thought, when thinking about that one experience is sustained over a long period of time, long enough to recall, describe, review details, and formulate the general meaning of that one event. As can be seen, several abilities are tapped.

The language of the nurse provides the prompters to the work the patient needs to do for her or his own therapeutic benefit. For instance, suppose a patient says to a nurse, "I had a rotten time in gym this morning." The nurse can evasively close off inquiry by saying, "That's too bad; better luck tomorrow." In this nurse–patient contact a few vague generalizations have been exchanged, nothing has been learned, and nothing useful has happened for the patient. Instead, suppose the nurse said, "I have fifteen minutes. There are two chairs over there; come talk about that experience." After sitting down, if the patient does not begin, the nurse could say: "What happened?" In encouraging focus and description of this one event the nurse would want to know: who was there; what went on; who said or did what; where in the gym; what the patient felt, and so forth. Needless to say, the nurse uses input stimuli to keep the focus. For example, if the patient changes the subject the nurse might ask "What does that have to do with the gym experience?" Only as the nurse listens to the patient and hears a full description can she first determine, privately, whether the phrase "rotten time" is a suitable generalization about this experience. Then of course, the nurse can ask: "What did you see that was rotten in the gym," and pursue that, requiring the patient to check accuracy of the generalization about the gym experience.

Patients tend to use vague generalizations rather than description, and often those generalizations do not fit the actual data. This occurs when there is inadequate data, frequently due to anxiety that has prevented the patient from noticing, taking in, and grasping most of what went on in the situation. Overgeneralizing is also an automatic pattern of behavior, like withdrawal, that in some earlier situation had great utility as a way out of a difficult spot. Overgeneralization as a pattern of language and thought behavior of patients, as with all other pathology, gets worse and spreads if left to its own path. However, in therapeutic nurse–patient relationships, generalizations of the patient can be checked out against described experience. Corrective efforts can be made. For purposes of discussion, behavior can be considered to include thoughts, actions, feelings, and patterns. In an investigative approach the nurse needs to recognize distinctions among these categories. Thoughts are ideas that can be expressed, formulated, and stated; actions can be shown, demonstrated, and described; feelings can be felt and named. Patients have difficulties related to these different aspects of behavior. A patient who is thinking about doing something might say, "I felt like slapping him." To help clarify, the nurse might say, "Name the feeling," for what the patient classifies as feeling is rather an intended action. The nurse's statement, as in previous instances, is a stimulus that *if heard, retained,* and *acted upon directly* serves to force the patient to think, to use words with accuracy as to their commonly accepted meanings, and to begin the process of ordering his or her disturbed method of communicating with other people. When improved communication is used by the patient, other people are more likely to listen, understand, take the patient seriously, and maybe even enjoy social conversation with the patient. All of these improvements also redound to the patient's views of himself and his feelings of self-worth.

Nurses can neither demand nor otherwise control the responses patients will make to nurse behavior during a relationship. The patient's responses are governed by the patient's perceptions of nurse behavior, and those perceptions are governed by the patient's needs, self-views, and anxiety, and are often automatic. Automatic, repetitive responses that occur without thought are characteristic of patients. The verbal stimuli of the nurse, as suggested in this paper, are unique, unfamiliar, and unlike what most others might say to patients. At first, these stimuli tend to evoke anxiety because they are unexpected, so the likelihood of evoking automatic responses of patients is considerable. However, when the nurse continues to use an investigative approach in his or her language, in many situations it begins to sound familiar; the patient's anxiety response becomes less likely; the nurse's words are heard, taken in, and subsequently acted on by the patient. Investigative language eventually forces thought in the patient. What is suggested here is not a repetitive use of a few inquiring phrases. The principle is to sustain the message (talk) but to vary the language (talk, tell, describe, say some more about the event, and so forth). The only control the nurse has, in the verbal interplay of nurse with patient, is over the nurse's language—the words used as inputs into the disordered communication system of the patient so as to evoke improvements for the patient's thought and language designation of experience. The nurse's words should be simple, clear, and the fewest possible to convey a direct and investigative message. Obviously, language facility, accuracy in word usage, rich variation with accurate use of synonyms, and selection of phrases appropriate to the nurse–patient verbal interplay in process are all aspects of competence of the nurse.

A modicum of detachment is required in professional work. Excluding discussion of personal needs and social life of the nurse has already been suggested. Without the exercise of self-discipline and appreciation of the significance of such detachment in the nature of psychiatric work, detachment becomes difficult if not impossible. But one of the traps of psychiatric work is unwitting participation in and therefore perpetuation of dysfunctional patterns of patient behavior, the route to chronicity for patients. Yet professional detachment is difficult, especially for young, newly graduated nurses, and for any nurse who does not examine his or her own part in nurse–patient relationships. Such examination includes reflecting on what might be the long-term effect for the patient of what the nurse said and did, repeatedly, in particular nurse–patient contacts.

Even so, divorcing the nurse's approach to patients from the nurse as a person is not easily accomplished and is never done totally. The best effort is to get major interferences out of the way. Use of gestures, winking, forbiddance, or seduction interferes. If the nurse is impatient, it is more difficult for a patient to think. If the nurse is oververbal, a great talker but a poor listener, the patient is likely to be put into a child role of listener. If the nurse is fearful of getting hurt, for instance, this too is communicated as hesitancy, tentativeness, and apprehension to patients. Anxiety of nurses is communicated empathically to patients, and often calls out automatic relief behaviors from both nurse and patient. Such interferences preclude therapeutic direction as an outcome in nurse–patient relationships.

Obviously, this is not a discussion about magic use of words by nurses. However, corrective effort directed by nurses at the language patients use to express and convey experience does benefit patients, but it is a long, slow process. Language influences thought; thought influences actions and feelings; all of these have impact on relationships with people. Depending upon the tenacity of patient's pathology, the payoff time for the nurse's effort may be short or long. The main factor is the willingness to sustain the effort, on the part of nurses and other professionals, despite setbacks and perhaps increasing anxiety as well as greater resistance to change shown by the patient. It is very rare to see a psychiatric patient who through heroic personal effort can get himself out of his own traps without the knowledge and help of others.

Among the many factors that get in the way of therapeutic nurse–patient relationships are the expectations of nurses. One such expectation is that because a nurse spent a whole hour with a patient, she or he hopes and expects that a certain change would occur—but then it does not. In one workshop a nurse spent five minutes with a withdrawn patient, pummeling him with questions, expecting the patient to talk, and when he did not, the nurse walked away. The pattern became that of mutual withdrawal. In working with psychiatric patients it is useful to hold the fewest possible expectations of them, if any, thinking instead, "I wonder what will come up in the next contact." Nurses should focus their energies on gaining theory and in polishing their investigative competence. Theory is important because it provides explanatory tools that sharpen the nurse's observations and provide understanding of human responses. Concepts such as anxiety, conflict, the self-system; knowledge about processes such as hallucinations; patterns of behavior and their many variants, such as withdrawal, ingratiation, incorporation, dependence, and the like provide explanations for patient behavior. (See Chapters 14, 16, 21, and 23, this volume.)

Investigative competencies are only touched upon in this chapter. The techniques of psychiatric nurses for helping patients to learn about and develop themselves to gain competencies for social living are largely interviewing techniques. Through such techniques patients are helped to produce their experiential data, to review it, to gain new perspectives about themselves, and to practice competencies for problem solving. There are facets not touched in this discussion: the matter of timing, the intrusive effects of anxiety and self-views of patient and nurse, the possible variations on verbal messages, the nurse inputs to get patients to work, and so on.

There is so much to know. The best way to learn is through supervised clinical practice, the supervisory review of clinical data being provided on a regular basis by a qualified psychiatric nurse. In work situations, where that may not be possible, at the very least regular meetings of staff nurses to learn from each other, by data and literature review, is a next-best possibility. It is a useful way to continue to learn more about and from nurse–patient relationships. As was indicated at the outset, professionals profess, and if nurses profess that they have expertise in human responses and in nurse–patient relationships, then keeping that expertise finely tuned is our responsibility.

One final note: There are signs that psychiatry is inching closer to a biomedical approach. The work of psychiatrists incorporates ongoing brain research, pharmaceutical research, and utilizes sophisticated equipment for forms of laboratory measurement, and study of within-body phenomena of psychiatric patients. It would therefore seem more urgent that nurses get on with full development of their area of interest—human responses of psychiatric patients.

REFERENCES

American Nurses' Association. (1980). *Nursing: A social policy statement.* Kansas City, MO: Author.

Hughes, E. C. (1963). Professions. *Daedalus, 92,* 655–665.

Sills, G. M. (1983). *The profession of relationships.* Unpublished paper, The Dean's Distinguished Lecture Series. School of Nursing, University of Pennsylvania, Philadelphia, PA.

CHAPTER 16

Investigative Counseling

Investigative counseling is an interviewing process that helps a person to investigate life experiences. Counseling is a serious, sometimes very difficult work for both counselor and patient. It is worth doing, for what is at stake is the further growth and development of a person. The work occurs in a climate provided at first only by the counselor; it consists of respecting and valuing patients simply because they are human persons—and for no other reason. The patient does not have to obey or please the counselor in order to merit respect.

Investigative counseling is the art and science of stimulating patients to change themselves. That change basically involves using energy ordinarily made available through experience involving anxiety, conflict, guilt, shame, and other emotions. Instead of merely relieving, discharging, or masking such energy, the counselor stimulates the patient to use it for purposes of learning something worth knowing by examining experiences. The changes that result are primarily intellectual and interpersonal competencies: instrumental behaviors that will continue to be invaluable in subsequent experiences, whether those experiences are anxiety producing or not. What the counselor uses, therefore, as outcome measures, is knowledge of such competencies: what they are, how they develop, how

Adapted from Lectures 14, 15, and 16, presented at the University of Leuven, Belgium, 1975. Schlesinger Library, Radcliffe College, Cambridge, MA. No. 87-M107 Hildegard E. Peplau Archives, carton 29, volume 1088. Copyright 1986 by Schlesinger Library. Adapted and edited by permission.

one uses them, and the interrelations between them. The outcome may include a change in health status, or even new ideological perspectives, but the content of these changes flows from the patient's use of the instrumental competencies that have been developed as the aim of the counseling sessions.

The authority of the counselor resides in knowledge about human processes and competence in developing them, not in position or role. Human processes are the same for all people; what is different is the degree of their development into usable competencies, the sociocultural experience out of which they were initially developed, and therefore the content of experience related to their use.

Counseling is a specialized form of educative experience in which the role of counselor is primarily that of change agent; the role is not pseudo-parental, pseudo-lecturer, pseudo-administrator, or pseudo-social. Unless the counselor is clear on the significantly different requirements and considerations of these various roles he or she will be unable to sustain a change-agent stance. In this stance, the counselor merely provides and sustains instrumental inputs to which the patient eventually responds by self-change. The counselor does not make change happen; he or she merely stimulates it.

The outcomes of counseling have a lot to do with the attitudes and beliefs of the counselor about how and under what conditions persons change themselves in favorable directions. The investigative approach is an open, noncoercive, nonadministrative approach. The counselor assumes that the patient is competent, acts accordingly, and provides inputs as if the patient had the competence to respond fully; and in time patients do meet these expectations.

In the counseling–patient relationship, the patient is an autonomous and free person. Nurses provide counseling to patients because it is a part of their work, because as nurses, they have an intense and inquiring interest in all problems of people related to health, and because they earn their livings this way. The patient does not have to be grateful, feel obligated, present tokens or gifts to the nurse, or otherwise repay the nurse.

All professional services expose the practitioner to the imperfections of humans, the lacks, gaps, and deficits in development, and the terrible interpersonal interactions that people have and perpetuate in personal relationships. That is the content of much of the work that professionals do—and more especially in counseling work. It is therefore necessary to develop a professional detachment, one that is unnecessary in social life; otherwise the counselor would become totally ineffective through continuing shock and feel burdened or overwhelmed by the facts of the lives of patients. A professional who sees only good and bad, black and white, perfection and imperfection, rather than degrees of gray in human behavior, ought not to engage in counseling activities. The burden of bad, black, and imperfection would be too much to bear. People become what they are as a consequence of life experience, and how they perceived it from their observational standpoint; counseling is a retrospective review of those experiences and perspectives, with newly evolving competencies with which to accomplish the review. It is a long, slow, up-and-down process and not a flip-flop from bad to good, black to white. A counselor therefore needs patience along with knowledge of the universal human processes and how they were shaped in experiences with people.

ASSUMPTIONS

Several assumptions apply in all forms of investigative counseling.

1. The form, quality, and content of the interview is guided by the interaction and purpose.
2. All behavior is purposeful, meaningful, and can be understood; that is, behavior has uses and significance that can be identified.
3. All behavior is relative—to a situation, a context, and/or a period in time.
4. Persons behave in the only ways known to them; that is, all habitual patterns of behavior have an experiential history.
5. Only a person can change his or her own behavior. Others provide potential stimuli, support, and a shared basis for understanding present behavior. New behavior comprises a change.
6. New behavior is generally awkward and inept until it becomes familiar, a part of oneself.

7. Anything that goes on can be talked about, described, analyzed, and understood in a professional–client relationship.

METHOD OF WORK

In counseling a neutral stance is taken. The counselor does not show approval, disapproval, or indifference verbally, in actions, or in gestures. These shaping patterns have already been amply used in social situations. The counselor allows the general direction to come from the patient, using such initiatives to pursue a focus and to secure description of events thus introduced by the patient. The counselor uses a one-way focus on the needs of the patient. The needs of the counselor are met outside the counseling situation.

The major function of the counselor is intense, active listening, hearing and grasping what the patient is describing and occasionally providing an input stimulus appropriate to what is going on. The counselor must be alert and focus intensely on the patient as a person working to review and understand personal experiences.

CHANGE AGENT

The counselor is first of all a model of a person who has and uses the competencies to be developed or refined by the patient. The counselor is also a model of a separate and autonomous person and the language used reflects that. The counselor takes responsibility for acting as a professional and therefore controls personal participation in the pattern integrations of counselor and patient that evolve; roles of parent are avoided because this converts the pattern integration into parent–child interaction.

The counselor privately applies theory or draws inferences to understand the nature of what is going on as a basis on which to determine interventions. Interventions are input stimuli that are consciously determined, from moment to moment, as the session is in process, and they become the guides to further work by the patient. Such inputs are in effect appraisals that are eventually internalized by the self-system. Recognizing the complexity of the self-system, the counselor does not expect instant use of inputs, but rather is patient and repeats them, varying the language but not the message, until internalization and action occur as inferred from the patient's response.

The counselor recognizes that the counseling process is a complex one, that progression through it is not linear, and that there are shifts from early to later aspects of the process (and the reverse). Expectations of progress, which the counselor does privately, are therefore less reliable than are session assessments and long-range comparisons.

In counseling, assessment and diagnosis are ongoing. Reliable diagnoses are recurring themes, problems, and patterns as seen in many variations across many sessions. Assessment is also an ongoing activity of the counselor, particularly assessment of developing competence. Equally important is the counselor's assessment of her or his own behavior in all sessions.

BASIS FOR CHANGE IN THE PATIENT

There are several easily recognized bases for change in investigative counseling.

The counselor as model provides an opportunity for the patient to experience a person who cares knowingly, which is different from caring emotionally. The modeling behaviors are emulated by a process of identification.

The patient develops latent capacities into competencies, as new understandings derive from the review of experience and are then used in gradually enlarging ways in more situations.

The counselor elicits trust and security through the continuity of time, place, purpose, method, and tested confidentiality. The patient comes to expect these trust elements to continue and thus become a basis for more intense work.

The patient gradually examines and changes the contents of her or his self-system by checking self-views against reality.

With increasing autonomy, the patient is freed from need for approval, disapproval, and/or indifference, and edits out supervisory personifications, taking personal responsibility for thoughts, actions, and feelings.

PURPOSE

The purpose of investigative counseling is to provide a place, time, and an opportunity for the patient to discuss and seek understanding of some facet of problematic experience. This is at first the counselor's purpose. It is told to the patient. As the patient hears, incorporates, and acts on this input, it becomes part of the self-system; when this occurs will vary with different patients and depends upon self-worth and anxiety of the patient, particularly with patients who have no expectation that anyone will listen to accounts of their situation as they see it. Nevertheless, as the sessions proceed, the patient will assess the counselor's behavior for deviations from the stated purpose, such as when the counselor does most of the talking or discusses personal experiences that are similar.

TIME

Counseling sessions are usually fifty minutes to one hour, one to three times per week. They begin and end at a designated time. Thus they are generally arranged in advance, scheduled at the mutual convenience of the patient and counselor, and, in nursing, scheduled into the nursing care plan. Brief situational counseling occurs usually in one session at the point when a patient's problem emerges. But even in these sessions it is useful to provide a time boundary. For example, the counselor might say: "You seem troubled. I will stay for one hour. Talk about what's happening."

In talking with patients it is useful to provide clues to time termination of contacts. "I have five more minutes before leaving." Such pre-warnings of the upcoming end of a session are also useful in scheduled counseling sessions. They permit the patient opportunity for "orderly closure" of an interpersonal transaction.

PLACE

Counseling sessions are usually held in the same place. This might be the nurse's office, the patient's bedroom, a quiet corner of a unit, or an unused room. The place should provide quiet so that counselor and patient can hear each other's communications. The place should provide privacy so that the patient's behavior (crying, for example) and communications will be safeguarded from the ears of other people. The place should be one that is free from interruptions and distractions, as from a phone, television, radio, and the demands of other patients; the place therefore should be one in which the designated time is for the full use of the patient, the counselor being wholly and unconditionally available and not subject to the demands of other business during that time. In brief counseling, the place is wherever the problem is presented unless it does not ensure privacy, in which case the nurse-counselor selects and suggests a suitable place.

ORIENTING THE PATIENT

In a first counseling session the nurse-counselor orients the patient to structure, purpose, and procedure. If the counseling sessions are nurse-initiated, the patient may question the selection. This is particularly likely among psychiatric patients who no longer expect such human concern for them and who can see that there are many other patients in approximately the same predicament. There is no really adequate explanation except one that includes such points as: (1) The patient seems to be troubled about something; (2) the nurse has the time and competence to help the patient to look at whatever seems problematic; and (3) the nurse is making the time available for the patient's use. It is a risky mistake to suggest selection criteria such as "I liked you best," "I'm interested in you," "You seem like a nice person," or some such statements suggestive of favorable or unfavorable comparisons with other patients.

Orienting the patient simply means providing information so that the patient will be familiar with what is about to happen. Such information should be given simply, clearly, forthrightly, and

directly, using simple declarative sentences. Assume that the patient can and will follow what is said, and will hear and use it, until
there are observations to the contrary. The following sequence of
orienting information (Table 16.1) has been found easiest for patients to follow when used in investigative counseling.

Once the orienting information has been given, the nurse uses an
opening remark to make it easier for the patient to begin: "This is
your time, begin anywhere, tell about your being sick" (or some
variation of that). If the patient asks for the orienting information to
be repeated (e.g., "When did you say you were coming again?" or
"What's the point of all this?"), repeat the information regarding
time or purpose.

Once an opening remark by the nurse is made the nurse waits—
for however long it takes—for the patient to start talking. If the
delay is overlong, ask something like "What are you thinking?" or
say, "I'm ready; begin anywhere"—then wait!

The first part of the interview is crucial in setting the pattern for
nurse–patient interaction. The desirable pattern is one in which the
patient does most of the talking, and the nurse listens and occasionally addresses a question about whatever the patient has just said.

During the first part of the interview patients may, and usually
do, try to change the relationship from professional to social by
asking for biographical information about the counselor. The
general principles are: (1) Confirm the self-evident. If you are
married, and wearing a wedding ring, and the patient asks, "Are
you married?" the nurse responds only with a yes. Or, if the
patient asks, "Did you say you were a nurse?" again the answer is
merely yes. (2) Avoid giving biographical data. The patient does
not need this information except to shift the nurse out of a counselor role and into a friend role. If the patient says, "Where do you
live?" the nurse can say, "Use this time to talk about you." If the
patient asks, "How old are you?" the nurse can respond, "This is
your time to talk about your life." Or if the patient asks, "Do you
have children?" the nurse could say "I'd be interested in hearing
about you and your children." To nurses who are accustomed to
other approaches, these are sometimes called "rude" techniques,
which is a misclassification; they are simple, direct, honest, and
they convey the message "The time is yours to talk about you and

TABLE 16.1 Orienting Information with Intervention and Rationale

Orienting	Intervention	Rationale
Name	I am Ms. ____, I'm a nurse. I've been given your name by the head nurse. It's Mr. ____, is that correct?	Treat patient formally, as a stranger. Do not use first names. Patient needs to know to whom (name and status) he or she is talking.
Purpose To discuss and seek understanding of problematic experience.	When I talked with you this morning, it occurred to me that you were troubled about having surgery. So I've made time available for you to talk about your reactions to the upcoming surgery.	The patient needs a very general view of the uses of information from counseling sessions.
Time Frequency Duration Termination date	I have arranged four sessions—two this week and two next week, Tuesday and Thursday, 1 to 2 P.M. Is that hour convenient for you? The last session would be next Thursday.	The patient needs time boundaries so as to organize the amount of work he or she will do in terms of time available.
Place Same for all sessions Quiet Private	This room would be a suitable place for the sessions. Or: I've arranged for a room down the hall that is more private—come with me.	The patient needs to know where the work will occur. The place should be one that affords quiet, privacy, and appropriate seating arrangements for both patient and nurse.
Confidentiality Tell the patient who else will have access to the interview data. Tell the patient how identifying data will be safeguarded.	I will be discussing what you say with your doctor. Or: I will not be discussing your data with anyone, but I will put a summary in your chart which I will go over with you first.	Before the patient talks about personal experiences he or she needs to know who else might see the data from the interview.

(*continued*)

TABLE 16.1 Orienting Information with Intervention and Rationale
(Continued)

Orienting	Intervention	Rationale
Note taking Hand written or tape recorded. Content consists of what nurse and patient say. Purpose is to study later.	I'll be taking notes (or using a tape recorder). I won't record name or address. Later on I'll study the notes carefully to learn as much as I can what patients like you experience when sick.	The patient has the right to know what the nurse will be recording. The patient may read the notes if he or she wishes.
Opening comment	Begin anywhere. I'll listen. Tell about being sick.	This further orients the patient to the session; the patient talks, the nurse listens.

your experience." The message suggests one-way, unconditional interest in the patient.

The nurse does not have to use obsequiousness, subterfuge, seduction, ingratiation, or pseudo-friend roles in order to extract information surreptitiously from patients about their lives. All professional relationships that focus on the tasks at hand tend to be direct, one way, and focused on the needs and concerns of the patient exclusively. Somewhere on the margin of awareness, patients know this; asking for biographical data about the nurse is a way of testing to see whether the nurse knows it too. Biographical data about the nurses changes the data a patient will give, which will be screened, compared, or matched with that of the nurse, in order to save face, to compete, to present self in a favorable light, and other such distortions.

The prevailing nurse tendency to give biographical data may be one basis on which a patient similarly expects the nurse-counselor to behave in the same manner. Therefore, it may be necessary to sustain many such attempts until the patient realizes that you mean what you said: It is the patient's time to talk about himself and his experiences. It is at that point of realization that patients will begin trust and continuity.

The consequence for the patient when the nurse does what she says she will do is a feeling of trust and safety. The trust results from experiencing adherence to specified time boundaries and stated purpose, and a one-way focus of interest and concern for the patient. Trust is generated from experiences in which people promise and then do what was promised; consequently they can be counted on to translate words into deeds.

SOME GUIDELINES

1. Patients do not die from interviews. They have many ways to manage any possible stress effects from the interview, and they are very likely to use these relief behaviors. What is likely to happen is some beneficial effect just from your sustained interest in the patient.

2. Make your mistakes openly; examine and fix them. After your first interview, review your notes, critique your verbal content, and fix it in the next interview. Use your mistakes to learn.

3. On the way to your interviews, each of them, check your expectations. That will keep your anxiety down. Do not expect anything. Go in to the interview saying, "I wonder what will happen; whatever it is I'll do the best I know how," not, "I expect ____."

4. It is likely that you will feel awkward and uncomfortable; that is always possible in a first experience before the method becomes familiar. Remember the first bath, hypodermic, or enema you gave! A first interview has the same newness and unfamiliarity about it. You will survive. The second interview will be somewhat easier.

5. Take some notice of the responses evoked in you by the patients in the first interview. Write these down as soon as possible after and outside the interview situation. These are clues to intentions and general interpersonal patterns of the patient, and they will be more evident in the first interview than much later on.

Table 16.2 provides information to assist you to recognize and control problematic counselor behavior.

TABLE 16.2 Problematic Counselor Behaviors and Reasons To Control Them

Behaviors	Why control them
1. Avoid smiling, nodding and other gestures.	May be misinterpreted as "laughing" at the patient or giving approval.
2. Avoid cliches: "That's fine" "that's nice."	Be a model for using clear language. Be flexible rather than use stereotyped phrases. Avoid non-cummunicative, mutual, cliched exchanges.
3. Do not take tokens or gifts.	They obligate, integrate, and change the relationship from professional to social. Say, "You keep it; give it to a friend. I do this because it's my work—if you found it useful, I'm glad."
4. Avoid defining the patient.	For example, do not say, "Did you feel guilty?" Ask, "What did you feel?" or do not say, "I'd say you were a good father," use "What was your view of yourself in that situation?" Let the patient define self—you'll know the patient's self-views that way.
5. Do not give opinion, advice, theory, or interpretation.	Use an investigative approach "What was your opinion?" "What advice did you get?" "From whom?" The patient should generate his or her own advice.
6. Don't fill in silences; sit them out, wait, maintain your attention and eye-to-eye contact with the patient.	Silences may be thoughtful; if so, you interrupt thought when you break the silence. They may also be angry or hostile, in which case you can say, "What's going on now?" Represent yourself as a person who can wait.
7. Don't predict, e.g., "You'll feel better."	You may be wrong.
8. Don't use approval, disapproval, or indifference.	These call out conforming behavior. Use an investigative approach instead.

Table 16.3 presents the major work of the patient and the counselor in each phase of the counseling process.

TABLE 16.3 Major Work Using a Counseling Process

Phases and aspects of counseling process	Major work of the patient	Major work of the counselor
I. Orientation: Establishes initial pattern and expectations of work	Does most of the talking	Arrange for sessions Meet own needs Provide orienting information Listens, hears, thinks about Gets to know the person Survives testing regarding: Biographical data Replicating Parataxic others Client evoking Annoyances Domination Orienting Promises
	Checks out counselor's premises, and competence, as well, as the seriousness of the work Names anxiety Incorporates and uses counselor input stimuli Sustains focus Describes one event more or less fully Gives evidence of beginning trust and security with counselor Begins to experience tenderness	Provides and sustains input stimuli to encourage observation, description, and self-expression Beginning diagnosis (private, not given to client) Apply theory Draw inferences Identify beginning themes and patterns Assess client competence

(*continued*)

TABLE 16.3 **Major Work Using a Counseling Process** *(Continued)*

Phases and aspects of counseling process	Major work of the patient	Major work of the counselor
II. *Working relationships:* Describes single events Describes several events of like kind Beginning analysis Seeing relations Contrast and comparison Generalizes patterns Formulation Meanings and significance Explanations Validation Testing and feedback of formulations	Enlarges description and continuities Ability to focus attention and describe one event Sustains focus on self and self–other interactions Introduces and connects data from previous session Notices and names anxiety Experiences tenderness Develops trust and security with counselor	Continues to apply theory Draw inferences Revise diagnoses Continue to identify patterns and theories Facilitate patient formulation of meaning of experiences Validate formulations
III. *Termination:* Client summary of major learning products	Uses new learning to achieve satisfaction and security in interpersonal relations	Counselor validation Revision Prescription for action

SUMMARY

Getting to know patients as human persons, unique in their experience but having universal experiences too, in common with all humans, is an attitude regarding nursing. Some nurses assume they know the patient based on exceedingly limited data, often as a stereotype of patients in some age group, social class, or diagnostic group. But they really do not. Getting to know a patient as a human person means talking with that person, in an investigative, purposive way, listening carefully, all the while being intellectually active and interested to know more. In these one-way talking sessions, both nurse and patient grow, change, and become more human persons as a consequence.

APPENDIX A:

Summary of Interview Techniques

To open the interview

This is the time to talk about *your* experience.
This is your time, begin anywhere.
Start anywhere, I'm ready.
What problem do you plan to work on today?
What's on your agenda for *this* hour of talking?
It's time to work on understanding your life; begin anywhere.

To start the stalled interview

Talk about what led up to your coming here.
Talk about the tough times in your life.
Talk about one difficult situation you were in.

To encourage observation and description

Of structure of events

Who was there?
Who else was there?

Adapted from University of Leuven Lecture 15, carton 29, volume 1088, and other notes, carton 30, volume 1103. Schlesinger Library, Radcliffe College, Cambridge, MA. No. 84-M107, Hildegard E. Peplau Archives. Copyright 1986 by Schlesinger Library. Adapted and edited by permission.

Who went with you?

When did this happen?

What year was it?

What time of day?

What was your age then?

Where did this occur?

Where were you at the time?

Where is your home?

Where did you work?

Of content of events

What happened?

Give the details of that experience.

What did you say?

Tell about that event—start at the beginning and tell all that went on.

What was it that you noticed?

What was the conversation?

To encourage description

Describe one time that you were. . . .

Talk about one day at home. . . .

Illustrate that. . . .

Describe one example. . . .

For instance—describe one time that happened. . . .

Describe one such experience fully—start at the beginning and tell all that went on.

Discuss that in detail—from the beginning to the end of your visit.

Say everything that happened that day—start when you got up in the morning.

Expand that.

Say some more about that time. . . .
Go on, then what happened. . . .
Talk about that one time fully. . . .
Fill in the details about that one experience. . . .
Tell all that occurred. . . .
Continue talking about that time. . . .
Was there anything else that went on at that time?

To encourage self-expression

Talk about yourself.
This is your time.
What was your part in that?
Tell about you and your life.
Review your experience.
What did you do?
What did you feel at that time?
Say what you thought.
What were you doing at the time?
What did you say?
What was your reply to that?
What did that have to do with you?
What was your thought about that?
Name your feeling.

When patient does not continue

Go on.
Then what?
Continue.

To deal with disguised communication

Translate that.
Are you talking in a private way?

Say that another way.

Tell me in other words.

Say that in a simpler way.

Decode that for me.

What does that have to do with you?

I'm trying to follow what you are saying.

Say some more.

Describe that fully.

Describe the whole experience; start at the beginning.

Fill in all the details.

To deal with unclear referents

Who is "we"?

Who are "they"?

Who is "he"?

Who is "it"?

Who is included in:

"Our"?

"Us"?

To get a focus on one event (from generalizations)

Tell about one time.

Stay with this one experience and describe it fully.

Give one instance of that.

Illustrate that.

Give an example.

Use the rest of the time to tell all about that one event.

Stay with that situation for the full hour.

To promote serial ordering of an event

Tell that step by step from beginning to end.

Say what came first, then second, then next.

Start at the beginning and tell what happened.
Put that in serial order—from beginning to end.

To deal with anxiety

Are you anxious?
Are you tense?
Are you nervous?
Are you upset?
Are you apprehensive?
Are you anxious now?
Are you tense at this time?
Are you upset at this moment?

To deal with automatic knowing ("you see," "you know")

No I don't see; tell me.
What is it I am supposed to know?
Are you assuming that I know something that I don't?

To deal with silence

Sit it out—keep eye-to-eye contact—wait.
What's going on?
Say what you are thinking now.
Are you tense at this time?
Are you upset at this moment?

To deal with voices

Tell about these so-called voices you say you hear.
Tell about those so-called voices of yours.
Describe these figures you say you hear.
Tell those so-called voices of yours to go away while I am here.
It seems to me the least these so-called voices of yours could do is
let you talk one hour with me.

Patient asks permission

That's up to you.

You decide that.

That's your decision.

How come you are asking me?

Patient asks for approval —Do you like ____?

What do you think?

What is your opinion?

What is your view on that?

What did you notice?

What is your idea about that?

Patient offers gifts to nurse

No, thank you.

If patient persists

You keep it, it's yours.

It's yours, give it to a friend.

You use it—it's yours.

What is your aim in offering me a gift?

If I need one—I'll get my own.

It's yours, you keep it—use it for yourself.

Patient leaves interview

The interview is from 9:00 to 9:50.

I'll be here until 9:50.

I'll wait here.

There are 40 more minutes of interview time.

At the end of 10 minutes of waiting, nurse goes to patient and says:

I'm waiting at the interview place.

There are x minutes left for talking (repeat every 10 to 15 minutes).

At the end of session, nurse goes to patient and says:

Time is up—I'm leaving now—I'll return on *x* date at *x* hour, same place.

Patient touches nurse or takes hand, etc.

Remove patient's hand gently and say:
What was that all about—talk about that.
Put that into words.
Say what that was all about.

Patient blames another

Describe that whole event.
What was your part in it?
What part did you play?

Patient comes late

Don't comment on lateness. If patient does, listen and say, "I was here at *x* hour."
The interview hour is from 9:00 to 9:50.
I'm ready whenever you are—start anywhere.
Start now—begin anywhere.
It's your time—use it now.

Don't show disapproval in word or gesture

Patient starts to hit or kick nurse —or others

1. Get out of the way.
2. Say loudly, "Stop that."
3. Get help to restrain patient.
4. Then say: "I cannot permit you to hurt anyone. Talk about that." Or "Put that action into words," or say, "What was that all about?"

Patient asks for biography regarding nurse

Don't give any, use:
Use this time to talk about your experience.
This is a time to talk about you.
This is your time to talk about your experience.
What do you need that information for?
What would you do with that information?
I'm here to hear about you and your difficulties in living with people.
How will that information help you solve your problems?

If patient persists over a long period, use:

I've said—my biography is not the point for discussion here.
If you persist the interviews will be terminated.
Warn 2 or 3 times, then terminate.

Feelings

Name the feeling you have now (or had).
Give a name to your feeling.
What name would you give to that feeling?

Thought

Say in words what you thought.
Put your thoughts into words.
State your thoughts.

Action

Describe what went on.
Describe that action.
Tell all about what you did and what the others did that time.

Patient says, "I can't think," use:

Something will occur to you—when it does, say it immediately.
You will—and when you do, put it into words.
What prevents you from thinking?
What gets in the way?
What stops you?
What are you thinking now?
Is that possible?
Say the last thought you have had.
When did you notice this about your thinking?

Patient says: "I can't remember, my mind's a blank"

You will.
Give it a try.
Make an effort to recall.
When did you first notice this difficulty?
Say whatever is on your mind now.
Did someone say this to you?
When did this start?

Patient derogates or belittles or curses the nurse

What is that all about?
What did you notice me doing that prompted your remark?
What did I do that evoked your comment?
Did I say or do something that upset you?
Are you anxious right now?

If patient derogates, belittles self

When did you decide that about yourself?
When did you first have that view of yourself?

Is this something someone else said about you?

What is the basis for that remark? Describe an instance.

When did you get that idea?

Who said that about you?

Use doubting tone.

Patient berates, derogates self or diagnoses self

When did you first decide that?

What's the basis for that idea about you?

Did someone call you that?

Did someone say that to you?

Illustrate that view of you.

Who else says that about you?

That's quite a statement about you—what is its origin?

Where did that label come from?

What is the source of the picture of you?

Use tone of disbelief.

CHAPTER 17

Professional Closeness

Professional closeness is an essential element in nursing situations. It is therefore incumbent upon the professional nurse to be aware of its essential characteristics, to be able to formulate these characteristics, and to know their meaning in nursing practice.

TYPES OF CLOSENESS

Professional closeness is a complex of behavior patterns that is learned in a professional school. It has characteristics which differentiate it from the other types of closeness that occur in family and other social situations, namely, physical closeness or intimacy, interpersonal closeness or intimacy, and pseudo-closeness. Of these, *physical closeness* is the easiest to attain. It can be illustrated by the physical act of a mother securely holding her infant or by sexual intercourse in marital life. It is sometimes demonstrated by physical touching—"laying on of hands"—and as such, is one ingredient of professional closeness. It is a nonverbal gesture that indicates shared concern or mutual regard or that conveys proximity or nearness. In professional work nonverbal gestures are best used when words cannot be found to convey the intentions of the professional person toward the client.

Reprinted from *Nursing Forum, 8*(4), 342–359. Copyright 1969 by Nursing Publications, Inc. Used with permission.

Interpersonal intimacy does not involve physical actions so much as it does verbal exchanges directed toward shared experiences. It does, however, include empathic linkages such as the communication of shared tenderness and of the interest one person has for another. In personality development it involves two persons of the same age and sex talking things over so as to check out the general meaning of their different experiences. Interpersonal intimacy is the outstanding characteristic of a "chum relationship" through which major abilities, such as the ability to collaborate, are exercised and learned. The nurse who makes the focus of the nurse–patient situation the description, analysis, and validation of meaning of the personal experience of both nurse and patient is putting the patient into the role of chum instead of treating him as a client.

Pseudo-closeness is represented by what goes on between casual acquaintances in which one of the persons uses praiseworthy comments to ingratiate himself with the other and to evoke more glowing approval from the other. Reassurances, sympathy, and cliché-laden remarks such as "That's too bad," or "Isn't that awful?" or "That must have been difficult," or "I am so sorry," are also in this category. These clichés do not further the grasp of the situation for either nurse or patient and, although they sound superficial, they are powerful devices that tend in the direction of closing off further discussion or inquiry.

Professional closeness has some points in common with physical closeness and interpersonal intimacy. In it, the professional person employs nonverbal gestures, such as occur in physical closeness, and empathic linkages, such as are associated with interpersonal intimacy. However, its focus is exclusively on the interests, concerns, and needs of the patient. The nurse is aware of her own needs, but sees herself as separate from the patient and detaches her self-interest from the patient situation so that she may act as stimulus to, and as an agent for, favorable change in the patient. The behavior of the nurse stimulates the patient to use and thereby to develop further his own competencies to understand situations and problems. The result for the patient is that from his predicament he learns something important to him; the result for the nurse is that she adds to her store of data from which facts that are universal in human experience can be abstracted and used to enrich the insights underlying the practice of professional nursing.

A nurse–patient situation described by McQuade and Goldfarb (1963) provides an illustration of professional closeness. The patient evidenced a need to control the nurse in order to cope with his own fear and feelings of helplessness. In this instance, the nurse temporarily yielded her need to control the nursing care and utilized a pattern of activity that permitted the patient's need to control to operate. Her activity included asking the patient what he wanted done and in what order. She could forego meeting her own need and yield her professional prerogatives in the situation because she was aware of the patient's need that was operating at that moment. This nurse action, by complementing the need and pattern of the patient, enabled the patient to evolve new needs which subsequently allowed for partial control of the nursing situation by the nurse.

It is this special kind of involvement with a patient, client, or family group which can be called professional closeness. It requires the nurse to observe not only the patient, but her own participation in the nurse–patient situation as well. It requires the nurse to utilize a matrix of theory for making some sense out of such observations. In the instance described, the nurse's task was to infer the interaction of need and pattern of activity of both nurse and patient. Having interpreted the situation, she made a clinical judgment as to the nurse activity that was more likely to further the interests of the patient before she took the nursing action.

THE PURPOSES OF NURSING

Professional closeness, based upon one-way interest in what is happening to another person, is a requirement for achieving the purposes of nursing, which are twofold. First and foremost, the nurse favors the survival of the organism. But recovery from an illness is not enough. When the life of the patient is assured, a second purpose guides nursing practices. The nurse aids the patient to grasp the meaning of his health problem and to learn from his current experience with it. Bruner (1966b) suggests that knowledge of "evolutionary instrumentalities" which enables the learner to "express and amplify his powers" is an inherent characteristic of man's long history. The nurse is one such instrument or stimulus in the life of a patient. And concern and capability in furthering the evolution of capacities of another person is a demonstration of professional closeness at its best.

The patient has reactions to illness, disability, or catastrophe, and he also attempts to cope with these stresses and reactions to stress. "Stress cannot and should not be avoided" (Selye, 1965). However, stress forces the patterning of behavior, and the nurse has an opportunity to utilize the nursing situation to stimulate such patterning in the direction of new learning and favorable change in every patient. As Bruner suggests, "You must get the perceptual field organized around your own person as center before you can impose other, less egocentric axes upon it" (Bruner, 1966a). This is particularly true of the patient undergoing stress; self-concern is almost the exclusive focus. The task of the nurse is not to sympathize with this self-concern, but rather to aid the patient to bring to bear—to develop through use—his competencies for seeing and understanding his predicament.

Through her help the patient can develop awareness of his reactions and coping behavior, thereby adding a dimension to the self-understanding which he already has and which every human being gradually evolves as a result of taking a look at current experiences. And the patient can evolve foresights which prevent recurrence of illness.

THE NURSE'S NEEDS

Nursing care occurs within an interpersonal relationship of nurse to patient. To understand professional closeness it is necessary to have some grasp of the interpersonal nature of the nursing process, for closeness is but one facet of nurse–patient interaction. Sullivan has defined a general principle called the theorem of reciprocal emotion (Sullivan, 1954). This principle states that "integration in an interpersonal situation is a process in which (1) complementary needs are resolved (or aggravated); (2) reciprocal patterns of activity are developed (or disintegrated); and (3) fore-sight of satisfaction (or rebuff) of similar needs is facilitated" (pp. 128–129).

This principle suggests the necessity for the nurse to observe her own needs and the patterns of activity that are called out by both her needs and her inferences regarding the needs of the patient. This task is not an easy one, since interactions change rapidly. The most that a participant in an interpersonal situation can do is to notice the significant among the many rapidly shifting signs and cues to what is going on. It is these cues that lead the nurse toward her inferences about the meaning of the situation.

The nurse, of course, has needs that run the gamut of biological and acquired needs (Peplau, 1957). However, some of these needs are not particularly useful in the nursing situation—for example, those that require the patient to call out needs and patterns of activity of his own so as to complement, and thereby to resolve or aggravate, the needs of the nurse. The nurse who needs approval, whose satisfaction lies in getting compliments, favors, or gifts from patients, will set up interactions to which patients will respond in a way that will satisfy these needs. In this case, the nurse is using the patient as an object for self-satisfaction, and a pseudo-closeness, rather than a professional closeness, develops.

On the other hand, the nurse who uses social situations or staff interactions to meet her own needs, and who can utilize profes-sional time with patients to focus exclusively on the needs, con-cerns, and experiences of the patient, demonstrates professional closeness. This nurse shows that she can put herself aside and can bring all of her capacities, talents, and competencies to bear upon the life of another person to the end that that person will grow a little, learn something new, and in effect be strengthened in a favorable direction (Peplau, 1964).

An awareness by the nurse of her own behavior is important, for it is all that she can change. Nurses do not "manage" patients; instead they manage the relation of the nurse to the patient vis-à-vis aware-ness and control of the nurse participation in the nurse–patient situ-ation. The nurse's behavior calls out responses in the patient. The nurse cannot change the patient's responses, nor can she demand responses that are different from those obtained. What she can do is to manage her own behavior as the stimulus to which the patient's behavior is a response.

Actually, the patient learns whether or not the nurse makes a point of guiding his learning. Most times he is oversensitized to the reactions of others and their behavior toward him and his problem. He watches and privately interprets what he sees and thinks nurses are doing in his behalf. The nurse who takes the stance that the patient is a learner and that the most critical focus of his learning is what is happening to him, will likely take more professional responsibility for the content of that learning.

To channel the patient's learning toward productive outcomes, the nurse stimulates the patient to observe and describe the events relating to the current difficulty. By encouraging the patient to respond to such questions as "What did you notice?" "What happened? Describe it," "What did you think?" "What did you say?" "What did you feel?" and so on, the nurse conveys interest in expressiveness by the patient. And, as the patient uses his powers to observe and describe, he not only develops them but he provides himself and the nurse with data from which, later on, meaning can be abstracted and formulated (Peplau, 1959).

What kind of stimulus behavior on the part of the nurse demonstrates professional closeness and tends to promote favorable change (growth, learning, and recovery) in patients? This is a central question for nursing educators and for nurse practitioners alike. Clearcut definitions are not easy to come by, for sometimes behavior that is not considered useful "stimulus" behavior is easier to state than are descriptions of constructive stimulus behavior.

First of all, it must be recognized that professional closeness is guided by consideration of what is "good" for the patient, and that the determination of what is "good" requires professional knowledge and judgment; it is not left to chance. Nor is the patient in a position to determine the most useful outcomes that he can achieve in terms of his present predicament. Hughes states: "Professionals profess. They profess to know better than others the nature of certain matters, and to know better than their clients what ails them or their affairs. This is the essence of the professional idea and the professional claim" (Hughes, 1963, p. 656). Barber suggests: "A sociological definition of the professions should limit itself, so far as possible, to the *differentia specifica* of professional behavior" (Barber, 1963, p. 671). Freidson indicates that "the professional practitioner claims that his skills are so esoteric that the client is in no position to evaluate them. From this stems his privilege to be somewhat removed from the market place and to accept the evaluation of his colleagues rather than of his clients" (Freidson, 1960, p. 375).

In speaking about the nursing care of patients who have had strokes, Ullman (1964) states:

> Proper nursing care for patients of this type rests in considerable measure on the nurse's ability to understand and interpret the nature of the patient's struggle with his illness as well as the level at which it is carried out by virtue of the degree of brain deficit that has occurred. The patient is attempting to preserve a sense of intactness as well as familiar relatedness to his environment . . . optimum results occur generally when we can accept the patient as he presents himself to us . . . we can only carry this out in practice if we have some understanding of how he experiences his illness, his disability, and how he communicates these changes to others. (p. 91)

These statements call for a relationship that is well beyond the nurse's "jollying" the patient into taking his medicine and seeing that his bedspread is neat. For the nurse to develop a relationship based on professional closeness she must have knowledge from the behavioral sciences and nursing science itself, plus a broad range of procedures for using such knowledge. Such knowledge aids in observation; it helps the nurse to know what to look for. In addition, knowledge explains observations—that is, a concept will aid the nurse to know the meaning of an observation. Knowledge also serves as a basis for action when it is applied to observations at hand.

Knowledge of this kind is in a continuous state of development. Therefore, professional closeness requires continuing inquiry on the part of every nurse in order that the common elements (universal) in similar nursing situations can be elucidated, the interventions can be continuously refined, and the relation between problem and nurse action can be formulated and explained. However, although the nurse is constantly looking for universals in cases or situations of like kind, she always starts by seeing the patient (or family unit) with whom she is working as if he were unique. Preconceptions derived from her theoretical knowledge or from other cases are constantly checked against the new data; and the results of these checks may alter previous views to a considerable extent. Therefore, the nurse must be a sensitive observer with many techniques of inquiry at her fingertips so that she can get to know the patient fully, in as many dimensions as possible, from data obtained directly from him.

In short, professional closeness is not simply a matter of being generous, kind, affable, and obliging to sick people, but rather one of being knowledgeable about the practices and problems of nursing care. It is not so much a matter of being "closer" to the person who is ill, but rather one of being "closer to the truth" of that person's current dilemma and of having the knowhow to use such understanding as the basis for effective help for the patient. And that knowhow includes interpersonal actions—enabling actions—through which the nurse gradually enables the patient to know and to help himself.

AFFECTIVE INVOLVEMENT

The question of affective involvement in nurse–patient situations is crucial to professional closeness. Daniels details different types of such involvement and reports a study of the manner in which medical schools seek to control it in the intern (Daniels, 1960; Becker, 1960). While suggesting that "affective neutrality" may lean too far toward complete detachment, the article suggests the possibility of "restrained involvement, controlled against the possibility of its becoming too intense or being expressed too freely" and of "evaluative considerations which not only rule inappropriate patterns out, but rule appropriate ones in."

Alpenfels has suggested: "Such factors as individual attitudes toward pain or illness, as trained observers in both fields [nursing and medicine] have pointed out, may interfere with therapy and well-being sometimes as effectively as the disease process itself" (Alpenfels, 1964). When nursing students learn to identify and manage personal attitudes toward pain, disfigurement, odors, and other phenomena seen in the nursing situation, they are helped to detach these nurse reactions and render them inoperative in the nurse–patient relationship. It is the task of the professional school to aid the student to recognize, formulate, and understand so as to control spontaneous reactions such as anger, disgust, and annoyance and yet to experience and express feelings of tenderness and concern in such a way that these are useful.

There are several types of clinical experience in which the nursing student is subjected to critical tests concerning "affective involvement." These situations include those in which a patient dies, in which there is gross disfigurement, in which a dead baby is born and the mother grieves, and in which a sick child must be separated from its mother on whom it has large dependence. In these instances the nurse can be devastated by sharing the feelings of the other, or she can develop a shell-like insulation or indifference to what is going on and carry out quite mechanically the necessary routines. Or she can avoid these situations entirely by assigning them to nursing students or to nursing assistants.

As a fourth alternative, the nurse can utilize professional closeness. In the instance of the grief-stricken mother, the nurse first of all has a theoretical grasp of the process of grieving. Then she uses this knowledge to clarify her interactions and observations of this patient and to structure the nursing actions which, in time, will help this mother to manage her grief and get on with living.

Professional closeness in such a situation requires a special kind of detachment: the nurse must be able to maintain a distance between herself and the patient and at the same time demonstrate concern, interest, and competence. Speaking of the "main themes of professionalization" Hughes makes the statement:

Detachment is one of them; and that in the sense of having in a particular case no personal interest such as would influence one's action or advice, while being interested in all cases of the kind. The deep interest in all cases is of the sort that leads one to pursue and systematize the pertinent knowledge. It leads to finding an intellectual base for the problems one handles, which, in turn, takes those problems out of their particular setting and makes them part of a more universal order. One aspect of a profession is a certain equilibrium between the universal and the particular. (Hughes, 1963, p. 660)

For the professional nurse to achieve "an appropriate equilibrium between detachment and interest," she must give some thought to the meaning of that nursing cliché "personalized nursing care." The nurse who views nursing as a personalized service may tend to think of herself more as a "choreboy of the client" and to do what the "customer" requests, rather than to determine, as a professional person, what is needed by the patient. For demands and needs are not necessarily synonymous. Putting the patient in the position of being a "customer"—a person who defines the services he wants and possibly gets—may even be detrimental. As pointed out earlier, Hughes claims that the client is not in a position to define the requirements of his case.

A report that sheds light on the meaning of "personalized care" to the patient states:

> We do not think that . . . the patients felt personalized care was a more important facet of total patient care than knowledge and skill. On the contrary, we postulated that being unable to judge the knowledge and skill of hospital personnel, patients used personalized care as an indication that their doctors and nurses were technically competent, dedicated, and interested in their patients. . . .
>
> Patients desired personal contact with hospital personnel because they needed attention. They wanted someone to talk to, to help pass the time, and keep them from feeling lonely, and to be kind to them and give them emotional support. Patients used this type of communication as a sign that not only were their nurses and physicians dedicated and interested in their care and cure and would not reject them, but also that these persons were technically qualified, possessing the knowledge and skill to get them well. (Skipper, Tagliacozzo, & Mauksch, 1964, p. 103)

What this report suggests is that in patient care situations the elementary learning that you can trust people who act as if they like you continues without revision and is used by patients as a sign or estimate of competence of personnel. However, this trust may not be justified in some instances. Surely there are better ways for a professional nurse to communicate competence, to evoke confidence in the patient, and at the same time to provoke the use and exercise of the patient's capacities as a person and thereby the further refinement of these capacities.

Some stocktaking is in order in terms of the question: When a patient assigns all or most all of the effort to others where does this lead him? Does it lead to dependence, chronicity, a blunting of ability? Is nursing merely a matter of meeting the needs of patients? Or is it instead an instrumentality through which a professional nurse aids a patient to recognize and formulate his needs, to cope with these needs more and more through his own efforts, and to take at least a tiny step toward further self-development. If personalized care, and not learning products, yields satisfaction for the nurse (because her need to please has been met) and serves as signs of safety for the patient (because he is not capable of judging professional competence), professional nursing is indeed in a sorry position.

No doubt all nurses would agree with Jeffries (1964) who says: "Of all the lifesaving equipment that helped me, the presence of another human being was the most essential. In this age of electronic computers and monitoring machines, the intellect and compassion of a nurse are still the best healing devices" (p. 77). A professional person needs to critically examine sweeping assertions, especially those that are pleasing to the eye and ear. Jeffries claims, "The nurse in her close association with her patient can do a great deal in these situations to relieve his anxiety. Understanding and interest, combined with good nursing, can spare him unnecessary apprehension and reinforce his courage during critical periods" (p. 77). However, she does not state criteria or define behaviors characteristic of "close association." Hence, although her article makes the reader "feel good" because it claims effectiveness, it fails to define the specifics in a form that is testable in many situations and therefore that might help the profession to move toward universals concerning "close associations."

In short, the article raises many questions. Who relieves the patient's anxiety? The patient himself does this as a response to specific nurse tactics. What nurse tactics were effective in the instance cited? On what theoretical grounds were they based? Would those grounds hold true in many similar instances of anxiety in patients? Professional nurses ought not to be satisfied with verbalized clichés about their effectiveness, but rather should seek to define the stimulus behavior of nurses that produces favorable effects on patients. Such definitions open up the possibility of testing and finding out whether in fact such effectiveness does occur in many nurse–patient situations.

There occasionally is the misconception that interest and emotional involvement are synonymous, as for example in the following quotation.

> To me, the art of nursing is the ability of the nurse to convey to the patient first of all her interest in his recovery, then her mastery in the techniques, and finally her willingness to contribute all she has of both interest and proficiency toward his rapid recovery. Many may protest that the nurse cannot become emotionally involved with every patient, but I say that if she does not have a high degree of interest in her patient's recovery, then the profession of nursing becomes a dead, mechanical, for-hire sort of thing. (Anonymous, 1964, p. 66)

In this quotation the manner in which interest is to be conveyed is not described. Furthermore, if the nurse focuses on recovery rather than on knowing the person who is the object of the nursing service and on understanding his problems in some depth, the imminent death of a patient leads only to sorrow rather than to more useful inquiry which may benefit the next patient in a similar circumstance.

The extent of emotional involvement with patient after patient in a day's work also requires consideration. Not only does emotional involvement of great intensity drain a nurse's energies, and particularly so in situations in which the extant problems may not be immediately amenable to solutions, but such involvement may also becloud the perceptual field and distort her observations.

Consider for example, the strains upon the nurse if she became "emotionally involved" with the variety of persons and problems mentioned in the following paragraph:

> Members attending the center seek out the nurse to talk about a wide variety of health problems. One member may be concerned because he wants a physical examination. Another reports a lump in her breast. They come to the nurse with nutritional, hearing, visual, and dental

problems. They come for interpretation of physician's instructions and with emotional problems associated with newly diagnosed physical ailments. (Bozian, 1964, p. 94)

Obviously, in these situations a variety of needs and feelings of the nurse could be evoked in a day's time if the nurse is unable to exert self-control and to sustain a one-way view focused on the concerns of the patient. Imagine what might happen if the concerns of the patients collide with the nurse's need to talk about herself, to obtain a satisfying audience from each patient, to respond spontaneously with whatever feelings each evokes in her. Do you provide more effective nursing services by listening, taking each patient seriously, grasping the importance of what the patient is saying, and finding the strategy that helps each patient to figure out what is problematic and how to use advice or information to solve the problem, or by sympathizing with these problems?

These characteristics of professional closeness are reflected in the characteristics of the professional nurse. The professional nurse works as a nurse because she has chosen this route for focusing and further developing her capacities, because she has beginning knowhow and genuine interest in furthering her knowledge through study of the phenomena requiring nursing, and because she earns (and may need to) her living this way. She has a genuine interest in the problems that confront the practitioner of nursing and engages in continuing study and definition of these problems and of effective nursing actions. When practiced by a person with these attributes, nursing is no longer an elementary practical art, but rather a professional service that contributes to the well-being of persons in this society.

REFERENCES

Alpenfels, E. J. (1964). Cultural clues to reactions. *American Journal of Nursing, 64*(4), 83–86.

Anonymous (1964). The art of nursing. *American Journal of Nursing, 64*(4), 66–67.

Barber, B. (1963, fall). The sociology of the professions. *Daedalus, 92,* 669–688. [or 669–688.]

Becker, H. S. (1960). Notes on the concept of commitment. *American Journal of Sociology, 66*(1), 32–40.

Bozian, M. W. (1964). Nursing in a geriatric day center. *American Journal of Nursing, 64*(4), 93–95.

Bruner, J. S. (1966a, February 19). Education as social invention. *Saturday Review,* 70–72, 102–103.

Bruner, J. S. (1966b). *Toward a theory of instruction.* Cambridge, MA: Belknap; Harvard University Press.

Daniels, M. J. (1960). Affect and its control in the medical intern. *American Journal of Sociology, 66*(3), 259–267.

Freidson, E. (1960). Client control and medical practice. *American Journal of Sociology, 65*(4), 374–382.

Hughes, E. C. (1963, fall). Professions. *Daedalus, 92,* 655–668.

Jeffries, J. (1964). The best healing device. *American Journal of Nursing, 64*(9), 74–77.

McQuade, A., & Goldfarb, A. I. (1963). Coping with feelings of helplessness. *American Journal of Nursing, 63*(5), 77–79.

Peplau, H. E. (1957). Aspects of psychiatric nursing: Therapeutic concepts. *League Exchange, 26* (section B), 44–45.

Peplau, H. E. (1959). *Principles of psychiatric nursing (American handbook of psychiatry,* Vol. 2). New York: Basic Books.

Peplau, H. E. (1964). Professional and social behavior: Some differences worth the notice of professional nurses. *Quarterly Magazine* (Columbia University-Presbyterian Hospital School of Nursing Alumni Association), *59*(4), 23–33.

Selye, H. (1965). The stress syndrome. *American Journal of Nursing, 65*(3), 97–99.

Skipper, J. S., Jr., Tagliacozzo, D. L., & Mauksch, H. O. (1964). What communication means to patients. *American Journal of Nursing, 64*(4), 101–103.

Sullivan, H. S. (1954). *The psychiatric interview.* New York: Norton.

Ullman, M. (1964). Disorders of body image after stroke. *American Journal of Nursing, 64*(10), 89–91.

CHAPTER 18

Themes in Nursing Situations

THE THEMATIC PHASE OF PSYCHIATRY

Three important phases in the continuing development of psychiatry have recently been identified (Ruesch & Bateson, 1951). The first phase is *descriptive psychiatry* in which peculiarities of behavior are listed and grouped into categories which are used in making diagnoses. The second phase is epithetic or *typological* psychiatry in which the primary focus is the identification of types of individuals, and placing them in such categories as schizoid, extroverted, ectomorphic, overactive, and so on. This labeling of "kinds" of people has also influenced lay and professional people's attitudes and has in some instances led to the use of these labels as epithets with which to derogate people. The third, the *thematic* phase in psychiatry, is a trend that has recently gained prominence. The psychiatrist, or any other worker, who is interacting with, and studying his relations with a patient, becomes concerned with the focal problems, recurring patterns, or central themes in the patient's past or present experience.

Each of these phases—descriptive, typological, thematic—is part of the gradual evolution of a mature theory in psychiatry that explains observations and guides practices in this area of health service. When another phase emerges that explains or guides psychiatric practices more productively, it too will be identified. This is the nature of theory—ever changing, being revised, reconstructed, and made more useful. Focusing on the thematic phase of psychiatry does not obviate the importance or simultaneous use of what is offered from the descriptive or typological phases, or of what is being produced in continuing explorations, such as in biochemical research.

WHAT IS A THEME?

A theme is a generalization, a summarizing characteristic, an abstraction of an event that actually consists of many details that are best summarized as this theme. The word is used in the thematic apperception test in which individuals are shown various pictures and asked to tell a story about each one. One of the values of this test is that it gives a general view of the abstract themes that recur and indicate the individual's mood, or thoughts, or actions.

In music we speak of a theme as a "melody constituting the basis of variation, development, composition, or movement." In the continuing nurse–patient relationship, do we find outstanding themes that occur again and again in many different variations? Do these themes recur so as to characterize either the process, or the event, or a substantial part of it? In dream analysis, the therapist may take the dream as it is told and the secondary elaborations of it and try to abstract recurring threads or themes, from the way the dreamer tells it, from the explanations he gives, and from the dream itself. These recurring threads indicate dominant concerns which the dreamer cannot reveal to himself directly; only under the conditions of sleep can disguised messages about these concerns be made available to him.

Anthropologists, in casting about for ways to study industrialized societies, are using the thematic approach. All institutions can be studied from the standpoint of universal themes such as *power*. Or particular institutions can be studied from the standpoint of particular themes such as the influence of *profit* upon production. Industrial engineers are interested in how the theme *compensation* affects labor unions, workers, and industrial management. These are recurring themes that characterize institutions and affect the interpersonal relations within them.

Perhaps the importance of a thematic approach can be made clearer if we touch on one theme that seems to affect psychiatric institutions, doctors, nurses, their patients, and the public. This theme is *hopelessness*. It seems quite apparent that many individuals view psychiatric patients as "hopeless." The public's apathy in providing funds for their care is probably one aspect of the effect of this theme. Of course, we do not have any all-out studies of its effect on institutional and public behavior, and so there are no specific data that we can use to combat it with a more productive theme such as *hope*. But certainly the recurring pattern of this theme in the behavior of nurses, doctors, patients, families, and others causes many of the stalemates in clinical practice. Does hopelessness overshadow our work in such an insidious way that it handicaps our therapeutic efforts quite seriously? How do we offer incentives that hold out hope of satisfaction and recovery for patients?

THE IMPORTANCE OF
RECOGNIZING THEMES

It is impossible for anyone to continuously recall or to keep in mind all of the intricate details of an interpersonal event. The mind of man does not work this way except for the few who have so-called photographic memories. We get instead a general impression—or theme—concerning what went on. If we merely characterize an interaction as "disappointing" or "good" we have no cue to remind us of some of the details out of which a theme arises.

One purpose for getting at the themes of interaction is to find out, qualitatively, what goes on between us. When we are aware of what goes on—and by awareness we mean, when we have taken in the details in such a way as to make more and more correct and useful inferences about them—then the situation becomes amenable to control. This opens up the possibility of creating favorable changes here and in other situations as awareness leads us toward shifts in the way we take part in these situations.

A second reason for wanting to know the themes of interpersonal events is the economical communication they afford. Much transpires in an interpersonal relationship, through both verbal and nonverbal communication. If we have some generalized inferences—or themes—about the situation, then we have a basis for recalling, expanding, and clarifying what needs to be remembered. We also have a basis for determining practices and for structuring modes by which the nurse intervenes in particular kinds of situations. For example, if the theme *dependence* characterizes a patient's participation in a situation with us, and if this theme occurs over and over again, its variations give us clues to what this patient needs. If, on the other hand, *mutual dependence* characterizes the nurse–patient relationship, then it becomes clear that the nurse must take a different part (Tudor, 1952).

This need to have inferences is likewise true in developing background information about patients. A case history reveals details of events as they have been recalled by various reporters and as they have been heard by various recorders. It also contains inferences, correct and otherwise, that have been made about those events.

There are, in state hospitals, reams and reams of case histories, and yet little is known about schizophrenia. Suppose we were to have a way of getting at the recurring themes that characterized the relationships of 100 schizophrenic patients with the significant persons in their lives—and also data about the interactions of nurses and these patients—from which themes could be abstracted. What themes would we find? At the very least, we would have something to work with that is not now available. We would also have an economical way to communicate and come to grips with the dominant features of these patients' past and present relations with people.

Using the interpersonal themes from a patient's past experiences as a hypothesis for studying his present relations, makes it easier for professional workers to study how their present responses might be reinforcing trends laid down long ago. It also permits them to steer away from traumatic events. It provides a frame of reference—which is open both to revision and validation—in talking things over with the patient and in making new observations. Helping the patient to discover the recurring threads in his attempts to relate to people is an important aspect of psychotherapeutic nursing, but to do this the nurse needs to have hypotheses with which to work.

A third reason for abstracting themes from interpersonal events is the basis they provide for comparing one situation with others. A blow-by-blow comparison of details is obviously unwieldy, and past experience shows that it does not help us much in finding out what we need to know. Our total impressions are more useful to us as a basis for referring back and forth from actual relations with patients to data in case histories, and for comparing what goes on in one situation with what went on in another.

A fourth, and perhaps the most important, reason for wanting to generalize from interpersonal data is that it provides us the opportunity to use our most human capacity—reasoning. Professional nurses operate in situations in which inferences and judgments must be made so that sound practices can be planned and carried out. Learning to make inferences is quite different from developing technical and manual skills, which much of our earlier nursing education focused on. The ability to reason and to arrive at useful inferences, judgments, or themes requires intellectual capacity that is developed slowly in a professional education program.

Judgments are the products of reasoning; they are abstractions from the details of a particular event or, from the details of a relationship between events. A professional person is able to formulate concepts from past and present observations and to infer the consequences of present actions in the foreseeable future. To become more creative in what we contribute in any relationship with people, it is necessary to make some judgments about what can be observed. This is true for each nurse–patient relationship. It is just as true for the relationships in a nursing team or for any other intraprofessional as well as interprofessional relations. In fact, we might say that it is the moral task of the maturing adult and the obligation of the professional person to make ever more useful inferences about what goes on in relations with people, and to use these inferences or themes to foster favorable changes in situations.

REFERENCES

Ruesch, J., & Bateson, G. (1951). *Communication: The social matrix of psychiatry.* New York: Norton.

Tudor, G. E. (1952). A sociopsychiatric nursing approach to intervention in a problem of mutual withdrawal on a mental hospital ward. *Psychiatry, 15,* 193–217.

PART V Concepts

Introduction

Since the early 1950s Hildegard E. Peplau has encouraged a phenomenological focus in nursing in general and in psychiatric nursing in particular. She has done so by example through her lectures and publications pertaining to concepts of concern in clinical work, and through her clinical and theoretical influence on national and international levels. Her imprint is noticeable on reports by the Group for Advancement of Psychiatry, the League Exchange Series publications, on the American Nurses' Association Social Policy Statement, and through the work of the World Health Organization. She has been a tireless contributor and facilitator of the conceptual development of nursing.

Concepts are central to Peplau's work, providing both structure and meaning to interpersonal events and intervention. In 1955, with trepidation, she published her first clinical paper, "Loneliness." She was, after all, from a culture, time, and profession where women could be covertly intelligent by being intuitive but were not supposed to be overtly intelligent, capable of rational thought. As she would say, such competence was at odds with her self-concepts, so it was incredible that such a paper materialized altogether and was published as the earliest, most definitive psychodynamic formulation of loneliness, predating the well-known Fromm-Reichmann paper on the subject. Peplau was one of only a few theorists who wrote on loneliness, and her publication represents a major contribution to the behavioral and applied sciences.

Learning, along with anxiety, are used as tools by Peplau to understand problematic behavior while intervening in it. Although her publication on learning appeared in 1963, her interest in learning theory dated from her student days at Bennington and Teachers College. In graduate school she came to disagree with the then-popular John Dewey, whose concept of learning was simply learning by doing. In addition, in 1956, when she formally developed the concept of learning as a phenomenon and a process to be used as a guide for the structure of the psychotherapeutic process, she did so in response and opposition to the stimulus-response conditioning/learning in vogue at the time.

Well into the 1940s and early 1950s, theoretical disputes regarding learning (a phenomenon of interest and research in American psychology) were at two extremes: conditioning theories of various kinds on one side and cognitive theories on the other. Responding to the restrictiveness of behaviorism associated with conditioning-response theories, and steeped in interpersonal theory showing the complexity of motivation and behavior and the obvious internalization of interpersonal events, Peplau developed the phenomenon of learning in such a way as to understand its operations and to use them to guide both therapist and patient. Too, without the restrictiveness of behavior approaches, conceptions of mental processes entered Peplau's teaching and clinical work—these were processes such as cognition, perception, and memory. Interestingly, Peplau's 1950s use of learning and cognition predated psychology's development of those concepts into formal theories concerned with mental processes. And Peplau's use of learning as a cornerstone of the therapeutic process predated by nearly two decades learning's coming to be seen as part of cognitive psychology. Her connection between thinking disorders and language in clinical work, and their link to intervention are unparalleled in the work of any theorist in the mental health disciplines.

Regarding the self-system, Peplau, who unquestionably was influenced by Sullivan, brings clarity and additional content to Sullivan's fledgling conceptual development of the self-system. Additionally, whether regarding concepts such as anxiety, the self, or hallucinations, clinical intervention is always linked to the operations of the concepts, making theory live and making sense out of the most obscure clinical data.

CHAPTER 19

Loneliness

Being alone in a situation may be a pleasant state, or an unpleasant one—or it may be unbearable. True loneliness—which is unbearable—is a clinical problem in psychiatric nursing practice, but it has received very little attention as such.

Before discussing the feelings of the person who is without company, it may be helpful for us to consider the differences between lonesomeness, aloneness, and loneliness.

Lonesomeness is a common experience. It implies being without the company of others but recognizing a wish to be with others. Lonesomeness can occur when an individual is isolated or it can be felt despite proximity to others in a group. The lonesome individual recognizes his desire to feel closer to others and, more often than not, he is able to state it as a feeling. Also he can usually express specific wishes, and take steps to relieve the feeling of lonesomeness.

Aloneness also implies being without company. It may signify a singular position, such as being alone in making certain kinds of decisions which affect living. Erich Fromm, for example, speaks of man's "moral aloneness" in reaching decisions of ethical significance. An individual is alone when he casts his vote in an election. Individuals can choose to be alone—to retreat temporarily from the activities with other people which customarily go on in the social stream. Being alone offers an opportunity for concentration, for focusing on and working through particular kinds of problems. Scientists, for example, often court aloneness. They find that it improves their productivity; it is a way to avoid distractions which would impede or delay their accomplishment. It is possible to be alone, without being lonesome or lonely, when retreat, seclusion, or protected isolation are recognized and chosen as desirable or essential for accomplishing specific purposes, for which plans can be made and acted upon.

Loneliness, however, is not a chosen state. Often the lonely person is not aware of the reason why he does what he does when he experiences loneliness. It is an experience somewhat different in character and in intensity from either aloneness or lonesomeness. Loneliness can be defined as an unnoticed inability to do anything while alone.

Often loneliness is not felt; instead the person has a feeling of unexplained dread, of desperation, or of extreme restlessness. These feelings are so intense, so unbearable, that automatic actions are precipitated. These automatic actions force other persons to come into contact with the lonely individual. Although he is not aware that loneliness is one of the feelings which govern him, his automatic responses recur and become patterns of living which may seem senseless to other people. One psychiatric patient referred to her pattern of response to loneliness as her "trapadaptation."

THE ROOTS OF LONELINESS

Loneliness is the result of early life experiences in which remoteness, indifference, and emptiness were the principal themes that characterized the child's relationships with others. Because it is an unbearable experience, loneliness is always hidden, disguised, defended against, and expressed in other forms. It may be expressed quite simply as homesickness, or it may appear as severe agitation, or in the form of alcoholism or drug addiction, and it is an important aspect of the schizophrenic pattern of living. In nursing situations, therefore, nurses do not deal directly with the patient's loneliness but rather with his defenses against experiencing the pain of loneliness—the plausible structure he has erected to cover up the problem and hide it from himself and from others.

Some general cues to the needs of lonely patients are available in the generic roots of the problem. When nurses can understand how loneliness has evolved, they can anticipate what kinds of relationships between the nurse and the patient would be similarly traumatic, and they can avoid acting in ways that might reinforce the problem.

Sullivan discusses loneliness as an acquired outcome of childhood situations (Sullivan, 1953). He points out that during early childhood each child makes an effort to secure the attention of adults—as active participants or at least as spectators—in activities which interest the child and stimulate his curiosity. However, these efforts are too often met with indifference, misinterpretation, or punishment which the child interprets as being due to failure on his part. Adults often interpret the child's attention-getting behavior as merely a device to distract and delay, and this interpretation serves as justification for their feelings of annoyance with the child.

The actual purposes of these initial efforts on the part of the child are varied. He seeks an audience so that he can see himself in relation to another person. This is how he first experiences the feeling of being related to others. He also needs an opportunity to exercise his growing ability to communicate what is meaningful to him during an experience. He seeks to check the meanings of his current observations and experiences with another person. Thus, he is exercising an important and much needed capacity which will serve, later on, to limit the importance which he attaches to his fantasies and to his autistic interpretations which are highly subjective and which are based on his fantasies, rather than on reality. Autistic thinking serves to gratify unfulfilled longings.

Childhood is a time when autistic invention—the capacity to invent and assign highly personal meaning to events—is most active. The child who seeks the attentive participation of adults but meets with indifference, remoteness, or even punishment instead, must somehow fill the gap. Otherwise, life seems empty of meaning, of skill, and of the feeling that he is related to others.

Alone, he has to find plausible explanations for what is happening to him. Feelings of smallness, helplessness, and longing for closeness give way to defenses against loneliness. The wish for the cooperation of adults in interpreting events is replaced by the use of fantasies and autistic invention. Later on, these cause enormous difficulty when the individual attempts to maintain a distinction between what is real and what is fanciful. One patient put it this way: "For me it is always a struggle to think clearly." The nurse asked, "You know when you are thinking clearly?" and the patient answered, "You feel that you are."

Without help and without skill, the child must resort to fantasies to explain current experiences. To adults, the new set of interpretations which the child makes seem to be falsifications and misinterpretations, and they are not appreciated for what they are any more than the initial efforts to secure active, direct interest were. To the child, the expansive distortions serve only to explain experience, but to adults, they may become proof that the child should be viewed as unmanageable, as a "liar," or as delinquent. The problem deepens and the child's sense of failure looms larger and larger.

This arrest in the socializing process at home does not prepare the child for contacts with peers in the next phase in development. Peers tend to poke fun at his ineptness, errors, and misinterpretations of the meanings of events. Not only the rebuffs of adults but now those of children, too, become a real and anticipated source of humiliation, punishment, and anxiety. Real or imagined threats, supported by the fear of error, deepen the sense of social isolation. The evolving need to be right, to be able, coupled with feelings of failure and of isolation from others, all help to nourish the developing loneliness.

PATTERNS OF DEFENSE

Sullivan tells us, however, that loneliness is so dreaded and so painful that it must be disguised; it is therefore dissociated, not noticed; instead, defenses against observation of it determine the individual's behavior. The patterns of defense are automatic and while the patient frequently can offer plausible explanations of what he is doing, the obvious purpose of the behavior escapes his notice. For example, a patient who drinks and then needs nurses to care for him during an alcoholic bout may offer many reasons for needing to have

nurses to care for him. But he misses the obvious interpretation—
that he is sorely in need of attention and contact with others, and
that this need has erupted as a momentary experiencing of loneliness and has thus brought on the episode of drinking.

Recognizing what the behavior of an individual who is defending
himself from bitter loneliness means may take sensitive observation, over a long period of time, but there are certain clues that
nurses can watch for.

Time-oriented complaints are often observed. The patient may experience the "endlessness" of each day, even though he may carry
out and complete his routine. He may have an aura of waiting, of
enduring, of "putting in time," so to speak. In considering events in
the future, the patient often observes aspects of the beginning and
also the goals or ends relating to the event, but he does not anticipate
the intervening steps—the transition points in the duration of the
event. For example, a patient who is planning to move may recognize
that the time to move has arrived and may consider the advantages
of the new location, but he has no concept of what is involved in the
preparation for moving and in the moving process itself.

With some patients, it often appears as if time were telescoped—
past events and present experiences are considered and lived as if
they were identical, fused together. While the person seems always
to wait for something to happen, when the thing he has been waiting
for is about to occur, he becomes impatient because he has to wait.
For example, one patient put it directly by saying, over and over
again, "I have to wait for the doctor and I can't." Another patient
could not say directly, but indicated through her dreams, that the
nurse was not noticing or attending to her needs in a complete way—
it was as if, by this means, she was trying to indicate the remoteness
of both her mother and the nurse by distorting time and telescoping
the mother-situation and nurse-situation into one.

The feeling of *familiarity* seems to be time-related and can be observed in patients who are fighting loneliness. The familiarity is
with things rather than with people and it seems more apparent
when the patient is experiencing great anxiety. One patient, for example, would occasionally state with conviction that she had heard,
read, or seen something before, although she was observing it in a
newly purchased book or a freshly published newspaper. Further

inquiry revealed that what was familiar was the feeling she had at being in that situation with the nurse, a feeling which she had experienced in an earlier situation. Another patient who was vomiting a good deal asked for a prescribed medication which was expected to relieve the vomiting and the discomfort associated with it. She was given the medication, but each dose was also vomited. As the patient became more anxious, a feeling of "everything seems familiar" developed and was expressed, in this instance, in relation to material in a newspaper she was reading. She then asked to test this feeling by having the nurse read from a new book which she was certain she had not read nor heard about, but here too "everything seemed familiar." The nurse wondered whether it was something in the nurse–patient situation which was being expressed indirectly in this way. Further discussion revealed that this patient had had a tonsillectomy at a very early age. During her hospitalization, her mother had brought her some lemonade, saying, "This will make your throat better." However, the tartness had increased the pain and discomfort, and now the medication for the relief of vomiting had also failed to work. This indicated what was familiar: an unfulfilled expectation that a trusted mothering person would bring relief from discomfort.

There is also a sense in which lonely patients seem to feel familiar with people; but on further inspection the chief characteristic of this feeling is that they view all other persons as *anonymous* beings. One patient may treat everyone as a welcome and known stranger; another automatically dislikes everyone except in rare instances when he finds one person he can like. However, in both patterns— anonymity-of-all and the rare-approval-of-one—the common factor seems to be the focus on the "weaknesses of others." In the first instance, all individuals are disrespected, indeed often feared and held suspect. In the situation where one person who is liked seems to be accepted, this acceptance is followed by a search for the familiar—the ever-present weaknesses in others. Then when a so-called weakness is located, the patient can feel threatened, anxious, and thus can automatically keep his own familiar pathology going. It is as if he had a continuing need to see himself as powerless, mistrusting, lonely—to feel this familiar, accustomed self and to feel more lonely and more threatened at the thought of change, of seeing himself differently.

Difficulties related to making plans are also observable. Some patients hesitate, vacillate, and are indecisive, not knowing whether to continue living with marked planlessness or to use exaggerated overplanning in the hope of improving their pattern of living.

With *planlessness* it is as though life were viewed and lived as one continual accident, based upon an expectation that something is going to happen, sometime; the person responds automatically to minor details that actually do occur, but does nothing to prevent or produce them. He endures the "long, empty, time-crawling days," as one person described them, and never contemplates making any effort to change the situation.

On the other hand, *overplanning* may also be observed. It may involve making extensive lists of things to be done—letters to be written, shopping to be completed, or clothing to be packed. It is as if the patient couldn't remember to carry out even the basic functions of living without something tangible, like a list, to remind him of what to do and when to do it. Or he may feel the directionless drift of his living and set up projects and deadlines to be met in order to avoid feeling frantic about the emptiness and disorder which surround him. His reasons for wanting direction are obscure to the patient.

Occasionally, overplanning can be observed as an emphasis on personal dressing for social appearances. It is as if the patient were arranging a carefully guarded and rarely displayed picture of himself—the social self—to present to some potentially humiliating, disapproving spectator. Usually such great care in dress is in contrast to a more careless, casual daily appearance.

EFFORTS TO ESTABLISH CONTACT WITH OTHERS

To the lonely person, the opposite of loneliness—closeness and relatedness to people—always appears to hold potential threat. People—adults who did not respond to him when he was a child and then, later, his peers—have been a continual source of possible humiliation and therefore of anxiety. But he continues to make efforts, often dramatic ones, to have contact with adults—that is, the more mature persons in his psychosocial situation. These efforts, however, can suggest many pitfalls for nurses.

Efforts to establish contact or proximity can be complicated by an inclination toward *worshiping others.* As I have already pointed out, occasionally one person may be selected by the lonely individual and invested with all the potential qualities for meeting his so-far-unmet wishes and needs. This presents little difficulty if the "worshiped one" has the skill and training to understand the situation. If a nurse who does not have such training is selected, however, or if she needs this kind of interest from patients—perhaps on the basis of her own loneliness—then the patient will soon come to recognize and exploit this, unwittingly, and to the discomfort of the nurse. Worshiping others is very often an obligating maneuver; it is a way by which, in the long run, the patient gets attention on his terms; it is a subtle way of establishing nonrational dependence on another person.

I have noticed that lonely patients tend either to lump nurses together—viewing all nurses as identical—or to identify one nurse whom they establish as being "different, better than the others." Often the relationship with the latter nurse develops so that the patient comes to make more and more demands, as if to test the genuineness of her interest. These maneuvers are also a way for him to test whether he actually can incur her disapproval. Often the patient will go to almost any lengths to do this, as if to make open and apparent the very deeply felt need for disapproval which he has acquired. When the worshiped person does show marked disapproval, then the patient mobilizes his anxiety as anger or hatred, often taking active steps to cut himself off from the relationship. It is as if proof of the worshiped person's not caring has at last been secured, and further effort on the part of the patient is unnecessary. In this situation the lonely individual must have help if he is to do anything to prevent the destruction of the relationship; he cannot do it by himself. It is up to the nurse to recognize what is going on and to sustain the patient's struggle with the problem, so that both he and she can clearly understand it.

Another kind of effort which these patients make at establishing contact, particularly in relationships with nurses, can be termed *role-reversal* —with the patient taking on the role-actions of the nurse while the nurse takes on some of the role-actions of the patient. An example of this was a situation in which the nurse became ill while caring for a psychiatric patient at home and, instead of signing off the case, permitted the patient to take over her nursing care— bringing meals, watching over her while she slept, and the like.

The patient talked about the feeling of worth and strength which she associated with helping the sick nurse; the feeling of interest and well-being that came to her when the nurse discussed her own problems. This no doubt is less apt to become a problem in hospitals, because the hospital system has too many checks on the actions of individual nurses to allow much reversal of roles. In private practice, however, where the nurse and the patient are together for many hours, it is much more common to observe the patient questioning the nurse about her personal affairs. There is, of course, a point at which this becomes one way in which the patient seeks to validate what he is empathizing from the nurse—testing to see whether she really understands. But what we are referring to here is unwitting behavior on the nurse's part, in which she chats about herself in response to the patient's questioning.

When role-reversal occurs, it can sometimes be used to begin a new and more useful type of relationship. The skillful nurse can observe when the patient is purposefully shifting the focus from his needs to hers. She can be quite direct with patients, asking "Are you interested in switching the conversation to a discussion of my personal living?" Often, this type of comment may be needed when the patient becomes quite repetitious in asking about the nurse's food intake, the comfort offered by the chair or the room she is using, the temperature of the room, and so on. The patient often uses these diversionary conversations to find out whether the nurse's needs can supersede his own. When the nurse can demonstrate that she is well able to look after her own needs and can assist the patient to do likewise, then something favorable may happen in the nurse–patient relationship.

A third type of effort to secure the contact with nurses to avoid loneliness may be called *somatic participation* and is based on the expression of bodily needs. A hypersensitivity to noise or to stuffiness in a closed room may lead the patient to open and then to close the windows innumerable times in one day. Or he may make frequent requests for snacks between meals but beg off eating at mealtime. Or he may complain of pain in an arm, his head, his stomach, or any other organ that can be called into service to indicate the "pain of loneliness." Minor illnesses, such as colds and sprains, seem to occur just in time to bring contact, protection, and nurture. One patient phrased it directly, saying "I'm hungry but not for food. I don't know what I am hungry for." Vomiting and belching often occur when the patient perceives the nurse as rejecting him, lacking concern and interest; or they may occur as a way of demonstrating the desire to "get rid of" directions from others when the nurse has given the patient some advice.

The lonely patient often has great concern about strength, frequently expressing its absence in such ways as: "I feel I have no strength today," "the treatment weakens me—it takes a lot of strength," "I can't talk much today, I am too tired," or "I have to save up my strength today because I may go out tomorrow." This dwelling on the conservation of strength may indicate great fear of bankruptcy—powerlessness and feelings of failure—as the outcome of its use.

"Being well" may be equated with being active and good, as for example, "I'm all worn out, I wish I was better, I guess I am not good any more." The patient often requires and insists on a great deal of rest. This is a valid demand—it is well known that conflict can incur even more fatigue and exhaustion than physical exertion. It is easier, of course, to talk about the strength one lacks than to put it directly and talk about the weakness one feels.

AVOIDING THE PAIN OF LONELINESS

Several patients have discussed what they call their "low tolerance of pain." Their whole living pattern reflects the great care they exert to avoid risk of any further injury, humiliation, and pain. Their familiar patterns of living—even though they are pathological, nonproductive, and essentially self-destructive in the long run—

seem to carry less pain than new experiences do. A relationship to a nurse who is a mature person—and who is interested and able to help the patient look at peripheral expressions of deeper problems which require psychotherapeutic intervention—may well be a new and painful experience. The old patterns are better known and thus more comforting for the moment than new ones are.

One form of ineptness that stands out in lonely individuals is their inability to observe themselves in action. Even though they function more as spectators—watching, waiting, hoping—than as organizers of their life experiences, they protect themselves by not recognizing their own failures. They may work hard to offer plausible explanations for a particular pattern of action but they always seem to miss the obvious meaning of what they are saying. For instance, these comments which one patient made indicate how an obvious meaning may not be noticed: "I certainly can get myself sick in a million different places. You think this is bad—the last time I had four nurses. They were so good to me; they never left me alone. All kinds of attention I have to have—so much attention I think I must be a queen. What did I have to get sick for? Anytime anything happens in the family, anytime they look at me crooked, I get sick."

The basis of this problem—the individual's inability to see himself in action—lies in his distortion of the self-concept. The patient may be unable to see himself as a clearly defined entity, separate from his environment, just as a baby cannot differentiate himself from his surroundings. The baby sees the mother as part of himself; the lonely patient retains this illusion. For example, one patient repeatedly apologized when I dropped my notebook—as if we were so "attached" that she felt that she had dropped it and I was the observer.

The problem may also be based on the limitation of the patient's self-concept—his concept being too shallow to embrace the whole self and to discriminate the borders clearly. Along with this lack of self-definition go such general attitudes as worthlessness, powerlessness, and uselessness. Typical comments from these patients are: "Life doesn't mean anything," "I guess I have no use for myself," "I have such wonderful children but they have no use for me," or "There is nothing I can do."

In some situations, the patient's emphasis is on proving points—
mostly proving what is not true rather than indicating what he is
actually experiencing. It is as if he could ward off loneliness by
proving that he is not dependent on others. This seems inherent in
role-reversal—with the patient intuitively using the nurse to prove
himself independent, powerful, worth something. Every one of
these patients seems to have spent his whole life in activities calcu-
lated to prove the falsity of what is real—that he is a dependent
lonely individual who has missed some vital experiences in the
process of growing up.

Sullivan indicates that one outcome of arrest in a child's socializing process is the extensive effort that he must always make
thereafter to maintain distinctions between the real and the unreal, between the actual and the fantasied, between the experienced and the imagined. Sometimes the nature of a patient's
problems readily reveal this difficulty. For example, insomnia and
intense interest in sleeping are usually observed together. Sleep
symbolizes relief from loneliness; it is the one form of relief that
the patient can achieve alone—if he can get to sleep. When he
cannot, a longing for contact emerges and with it great anxiety
which, in turn, insures his keeping awake. The patient may try
sedation to get relief but sleep induced by sedation often brings
with it terrorizing dreams which may repeatedly spell out the
wish for closeness and interest from others.

We might speculate that loneliness is a *felt* component of a larger
problem—emptiness. Emptiness might well be an over-all concept
embracing a constellation of interrelated experiences. Emptiness
must be so devastating that no one actually can experience it—it is
nothingness, barrenness. Aspects of it can be observed, however,
in patients whose lives are barren of friends, who have sustained
no role in the world of work, and who have been unable to fill any
such social role as wife, husband, mother, friend, neighbor. The
fixed points in the patient's sphere are all things—money, prop-
erty, possessions—rather than persons. An ethical or philosophical frame of reference is lacking. As one patient put it, "There is no
one and nothing to tell." Eventually, the patient may even restrict
his movements to one room. He seems to feel tremendous need to
keep feelings in a "deep freeze." It is not possible to feel such total

emptiness; only the defenses against its variations—of which lone-liness is one—can be endured.

Some lonely patients seem to have made early efforts to ward off the evolving pathology of loneliness. They have tried to fore-stall the consequences by substituting non-personalized transac-tions with knowledge, or with things, for relations with people. Reading copiously is one way of reducing autistic—or overly sub-jective and unreal—thinking; it is one way to "fill up" with the least risk of humiliation, failure, and disapproval. One patient recalled this when he said, "In college I think I felt that I was leading a life quite alone. I didn't have anyone to discuss anything with. I hated my teachers and the subjects but this didn't interest the family. They were like dead weight and I was in a hurry to get a degree. I wanted to compel my family to be interested. They encouraged the idea of college but they didn't encourage me."

THE NURSING CARE OF LONELY PATIENTS

The care of lonely patients requires the nurse to understand the generic development of the problem, its variations in the clinical situation, and its relation to the social structure of the ward situa-tion. Riesman explores some of the shifting elements in our social structure which drive the individual to desperate pursuits as a "lonely member of a crowd" (Riesman, 1950). He points out that the present generation is different from earlier ones in one important respect. The modes of conformity that individuals use and the qualities of feeling they have are developed in response to the evaluations of their peers rather than to concepts of authority which they acquired in the mother-child relationship. The earlier generation placed less emphasis on the individual's identification with a group, so the individual experienced loneliness more in relation to "internalized or illusory figures" than to his peers. The individual's relationships with his peers and their evaluations play a very large part in contemporary loneliness, however. Yet the need to conform, to be like others, to distort and destroy or deny human differences is one of the leveling factors in both generations, and therefore it is a basic factor in loneliness. The hope of autonomy, of self-directed constructive use of capacities, lies beyond conformity. The realization of this hope is impeded for the earlier generation by internalized authority figures; for the present generation, it is obstructed by the need for status and approval in the peer group.

When a patient in a hospital has the underlying problem of loneliness, he tends to think of his fellow patients as his peers. Each patient, being more or less trapped by a need to belong, tends to form relationships with other patients. These relationships are based on "mutual loneliness"—pathological pull of the familiar—rather than on conscious choice. Caudill reports findings regarding the structure of closely knit groups of patients and its effect upon them (Caudill, 1953; Caudill et al., 1952; Caudill & Stainbrook, 1954). We are greatly in need of data to help us determine whether nurses could render these situations more favorable for patients' emotional growth.

In private practice, where the patient does not have a peer group available to him, dependence on the nurse develops quickly. This dependence can have the qualities of a mother-child relationship or of a peer relationship. Since loneliness implies an early developmental arrest, dependence is to be expected and accepted, and the patient should be helped to use it as a step toward independence and interdependence.

It is useful to specify the limits of the relationship. A clear statement of fixed points helps the patient to recognize the necessary boundaries of a useful relationship. These limits need to be specific and to be stated simply, and they need to be adhered to because the patient will test them over and over again to check and recheck the sincerity, honesty, and integrity of the nurse.

In addition to providing contact and constant limits, each nurse ought to be able to offer the patient a procedure for working on the problems that arise in relation to the nursing situation. The nurse who spends eight hours with a patient will hear a good deal about his difficulties, hopes, and dreams. She cannot sit silently without responding in a human way. Her responses to the patient, verbal and otherwise, will therefore have a great deal to do with the alleviation or intensification of his problems. Procedure cannot be discussed adequately in a paper of this length, but I can say that there are opportunities to give constructive help to patients in all that goes on in a nursing situation: in the management of the situation; in the use of such customary nursing activities as bathing, feeding, dressing, and the like; in such socializing activities as conversing, card-playing, and the like; and in the therapeutic handling of terror, desperation, nightmares, hallucinations, and so on.

An understanding of the problem of loneliness suggests that what the patient needs is:

1. To experience and, therefore, to come to feel and know the active interest of mature persons and their attentive participation in his activities.

2. To secure the assistance of persons who are more mature and skillful than he is as he learns how to struggle with his problems.

3. To have a variety of opportunities to describe, interpret, and validate what is happening to him in a current situation.

4. To have contact with persons who can help him get in touch with other human beings, feel related to them, and work collaboratively and live productively with them.

REFERENCES

Barnes, D. (1937). *Nightwood.* New York: Harcourt, Brace.

Caudill, W. (1953). Applied anthropology in medicine. In A. L. Kroeber (Ed.), *Anthropology today* (pp. 771–806). Chicago: University of Chicago Press.

Caudill, W., Redlich, F. C., Gilmore, H. R., & Brody, E. B. (1952). Social structure and interaction processes on a psychiatric ward. *American Journal of Orthopsychiatry, 22,* 314–334.

Caudill, W., & Stainbrook, E. (1954). Some covert effects of communication difficulties in a psychiatric hospital. *Psychiatry, 17,* 27–43.

Fromm, E. (1955). *The sane society.* New York: Holt, Rinehart, & Winston.

Parsons, T. (1951). *The social system.* Chicago: Free Press.

Riesman, D., Glazer, N., & Denny, R. (1950). *The lonely crowd: A study of the changing American character.* New Haven: Yale University Press.

Roth, L. (1954). *I'll cry tomorrow.* New York: Fell.

Ruesch, J., & Bateson, G. (1951). *Communication: The social matrix of psychiatry.* New York: Norton.

Sullivan, H. S. (1953). H. S. Perry & M. L. Gawel (Eds.) In *The interpersonal theory of psychiatry.* New York: Norton.

CHAPTER 20

Theoretical Constructs: Anxiety, Self, and Hallucinations

In this paper, three key constructs—anxiety, self, and hallucinations—are explored within the theoretical framework of interpersonal relations (Peplau, 1987). Connections among these concepts are shown. Applications to clinical practice of nurses in psychiatric hospitals are described. These concepts pertain to phenomena commonly observed by nurses during their relationships with psychiatric patients. The nursing practices that psychiatric nurses provide are more likely to be remedial in intent and outcome when guided by theory.

BACKGROUND

Definition of Nursing

The definition of nursing that pinpoints the work of nurses and underlies this presentation is: "the diagnosis and treatment of

Original title: "Interpersonal Relations: Theoretical Constructs and Applications in Psychiatric Nursing Practice." Chapter 6 in Cormack, D. & Reynolds, W. (Eds.). (in press). *Psychiatric and Mental Health Nursing: Theory and Practice.* London: Chapman & Hall. Reprinted by permission of the publisher.

human responses to actual and potential health problems" (American Nurses Association, 1980). Thus, the emphasis is on problematic, psychosocial, behavioral, human responses of patients rather than on diagnostic categories of mental illness that are diagnosed and treated by psychiatrists. The theoretical concepts presented in this chapter refer to human responses of psychiatric patients that arise in day-to-day nurse–patient relationships, and that call for responsible, helpful nursing actions.

The Nursing and Medical Professions

Psychiatric nursing is different from psychiatry. Both are branches of their respective professions. Although both professions share the common mission of promoting health and work collaboratively toward its achievement, each profession has a separate sphere of responsibility. The definition of nursing provides the focus of the nursing profession's work and the area of the expertise of nurses.

Psychiatric nurses have as a *primary* responsibility nurturing and aiding psychiatric patients in their personal development through nursing services. The public expects psychiatric nurses to understand the human responses of psychiatric patients and to use nursing practices that will help guide patients in the direction of understanding and resolving their human dilemmas. Nursing research, concerning the nature of those human responses that are within the purview of nursing, provides theoretical constructs nurses use to guide their observations, inferences, and practices.

Psychiatric nurses also have *secondary* responsibilities that include cooperative work with physicians who prescribe psychiatric treatments for patients. Nurses voluntarily assist in the work of psychiatrists. For example, nurses assist in carrying out various medical procedures; they give medications, monitor reactions, record effects, and recommend adjustments in drug dosages; they discuss cases, share data, and plan together so that the patient's total program makes sense and is as constructive as possible. Nurses know that in addition to human responses, there are physiological and biochemical reactions that occur automatically, for example, when a patient experiences pervasive, recurring anxiety or terror. The medical treatments of these reactions by giving various pharmaceuticals, electroshock, or other treatments prescribed by psychiatrists are not included in the discussions that follow.

About Theory for Nursing Practice

It is the contention in this chapter that each profession selects and defines its theoretical constructs in ways most relevant for that profession's work, using the best available scientific knowledge. In nursing, that knowledge is obtained from two sources: (1) from nursing research, both empirical (clinical) and controlled; and (2) from the research findings published by all other basic and applied sciences.

Knowledge selected from these two sources comes in the form of facts, principles, concepts, processes, models, general information, and the like. All these forms assist nurses to know as much as possible about the particular phenomena within the scope of their clinical work. For application of theory in direct clinical practice, however, at least for novices in the profession, a particular format seems useful.

The three theoretical concepts in this paper are described. They are also shown in a serial order format that indicates two sequences: (1) the consecutive order in which the essential characteristics of the phenomenon occur, and (2) the sequence of nursing actions addressed to the various steps in the emergence of the phenomenon. Of necessity, these are sometimes two different sequential orders. The three constructs and suggested nursing practices were drawn from clinical data and scientific literature and were tested, clinically, by many nurses for several decades. Nevertheless, the reader is strongly advised to learn the concepts and personally test them for effectiveness by reflection on personal experience and in clinical nursing of psychiatric patients.

Interpersonal Relations: The Theoretical Framework

Theory of interpersonal relations is of particular significance to nursing practice. Sullivan (1956) defined this framework as the study of what goes on between two or more people, all but one of whom may be completely illusory. Hallucinations, in this context, are to be viewed as interpersonal interactions between a real person and one or more illusory figures. Moreover, because nursing actions have consequences for patients, especially in terms of their impact on presenting psychopathology, nurses have a responsibility to study what goes on in their nurse–patient relationships. The results of such continuing study and the application of theory during practice afford choice rather than unwitting or "routine" nurse responses during interactions with patients.

Nurses lay claim to around-the-clock nursing care of inpatients. Their interactions with patients tend to occur with greater frequency, are of longer duration, and have more continuity than is true of the relationships patients have with all other health professionals. The potential is great for therapeutic benefits, as well as for illness-maintenance (Peplau, 1978). Interpersonal relations theories throw light on the quality of interactions (Peplau, 1988). Applications of interpersonal constructs enable nurses to become aware of, reflect on, and consider the possible consequences of the quality of their participation in nurse–patient relationships (Peplau, 1987). Thus, nurses gain a basis for choosing the behaviors they will use with patients in subsequent day-to-day interactions.

Uses of Concepts and Information in Practice

Theoretical constructs are among the major tools psychiatric nurses use during their work. At their best, such constructs describe and explain the origins and nature of the phenomenon or phenomena to which they pertain. Concepts also assist in making observations, by providing a general name under which certain raw data that have been noticed can, at least temporarily, be classified. For instance, on observing restless pacing in a patient, the application of the concept of anxiety would be considered. Concepts assist in making assessments, in that they supply, in their definition, cues to what to look for or to inquire about. The subsequent nurse observations or patient descriptions provide data to confirm or disconfirm to the nurse the appropriateness of the particular concept chosen for use at that time. Nursing diagnoses of the human responses (needs, problems, dilemmas, etc.) of patients are also concepts. The current trend in this within-profession development is to identify, name, and describe indicators for each diagnostic category (Kim, McFarland, & McLane, 1987). Theoretical concepts used to define a phenomenon can also be used to infer and design the nursing actions most likely to be corrective, remedial, or preventive of that phenomenon. Concepts are also used in planning nursing care, both the plan and the relevant constructs being further used in periodic and final evaluation of outcomes of nursing care for particular patients.

In addition to theoretical concepts, nurses need information. Effective nursing care is dependent on nurses having maximum information about patients, which requires that nurses have full access to case history data contained in the hospital record, treating it with professional confidentiality. Additionally, a nursing history should be obtained. This instrument is constructed to obtain data directly pertinent to nursing's focus, as specified in the definition of nursing and amplified in a taxonomy of nursing diagnoses (Gordon, 1985; McLane, 1987). This information provides background data, facts that supply a context for inquiring about the life of the patient. These facts inform the nurse; however, if supplied by informants other than the patient, they may not be wholly accurate.

Theoretical constructs, diagnostic terms, and life-history information are sometimes misused by professionals to the detriment of patients. The purposes of these data are to instruct and guide the private, professional, and intellectual activity of nurses in determining the nature of dilemmas patients present to them, and in choosing the therapeutic work that is necessary. Theoretical terms, diagnoses, and case history data are not labels or information to be used to intimidate, browbeat, stigmatize or label patients.

The tendency of all human beings is to seek explanations for their troubling experiences. Such explanations, however accurate or inaccurate, provide a modicum of comfort; at last the dilemma has a name or a reason for it. Research suggests that people are more "curious about causality when something unexpected or unusual happens" (Sears, Peplau, Freedman, & Taylor, 1988, p. 121). Psychiatric patients are not exceptions in this matter. For them, explanations for their dilemmas given to them are often heard as epithets, and they prematurely close off further work, which psychiatric patients must do in order to move toward and eventually achieve in order to understand and resolve their difficulties.

The Nurse–Patient Dialogue

Psychiatric nursing practices are primarily verbal. They consist mainly in talking with patients informally or in scheduled individual, group, or family interview sessions. Talking that occurs during these nurse–patient interactions serves such purposes as therapeutic work, teaching, planning, or review of patient programs or schedules, as well as planning for discharge from hospital. All contacts nurses have with patients are potential learning experiences for both parties: Nurses enrich and refine their expertise, and patients expand and improve their competencies and their self-knowledge. In this sense, nursing care of psychiatric patients can be viewed as the provision of highly specialized learning events, in the verbal mode, that in a very personal way are educative for patients.

Psychiatric patients are embarked on a search for truth about themselves and their life experiences. This search is *not* for the literal, factual truths but rather for the inner truths about their perceptions and attributions of their experiences and the consequences in relationships with people. The term *attributions* refers to "the process by which people arrive at causal explanations for events in the social world, particularly for actions they and other people perform" (Sears et al., 1988, p. 117). Attributions about past events tend to influence expectations related to present and future events, and they also determine feelings, attitudes, and behaviors.

Psychiatric patients are lacking in the intellectual and interpersonal competencies so necessary for the work involved in their search for self-understanding. It is the quality of the verbal participation of nurses in their interactions with patients—listening and posing investigative questions—that slowly but surely stimulates the development of these competencies in patients (Field, 1979). Competencies develop when latent capacities are used by patients. Tapping into and thereby forcing patients to use these capacities is an aim of nurses when talking with patients.

Talking with patients in a professional mode is substantially different from customary social conversations, such as a nurse might have with personal family members or friends (Peplau,

1964). Nurse–patient discourse has as its purpose aiding a patient to gain the self-understanding and competencies required for living in the community outside the hospital. Therefore, the focus is one way, on the needs, concerns, and experiences of the patient; in friend-to-friend relationships the focus is reciprocal, on the needs of both parties. Considerable self-discipline is required of nurses in order for them to accomplish a shift from a customary social mode of talking to a professional stance.

Nurses are sometimes reluctant to seek maximum information from patients for use within the nurse–patient dialogue. They consider this to be prying, which it would be in social situations with friends. Nurses have often been advised to be subtle and indirect in talking with psychiatric patients, who already have problems with ambiguity and lack of forthrightness in interpersonal situations. It is more useful when nurses are open, clear, simple, forthright, and direct with patients without being directive, autocratic, and controlling.

Work of nurses with patients proceeds on the basis of information made available by the patient during nurse–patient relationships. In this regard, a *general principle* applies: Anything that is going on, or that has occurred in the life of a patient, can be talked about openly and fully, reviewed, eventually understood, and then filed in the backlog among the patient's other past experiences. Conversely, anything that is not talked about and is instead merely acted out is not likely to be understood by a patient. This principle suggests, for example, that when patients act out aggression the most constructive nursing interventions are: (1) Stop the aggressive action; and (2) immediately sit down with the patient and require discussion of what went on by asking, "What was that all about?" With patients who are withdrawn, isolating themselves from others in the inpatient hospital unit, the principle suggests that periodically, every day, a nurse should be assigned to sit down next to the withdrawn patient. The nurse might initiate talking by saying: "I have a half hour to talk with you," and then wait for a response. Later on, the nurse might ask: "What are you thinking? Say your thoughts out loud." When the promised time period is up, the nurse announces her departure and says when another half hour of nursing time will be provided. Eventually, as the nurse's presence becomes familiar and expected, withdrawn patients will begin to talk, but they very rarely initiate such effort. In other words, from the moment of admission to the hospital the entire nursing staff ought to build in the expectation that patients are there to resolve their problems, which requires talking about their experiences, the nurse listening and being helpful as patients do their work.

Giving advice to patients is not what is being suggested here. To give advice is, in effect, to tell other persons how to live their own lives and is rarely welcomed or used. It can be assumed that psychiatric patients have already been given much advice and to no avail. Nurses who are overeager in giving advice serve as reminders to patients of previously ineffectual advice givers who most often were figures of authority.

Listening to patients attentively, all the while being intellectually active and considering privately which theoretical constructs help the nurse to grasp the import of what a patient is saying, and then posing a question that furthers the patient's effort, is the nurse's work. However, words used in the nurse's questions do not magically produce constructive changes in psychiatric patients. Verbal interventions of nurses, intended to be corrective of the observed like-kind phenomena to which they are applied, must be repeated, sustained over time during recurring contacts with a given patient. In some instances considerable periods of time may be involved, thereby testing a nurse's patience and resolve. Furthermore, repetition can become monotonous for nurses, if not annoying for patients. Ingenuity, imagination, and flexibility in the use of words and their synonyms is indicated. The *general principle* is: Vary the language but sustain the intended message. In this regard, a very useful exercise to illustrate the principle particularly for nursing students is to have them prepare a written list of all the different ways to ask a patient, "Are you anxious?"

The questions that nurses pose to patients serve the purpose of investigation, aiding patients in their search for self-knowledge. Questions that begin with *who, when,* or *what* are to be preferred; *why* is an intimidating word in that it assumes that patients have reasons for their actions or experiences rather than being engaged in a search for them. The term *can you* questions a patient's ability to respond; *will you* suggests the possibility of willful stubbornness if the patient does not respond. The point being made here is that the language of the nurse conveys meaning, and all too often patients are sensitively tuned to nuances of language, which they hear as references to them personally.

It is quite useful for nurses, particularly nursing students, to record on audiotape several sessions in which they talk with psychiatric inpatients. Review of these tapes afterwards provides an opportunity for nurses to hear and become aware of their habits of speech, and to consider the short-term and long-term impact of their words on the perceptions of patients. Exercises such as these provide a basis for nurses to begin to shift their mode of language usage from a social to professional mode, and therefore to begin to audit and edit their verbalizations during nurse–patient dialogues.

The verbal nursing actions suggested later in this chapter are primarily investigative. They are used to encourage the patient to do the problem-solving work in order to move toward resolution of difficulties in living with people in the community, outside of the hospital. The assumption is that the patient, and only the patient, has the data concerning his or her dilemmas. What the patient does not have is access to this data, nor methods for reviewing and making sense of it. Therefore, most psychiatric patients cannot extricate themselves from their difficulties without professional help. The professional nursing assistance to patients proposed in this chapter helps patients investigate their circumstances and gain both new perspective and interpersonal competencies resulting from that effort. Two major instruments nurses use in this work are verbal facility and theoretical constructs that explain the phenomena problematic to the patient.

ANXIETY

The twentieth century is often called "the age of anxiety." The history of anxiety as a human experience is much longer. A recent publication devotes an entire chapter to anxiety as experienced by Calvin throughout his life in the sixteenth century (Bouwsma, 1988). Calvin recognized anxiety, his own and that of others, as a human condition. He discussed it often, and the energy anxiety provided was a driving force in his lifelong productivity as a religious reformer.

During the decade of the 1970s considerable research related to anxiety was conducted as reported in a conference report (Tuma & Maser, 1985). This publication raises important unresolved issues: What is the relation between fear and anxiety? Are there differences in the quantity and quality of general versus pathological anxiety? Does anxiety occur along a continuum or does a discontinuity paradigm pertain, panic being a unique episode rather than the extreme end of a continuum of anxiety? While the papers in the Tuma and Maser publication (1985) point to some areas of consensus, taken as a whole they suggest that theories explanatory of anxiety are as yet far from reliable and valid and that much more research into the nature of anxiety is urgently needed.

Laypersons and professionals often use the same terms but in different ways. Commonly, the laity use the word *anxious* when *eager* is what is intended. *Panic* is a lay term to indicate being *jittery* or *nervous*. A characteristic of professionalism is precise definition of constructs that refer to phenomena within the purview of work of the profession and from which remedial interventions can be derived.

General Characteristics

Anxiety is a universal phenomenon. Everyone experiences the discomfort of anxiety in some degree at some time throughout life. As a universal experience there are some general characteristics of anxiety that apply in all cases.

Anxiety is a subjective, affective experience; it is *felt* as an unpleasant uneasiness, as apprehension, dread or uncanny sensation.

Anxiety is an *energy,* and therefore it cannot be observed directly; what can be noticed are the effects of anxiety—the transformations of the energy into physiological reactions and behavioral responses that are the clues to the presence of anxiety.

Anxiety is *triggered cognitively* by an input of real or imagined, internal or external, personal or situational information perceived as a threat to one's status or prestige or to attributions, beliefs, and expectations about oneself and one's world. Anxiety can also be triggered when a person feels the anxiety another person in the same situation is then experiencing; this transmission occurs by way of *empathic observation,* the ability to feel in oneself the emotions of another person during an interpersonal relationship.

Anxiety triggers an *immediate physiological reaction,* automatically, as evidenced by increased heart rate, sweating, trembling, irritability, vertigo, and so forth. It may trigger a sense of foreboding, uncertainty about what might happen, anticipation of loss of control, or an inability to cope or to survive.

There is an *awareness* of apprehension, felt discomfort, and of physiological reactions; but most often there is *unawareness* of and/or inability to formulate and verbalize the precise nature of the triggering cognitive input.

Anxiety is *adaptive* in that it serves as a warning signal of impending threat to the organism's survival, particularly to the survival of the self-system. An immediate human response (other than physiological reaction, which is automatic) is required to reinstate comfort and ensure survival. In this discussion these responses are called *relief behaviors.* The intention of relief behaviors is to reduce, relieve, and to prevent escalation of anxiety. Psychiatric inpatients have many relief behaviors that are used automatically, without conscious thought.

Anxiety occurs in *different degrees,* ranging from mild, to moderate, to severe, and to panic (terror, horror, awe, dread, uncanny sensation); escalation from lesser to greater degrees of anxiety can occur when the anxious person empathizes with the anxiety of another or other persons in the same situation, and/or when the relief behaviors employed fail to work as intended.

There may be a *predisposition* to anxiety within particular families.

The foregoing universal characteristics of anxiety include those common elements, regularities that occur across cases irrespective of ethnic and cultural factors. These latter factors and the particulars of a person's experience of anxiety, are inherent in the style, content, or behavioral acts illustrative of patterns of relief behavior. The personal characteristics are also intrinsic to descriptions of the experience given by patients.

Definition of Anxiety as a Clinical Construct

The essence of anxiety, abstracted from the foregoing general features, and confirmed in empirical-clinical psychiatric nursing research, has been formulated into a theoretical construct of this phenomenon (See Table 20.1). Nurses need to know the universal characteristics, as many facts and as much information as they can obtain about anxiety as a human condition. However, for purposes of application during nurse–patient relationships, a succinct, practically oriented, easy-to-recall, theoretical construct is required.

The concept definition in Table 20.1 asserts that anxiety is triggered when *expectations* that are operative, up front in mind, with or

TABLE 20.1 A Concept of Anxiety

Definition: Sequence of steps in development of anxiety	Information needed to understand a person's experience of anxiety
1. *Expectations* are held, up front, in mind.	What expectations? Origins? How long held? How important? Can they be changed or given up? Was the expectation reasonable—capable of fulfillment?
2. *Expectations* held are *not* met.	What interfered? What happened instead? Who was to meet the expectation, when, how, what evidence?
3. *Discomfort* is felt.	Experienced in what part of the body? What degree? What was noticed by patient?
4. *Relief behaviors* are used.	What behavioral act or acts related to what pattern?
5. The relief behaviors are *justified* and rationalized.	

without the full awareness of the person, in a given situation, are *not met*. *Felt discomfort* is followed almost immediately by behavioral acts that provide *relief*, by reducing or preventing more anxiety, and that subsequently are justified or rationalized. The essentials in this concept, to be recalled and applied in clinical practice, albeit in a different order as shown in Table 20.2, are italicized.

The term *expectations* is a general classification that includes such similar but not identical cognitions as assumptions, preconceptions, attributions, wishes, wants, beliefs, values, hopes, desires, needs, goals, self-views, and the like. The term *expectations* simplifies the nurse's conceptual task of recalling one overall

TABLE 20.2 Concept Application in Psychiatric Nursing Practice[a]

Nursing aim	Nursing verbal interventions[b]
3. Get the operative expectations formulated and stated by patient.	3. After the patient is clearly aware of the relation between 1 and 2 below, then ask, "What were you thinking about *before* you felt upset?"
4. Get a formulation and recognition of the connection between expectations held and what happened instead.	4. When the patient has clearly formulated an expectation, then ask: "What happened instead?"
5. Consider which factors in the sequence are amenable to control.	5. Then discuss what change in 3 or 4 above might be possible.
1. Get patient to become aware of and name anxiety.	1. Ask the patient: "Are you anxious?" "Are you nervous?" "Are you upset?" "Are you tense now?"
2. Get the patient to become aware of and state the connection between the named anxiety and the behavior used to relieve it.	2. When a yes answer has been obtained to 1, ask the patient: "What are you doing now to relieve being nervous?"

[a]Note that the sequence of steps here is different from those in the definition in Table 20.1.
[b]Vary the language but not the message.

rubric during clinical work. The following examples illustrate aspects of the essentials that define the concept:

A person assumes that the earth will remain firm; suddenly, unexpectedly, an earthquake occurs; immediately the individual is awash with terror.

A patient feels a pressing need for a show of affection from her mother, who heretofore has demonstrated a remarkable inability to express love to her daughter; the daughter telephones her mother thinking, "This time she will be nice to me." On answering the phone, the mother berates her daughter for this interruption in her day; the daughter cries, feels helpless, and berates herself for bothering her mother.

A psychiatric patient who has a very beautiful face claims loudly and frequently that she is "ugly." Nursing personnel counter and rebut the patient's operative self-view and tell her, "No, you are so beautiful," or "I wish I had your lovely face." The patient, using a razor blade, slashes her face, which both confirms the operative self-view by the effect of this action and relieves the anxiety evoked by the unmet expectation.

In therapy, a patient, with a rush of feelings of anger and rage, tells the therapist, "My father hated me; my mother couldn't stand me; my sister was always disgusted with me; all my life nobody loved me." The therapist then said, "Well, I love you," at which point panic ensued; the patient ran through the unit screaming, smashing furniture, and finally was restrained, taken to a closed unit and put into a seclusion room.

Not all unmet expectations lead to crippling anxiety. The energy of mild degrees of anxiety may rapidly be converted into disappointment, providing sufficient relief as well as a clear understanding of the expectations that were not realized. The use of annoyance and anger, in similar fashion, as energy transformations that afford relief is quite common. However, "apparently" minor incidents, often involving only marginal awareness of the operative expectations, do sometimes produce quite severe anxiety (see Table 20.3).

TABLE 20.3 Degrees of Anxiety

Degree of anxiety	Effects on perceptual field and on ability to focus attention	Observable behavior
+ Mild	Perceptual field widens slightly. Able to observe more than before and to see relations (make connection among data).	Aware, alerted, sees, hears and grasps more than before. Usually able to recognize and name anxiety easily.
++ Moderate	Perceptual field narrows slightly. Selective inattention: does not notice what goes on peripheral to the immediate focus but can do so if attention is directed there by another observer.	Sees, hears, and grasps less than previously. Can attend to more if directed to do so. Able to sustain attention on a particular focus; selectively inattends to contents outside the focal area. Usually able to state "I am anxious now."
+++ Severe	Perceptual field is greatly reduced. Tendency toward dissociation: to not notice what is going on outside the current reduced focus of attention; largely unable to do so when another observer suggests it.	Sees, hears, and grasps far less than previously. Attention is focused on a small area of a given event. Inferences drawn may be distorted due to inadequacy of observed data. May be unaware of and unable to name anxiety. Relief behaviors generally used.
++++ Panic (Terror, horror, dread, uncanniness, awe).	Perceptual field is reduced to a detail, which is usually "blown up," i.e., elaborated by distortion (exaggeration), or the focus is on scattered details the speed of the scattering tends to increase. Massive dissociation especially of contents of self-system. Felt as enormous threat to survival.	Says, "I'm in a million pieces," "I'm gone," "What is happening to me?" Perplexity, self-absorption. Feelings of unreality. "Flights of ideas" or confusion. Fear. Repeats a detail. Many relief behaviors used automatically (without thought). The enormous energy produced by panic must be used and may be mobilized as rage. May pace, run or fight violently. With dissociation of contents of self-system, there may be very rapid reorganization of the self usually along pathological lines, e.g., a "psychotic break" is usually preceded by panic.

The expectations a person holds at any given time may be unmet for many reasons. External circumstances may change suddenly, as in earthquakes, tornadoes, fires, car accidents, or sudden death of a family member. An individual may hold expectations that, for their realization, involve competencies or capacities that he or she is lacking. Psychiatric patients particularly have sets of nonrational expectations of which they are largely unaware, which nevertheless gain expression in their behavior. Expectations are personal, situational, and sociocultural, or mixtures of these. Although hospital personnel can make guesses as to what expectations are held by particular patients, the accuracy of these estimates is debatable until a patient becomes aware of, formulates, and expresses his or her own experiences. Some of these patient formulations may validate the guesses that staff have made.

The discomfort of anxiety is *felt* in some part of the body, as are physiological effects. The extent of the discomfort is dependent on the degree of anxiety. Where the discomfort is felt can only be determined by asking the patient. Some patients feel the discomfort in their "gut," others in their genitals; some complain of "feeling funny" in the head or of blurred vision. Psychiatric patients tend not to connect these felt discomforts with being anxious. Similarly, the automatic physiological reactions, which are both felt and observable, are sometimes misnamed by the sufferer as a medical problem.

For example, with severe anxiety or panic there is a sudden rush of adrenalin-related chemicals into the body accompanied immediately and automatically by various physiological reactions. Increased heart rate, felt constriction in the chest or throat, sudden dryness of the mouth, flushing and sweating, trembling of hands and legs, and dizziness are among the more common physical reactions. Panic can be felt as "a blow on the head." Severe anxiety may precipitate urinary urgency or activities involving the genitals—or an organic like mental confusion can be experienced. These physiological effects are not specific for anxiety but may also be early warnings or symptoms of various diseases such as heart disease, stroke, or diabetes. On those occasions when heart attacks and panic occur simultaneously, the general nursing background of psychiatric nurses informs their observations in this matter.

The definition of anxiety indicates that the energy of anxiety, signalled as discomfort, is more or less immediately transformed into behaviors that are intended to reduce, relieve, or prevent more anxiety. In most textbooks, these behaviors are called *defense mechanisms* or *coping behaviors*; in this paper the term *relief behaviors* is used because this designation pinpoints the functions served by the energy transformations. Psychiatric nurses who have witnessed sudden rage and violence of patients need to recognize that severe anxiety or panic are antecedents of these relief-giving outbursts. The rage and violence simultaneously relieve the antecedent anxiety, whereas the staff response may evoke more terror.

Patterns of relief behavior sort into at least three different major areas. (1) *Psychiatric* classification categories; this includes such diagnoses as neuroses, psychoses, and antisocial acting-out. (2) *Psychosomatic* complaints, in which the body as a whole, a body part, or an organ are used to transform the energy of anxiety into expression of symptoms of a physical illness, perhaps as a symbolic expression of a personal dilemma. Commonly, there are one or more complaints of physical dysfunction for which no hard evidence obtains after thorough medical investigation. (3) Generating *learning* products, by using the energy of anxiety in examining anxiety-evoking experiences in order to learn from them. This means being aware of and recognizing anxiety when it occurs, being willing and able to manage the discomfort while transforming the energy into actions and use of resources, as required, for investigation of the personal and situational antecedents of anxiety (Peplau, 1963a). Performing artists have long known that the energy of their preperformance anxiety, if sustained and not masked or blotted out by some immediate relief-giving action, can be used to heighten their sensitivity and thereby enhance their artistic performance.

Adaptation and Learning

The first two areas—psychiatric and psychosomatic—cover adaptive responses; the third area has to do with learning. Adaptation and learning are two different human processes that persons employ when coping with the inevitable dilemmas of living. Synonyms for *adaptation* are to *adjust*, to *fit*, to *conform* to environmental conditions or to new stimuli. The physiological reactions to anxiety—signals warning of a threat to survival—are immediate, automatic, and adaptive. *Learning* is variously defined in the literature. For the purposes of psychiatric nursing practice the common meaning of this term is most useful. The synonyms for learning generally include to *find out about,* to *ascertain,* to *study* and to *obtain knowledge or skill,* and to *gain understanding by investigation.* The descriptors of these terms define two processes that have significant differences. They differ in the extent of the cognitive effort employed, in the patterning of energy transformation, and in the immediacy or delay in gaining relief from anxiety. Anxiety influences both processes. It supplies energy, the quantity being dependent upon the degree of anxiety that occurs. That energy must be and is transformed, either rapidly, into adaptive behaviors providing immediate relief, or more slowly, into cognitive, problem-solving behaviors; the discomfort of anxiety is sustained during a search for necessary information and until the learning products obtain and eventually provide relief.

It is instructive to notice how quickly psychiatric inpatients adapt to institutional requirements of them. The position taken in this chapter is that psychiatric hospitals ought to be seen as special educational institutions that provide personalized programs of educative events so that patients learn about themselves and gain enduring competencies for social living.

Relief Behaviors of Psychiatric Patients

Anxiety is not in and of itself pathological. Symptoms connected with pathology that is called mental illness are evolved, initially, as coping behaviors. These often are, at first, actions taken consciously in anxiety-laden situations perceived as threatening to the self-system. Persons who experience anxiety, particularly in a severe degree—either their own or the anxiety of others with whom they empathize—tend toward avoidance. They move away from people and out of situations that seem to evoke anxiety. This is an adaptive reaction.

For example, withdrawal, a common pattern of behavior observable in psychiatric inpatients, is at first a conscious decision an individual makes to remove himself or herself physically from an anxiety-provoking situation. Such behaviors are effective in terms of relief from anxiety. However, and especially in persons who are psychologically vulnerable in ways other than recurring anxiety, such behaviors tend to become ineffective for problem solving and learning. If, for instance, withdrawal is used repeatedly as a coping behavior, then the problem solving that is attempted during withdrawal becomes a highly private matter. It consists of autistic rumination about anxiety-laden experiences in which the individual not only has control over determining all dimensions of those experiences, but also has the control under the condition of the limiting effects of anxiety, on limited observation of what occurred during those events. The tendency is toward distortion of what was noticed, in the direction of self-interest and need. Moreover, the individual's perceptions and conclusions are unchecked, unverified, and unvalidated by discussion with another observer. The withdrawal, rumination, control, and distortion serve, unknowingly, to relieve the discomfort of anxiety, which, incidentally, is the unwitting immediate aim of the withdrawn individual. What goes on during withdrawal is more significant than is the pattern per se.

Withdrawal and other such behaviors are called *relief behaviors* because of their overriding purpose. The term is in keeping with the interpersonal theoretical framework. In an intrapersonal framework, such as that of Freud and others, these phenomena are called *mechanisms of defense*. Relief behaviors have three main characteristics: (1) they have overall patterns, (2) they are involuntary, and (3) they fail to work at some point.

OVERALL PATTERNS

Overall patterns occur, each pattern having many separate acts containing the same theme as in the pattern. For example, although withdrawal is one pattern, there are many ways to withdraw. Often there is a sequence of separate acts sometimes used in a particular serial order. When one action is challenged, another will go into play. For example, a patient does not answer a question of a staff member who comments on that; the patient does not respond to the comment and looks away, then moves out of the situation—and then isolates himself or herself from others as totally as possible. Psychiatric patients tend to have fewer patterns of behavior than do healthy persons. In repetitive monotony, most mentally ill patients tend to go around and around a circle of many acts related to few behavioral patterns. One patient, on recognizing it after considerable therapy, called this her "trapadaptation," a very apt neologism.

Virtually any behavioral act can be used for giving relief. Consider the commonplace: "I'm sorry." At first the phrase was acquired consciously, usually in childhood with prompting from adults. Then it becomes an automatic relief-giving verbalism used in many later situations in which anxiety is evoked when inadvertently, unexpectedly giving offense or injury to another person in a social situation. The phrase, once uttered, provides relief and closes off inquiry into the circumstances. At the other extreme, a delusion serves similar purposes. A *delusion* is an inadequate conclusion, inferred from insufficient data about an event observed and experienced under the conditions of panic, which at that time provided desperately needed explanation and relief from self-system disintegration consequent to panic. Patients resist investigation into their delusions because they urgently need them to prevent recurrence of panic of which they are unaware. The way back starts with recognition of anxiety (see Table 20.2).

Psychiatric patients tend to have many anxiety-relieving behavioral *acts* as sets related to a few such patterns as: blame (self-blame or blame-avoidance), scapegoating (taunting, bullying, intimidating), helplessness, dependency, concealment, shame and/or embarrassment, envy and/or jealousy. For each pattern there is generally a characteristic repertoire of separate behavioral acts often used in a particular sequence. When one fails to work, another action automatically comes into play. For instance, an overall pattern of aggression can include, in an escalating order, annoyance, idling hostility, passive aggression, resentment, overt anger, rage, and impotent rage.

The language-thought process is quite frequently used by patients to evolve language-thought patterns that initially relieve anxiety. Anxiety disorganizes thought, a frequent occurrence in the prehospitalization experiences of psychiatric patients. Consequently, language-thought disorders are commonly observable and in need of remedial assistance, which nurses can provide (Field, 1979). For example, a pattern of *overgeneralization* can be noted in such separate language behaviors as global vagueness ("everyone does that"), erroneous classification, stereotypical cliches ("time will tell"), use of global, nondescriptive adjectives (good, bad, happy), and the like. *Automatic knowing*, in which the patient assumes that another person knows something the patient has not expressed, is the pattern of such phrases as "you know" or "you see." Anxiety also wipes out thought, as in *blocking* or *blanking*. All of these anxiety-related difficulties are relief behaviors, which, by accretion, form the syndrome called *language-thought disorder* so common in patients diagnosed as having schizophrenia.

Involuntary Nature

A second characteristic of relief behaviors is the eventual *involuntary nature* of the behaviors following repeated use at the slightest felt discomfort related to anxiety. Such behaviors were at first consciously taken. By the time of hospitalization, psychiatric patients tend to be unaware of their original intent or use, their current utility, their self-limiting nature, or their original connection to anxiety, currently or in the past. Becoming aware of these points is part of the serious work patients need to do, with the help of nurses.

Failure To Work

A third characteristic of relief behaviors is the tendency, at some time, for the behaviors to *fail to work*, at which point severe anxiety or panic is experienced. Massive failure of sets of relief behaviors in providing the assumed relief during panic precedes a psychotic episode.

Application of the Construct

Anxiety quite probably cannot be eliminated from human experience, yet it is a powerful energizer that demands transformation into behavior that can be either in the direction of learning and personal growth or toward pathological adaptations, as in symptoms of mental illness. Anxiety, however, can be amenable to personal control. The first step in that direction is to be aware of the presence of anxiety at the point of feeling the initial discomfort it produces. Most psychiatric patients do not have this kind of control. Helping psychiatric patients to recognize and name anxiety as such, when it is occurring, is a learning experience psychiatric nurses can provide (see Tables 20.2 and 20.4).

The learning experience may proceed somewhat in this sequence. The nurse will observe that a patient with whom she or he is talking is showing a physiological effect of anxiety, such as flushing or hard breathing, or is using a relief behavior, such as restlessness, over-talkativeness, or changing the subject of the conversation. At that point, it is useful for the nurse to ask, "Are you nervous now?" or some language variant of this message. If the patient says yes, the nurse can then ask, "What are you doing now to relieve it?" This question forces the patient to *begin* to notice the relief behavior the nurse has observed. If the patient says, "I'm breathing hard and I'm restless," then obviously the patient has made the connection between the felt discomfort of anxiety and the transformation of the energy of anxiety into the behaviors both the nurse and the patient have observed. The nurse can offer validation, as in saying, "I noticed that too."

What is more likely to happen, particularly with long-term psychiatric patients, when the nurse asks, "Are you tense right now," is that the patient's response will be a vigorous no. If the nurse persists and asks about anxiety in subsequent nurse–patient contacts, over as long a period of time as it takes, eventually the patient will give a yes response. The usual sequence in getting to this affirmative response is: (1) *unawareness:* not noticing, the patient saying no in various ways; (2) *selective inattention:* self-doubt, the patient responding variously with, "Once I was," "Maybe I am," "Perhaps a little," and, finally, (3) *awareness:* the patient saying "Yes, I am."

No substantial therapeutic work can be accomplished until step 3 is reached. This is because the self-system (see Chapter 20, this volume) is an anti-anxiety system that always operates to prevent anxiety, such as is involved in the therapeutically oriented self-disclosure work that patients must do in order to heal themselves. The very first step in such work is to have control over anxiety and its unwitting escalation by recognizing and naming anxiety when it

TABLE 20.4 Nursing Interventions Related to Degree of Anxiety

Degree of anxiety	Nursing interventions
+ Mild	Learning is possible. Nurse assists patient to use the energy anxiety provides to encourage learning. See Table 20.2 to apply in nurse–patient interaction.
++ Moderate	Nurse to check own anxiety so patient does not empathize with it. Encourage patient to talk: to focus on one experience, to describe it fully, then to formulate the patient's generalizations about that experience.
+++ Severe	Learning is less possible. Allow relief behaviors to be used but do not ask about them. See Table 20.2 to apply in nurse–patient interaction. Encourage the patient to talk: Ventilation of random ideas is likely to reduce anxiety to moderate level. When this is observed by the nurse, proceed as above.
++++ Panic	Learning is impossible. *Thereness:* Nurse to stay with the patient. Allow pacing and walk with the patient. No content inputs to the patient's thinking should be made by the nurse. (They burden the patient who will distort them.) Use instrumental inputs only, the fewest possible and the least number of words: e.g., "Drink this" (give liquids to replace lost fluids and to relieve dry mouth); "Say what's happening to you," "Talk about yourself," or "Tell what you feel now" (to encourage ventilation and externalization of inner, frightening experience). Pick up on what the patient says: e.g., Pt: "I'm in a million pieces," N: "Talk about that," or Pt: "What's happening to me—how did I get here?" N: "Say what you notice." Short phrases by the nurse—direct, to the point of the patient's comment, and investigative—match the current attention span of the patient in panic and therefore are more likely to be heard, grasped, and acted upon with the patients responses gradually reducing the anxiety in a helpful way. Do not touch the patient; patient's experiencing panic are very concerned about survival, experiencing grave threat to the self, and usually distort the intentions of all invasions of their personal space. When the patient's anxiety is very obviously greatly reduced then apply Table 20.2.

is felt. But initially, when a nurse asks, "Are you nervous now?" the patient's anxiety will increase. However, as the unfamiliar question and its requirement that the patient notice anxiety become familiar, the patient will hear the question, take it in, and make an effort to act on it.

In working with psychiatric patients it is generally not useful to point out or to challenge their relief behaviors (or symptoms), especially in view of the unawareness of the patient and of her or his great need of these actions. Unawareness means that the patient is unable to notice these behaviors and that to do so would increase anxiety—which sometimes can escalate into panic. When a nurse asks (as in step 2 of Table 20.2), "What are you doing to relieve your nervousness," the patient's response will indicate the patient's ability to notice his behavior. If the patient says, "Nothing," then quite obviously he or she is not observing the pacing, trembling, or other relief behavior the nurse observes. The nurse may ask, "What do you usually do to get comfortable" or, "When upset in the past, what did you do then?" Again, the patient's response provides a clue to the patient's awareness. When the nurse persists with investigative-type questions, as indicated above, in several contacts over time, eventually the patient will *begin* to notice his or her relief behavior.

The nurse's questions do not challenge or question the patient's ability as would such phrasing as "Can you tell me?" or "Will you tell me?" or still worse, "Why don't you tell me?" which is a question that is intimidating and a reminder of authoritarian persons known in the past; *why* questions are often heard as accusatory by psychiatric patients. The phrasing of questions from nurse to patient are, in effect, input appraisals, which must be heard, internalized, and then acted upon by the patient (see Chapter 20, this volume, on self-system).

Rationale for the Nursing Application

In Table 20.2, the sequence of nurse application of Table 20.1 is *first* to promote awareness and naming of anxiety by the patient. Naming—people, places, objects, events—is a very old competence, learned very early in life, as in naming "mama," and is rarely lost in psychiatric patients. *Secondly,* nurses ask patients to notice, name, and connect the relief behavior being used in relation to the named anxiety. Identifying the relation between a current circumstance (relief behavior) and its immediate antecedent (discomfort of anxiety) involves the competence known from childhood that is involved, for example, in observing and feeling a soiled diaper and having it changed.

The *third* step in nursing application of the construct of anxiety requires the 'patient to see and to state a more complex relation. The patient has to notice the connection between felt discomfort and relief behaviors, *and* between the antecedent unmet expectation and the consequent effects—a cause–effect relation. For psychiatric patients, this third step is complicated by their tendency to have "fleeting thoughts" rather than clearly formulated cognitions, for example, about their expectations. Much effort is usually required on the part of the nurse in asking investigative questions such as, "What were you thinking of at the point you felt nervous?" (or "felt anxious and then as you said, got restless"). Such questions serve as stimuli that in time encourage the patient to retain, notice, formulate, and state the fleeting thoughts. The sequence of nurse application shown in Table 20.2 is based on the foregoing rationale.

SELF

Revision of the contents of the self-system is a crucial part of the self-development work psychiatric patients must do. Problems related to self and to anxiety pervade the psychopathology of patients for which treatment programs are to provide remedial assistance.

Currently, in the social sciences, there seems to be renewed interest in the self-concept. Gecas (1982) has provided a comprehensive review of conceptions of self, beginning with the work of Cooley (1902) and including contemporary research as well as an extensive bibliography. Wylie (1974) has also published a review of research on self.

The nursing literature on this phenomenon is not as extensive as this important aspect of nursing's work would suggest. The American Nursing Association (ANA, 1989) has a publication on nursing diagnoses, in line with the definition of nursing cited earlier, which includes classifications of self-concept problems such as self-esteem, body-image, identity, and the like. In the work of various nurse theorists (King, 1981; Roy, 1984) self-concept is included.

General Considerations

The self-systems of nurses and those of their patients are at interplay in all nurse–patient encounters. Moreover, psychiatric patients who are hospitalized invariably hold self-views that are crippling, dysfunctional in social terms, and therefore central among their many psychosocial problems. Nurse–patient interactions provide nurses with many opportunities to be instruments for constructive changes. Nurses have the function of helping psychiatric patients revise their self-views more in accord with inborn capacities and in the direction of views that enable living comfortably and productively with other people in the community. This nursing responsibility is accomplished when nurses have and use a viable theoretical construct concerning the self-system, as Sullivan (1956) called it. Nurses need theoretical understanding about what the self is, how one develops a self-system in the first place, how it functions and what purposes it serves, what the observable phenomena of self are that are involved in mental illness, and, finally, how such theory informs and guides the nursing interventions during nurse–patient relationships.

To be helpful to patients, nurses need to obtain a general idea of the nature, dimensions, and general orientations of the contents of the self of each patient. However, it would be a serious error to believe that complete knowledge can ever be secured about the total contents of any person's self-system. At best, only an approximation can be obtained. This caveat applies to work with psychiatric patients especially, for they tend toward private thought and concealment rather than toward public expression and self-disclosure. According to Sears et al. (1988, pp. 269–273), self-disclosure serves such uses as expression, self-clarification, self-validation, social control, and relationship development. Psychiatric patients need therapeutic help in order to attain these purposes.

Psychiatric patients do make comments about themselves and others from which the general tendencies in their self-system contents can be inferred by nurses. Nursing's work cannot proceed effectively without some general hypotheses about the self-views of patients. Such working hypotheses can be obtained by nurses from data that patients present to them in nurse–patient talks, on admission to hospital, and within the first few days thereafter. It is useful for nurses to notice and write down verbatim statements patients make with reference to themselves. These concrete items can then be classified into "I," "maybe me," and "not me" self views along lines of Table 20.5. These data can also be sorted further into those pertaining to family, friends, strangers; one's intelligence or competence; or into major patterns the language used suggests: derogation, accusation, belittling, blaming, concealment, and so forth.

Developing a *working hypothesis* of the contents of self of each patient can be a staff effort that generates a shared understanding as a basis for the joint, remedial verbal nursing approaches to be used. It is difficult to see how patients whose self-views are primarily derogatory can be helped without the nursing staff's having an understanding that such is the case, and without their knowing the what and why of remedial nursing interventions. Nurses, of course, do not change the self-views patients hold—only patients can do that; nurses, however, through their verbal approaches in nurse–patient dialogues, do provide instrumental inputs intended to stimulate patients to do the necessary work of self-change.

What Is the Self?

The self is an abstraction; it is a convenient way of describing a function of the total person. It is not a thing, nor a body part, nor a place in the "mind." The self is a function of the mind, which is a more comprehensive function of the entire human organism. The self is something like a theoretical framework in that it serves as an organizing structure through which experiences, events, and people are perceived and known, accepted, or rejected. The self is a conceptualization of one of the most important human functions.

In the literature, the self is alternatively referred to as *ego, personality, identity,* and such. These conceptions are not precisely synonymous with *self-system* as defined in this discussion. The construct provided below is presented in a format considered to be most useful for purposes of both observation and intervention in psychiatric nursing practice. The self is viewed as a system because of the interlocking nature of its many functions and the tendency toward maintenance of equilibrium or stability. As with all systems, a change in one self-system function, constructive or otherwise, has an impact on all other functions. It is for this reason that helping patients revise handicapping self-views and aiding them to embrace constructive ones in accord with their capacities is a most difficult, time-consuming, piecemeal task.

Parsons (1961, p. 38) in another context, identified four "essential functional imperatives of any social system: pattern-maintenance, integration, goal attainment, and adaptation." These formulations apply as well to the self-system. The self expands, contracts, changes, and is otherwise revised as it functions, particularly in maintaining security. Security obtains through intellectual activity and interpersonal "security operations" (or relief behaviors), which *simultaneously* sustain system integration and prevent anxiety.

When a psychiatric patient who is experiencing panic and/or terror says, "Where am I? I'm all over the place—in a million pieces," that patient is saying that integration of the self-system has been gravely threatened or is being lost. Security of the self-system, which is assumed, and is felt when the interlocking functions are maintained, is—during panic and terror—replaced by enormous, felt insecurity, disintegration and dysfunctioning of the self. The security operations (relief behaviors) that previously worked successfully to maintain system stability now fail. Terror arises during this shift from expected integration to perceived disintegration of the self. Panic and terror cannot be sustained for very long, for in effect the individual is for that duration without an integrated self-system. Therefore, the self reorganizes swiftly, and if the person is unaware at least of the anxiety experienced at that time, or if the interventions others in the situation provide are not cognizant of the nature of terror and act accordingly, the reorganization will be along lines of psychopathology. Panic precedes a psychotic break (see Table 20.5).

Sullivan (1956) defined the self as an anti-anxiety system. In this regard, beginning in infancy and continuing throughout life, the

TABLE 20.5 Dimensions of the Self

In awareness: "I"	Selectively inattended: "Maybe me"	Dissociated: "Not me"
Up front in mind.	On or near the margin of attention and awareness.	Excluded from awareness.
Easily recalled, noticed, talked about.	Can recall if attention is directed to do so.	Unable to notice or accept these self-views without experiencing severe anxiety or panic.
Fully accepted self-view.	Only partially accepted self-views. Doubt.	Unacceptable self-views.
Views are "owned" and presented in using such pronouns as *I, me, my,* and *mine.*	Views are "partly owned." Views presented with qualifiers such as "Maybe me," "sometimes I," "once I was."	Views are "disowned." Prefixes to convey exclusion include negatives such as "not me," "at no time," "never did," "no way."
Anxiety: None.	Anxiety: Mild to moderate.	Anxiety: Severe to panic
These views are reflected appraisals deriving from input appraisals from people and experiences that were the most *frequently recurring* designation, definitions of self and *perceived* as "me"—i.e., approved.	These views are reflected appraisals derived from input appraisals from people and experiences that were infrequently occurring designations, definitions of self and *perceived* as disapproved.	These views are reflected appraisals from input appraisals from people and experiences that occurred rarely, were connected with great pain punishment or panic and *perceived* as aspects of self to be ignored or be indifferent to.
In psychiatric patients these views tend to be mainly derogatory, destructive to self-development.		In psychiatric patients these views tend to be ones in accord with capacities for self-affirmation and for constructive self-development.
Sets up situations to confirm and get affirmation of others of these self-views.		Sets up situations to maintain exclusion of these views from awareness.

self, in accord with the stage of intellectual and interpersonal development, polices its owner's behavior in interpersonal situations. This vigilance occurs in the interest of maintaining security and the previously mentioned functions, and in order to reduce, relieve, and prevent more anxiety. For example, the self audits and edits out errors of speech or slips of the tongue so as to prevent anxiety, subsequent humiliation, or embarrassment, and therefore loss of prestige (See Table 20.6).

The self-system is a product of socialization, a function in humans that evolves and is revised along constructive or destructive lines during interpersonal relationships throughout life. Mead (1934) suggested that "selves exist only in relation to other selves," that individuals have within-person concepts, the "generalized

TABLE 20.6 Major Components of Self-Systems

Interrelated functions	Contents
Sustain integration of self-system	Self-views
Maintain equilibrium and stability	Self-images
Prevent anxiety	Self-worth
Police attention; audit and edit errors and "slips of tongue"	Self-respect Self-esteem
Monitor relation between focal attention and "security operations" (patterns of relief behavior)	Stature Status
Manage incongruence, i.e., conflict among self-system contents	Prestige
Maintain boundaries between self-in-awareness, selectively, inattended contents, and dissociated contents of self	Supervisory personifications (if not edited out)
Allow acceptable incremental revisions and avoid massive change in self-system	
Monitor self in interpersonal interactions to gain confirmation of self-system contents and to maintain exclusion of dissociated self-views	

other," by which they imagine the views and reactions of others to their own behavior. This conception is in accord with Sullivan's (1956) later definition of interpersonal relations. The lonely isolate who hallucinates invented figures does so, in part, so that the other self-system relation to "other selves" can be maintained, and characterizations of the figures are drawn from the incorporated "generalized other."

Origins of the Self-System

Infants are not born with a self-system, because the self-system is an anti-anxiety system evolved as a product of socialization. Infants do bring their own resources—inborn capacities and tendencies—into the interactions they have with socializing agents, the first of which are their primary caretakers. These resources include genetic endowment, gender, temperament, body characteristics and body build, bodily rhythm, level of capacity for intelligence, various capacities such as those for speech, hearing, vision, and bodily movement. In a self-system that functions constructively there is, at least in childhood, awareness and acceptance of the nature of one's resources and a match between them and operative self-views that are held in awareness. At birth, however, these resources are merely potentials, capacities that are transformed (or fail to be) into interpersonal, intellectual, and other social competencies required for social living within a community.

At birth, the most important ability an infant has is the ability to cry. This prespeech instrumental ability is the only one the infant has use of in order to call the attention of others to his needs for food, warmth, and other forms of comfort. The responses to the infant's cry, of the "mothering one," "parenting ones," "primary caretakers," and/or "significant others," begins the process by which the infant evolves a self-system.

The structure of the self-system process, its phases and steps, are of particular interest to psychiatric nurses. When nurses assist psychiatric patients to become aware of and to revise the contents of their self-systems, the same structure and the same sequence of its phases as those evolved in infancy are utilized. The processes evolve in the manner described in Table 20.7.

TABLE 20.7 Components of Evolving Self-Systems: Process and Nursing Applications

Process components	Nursing applications
1. Felt relations: Infant feels satisfaction and shares mutual satisfaction with mother in feeding situation.	Nurse evokes trust in patient, as a *felt relation*, as the patient perceives that the nurse does what she promises the patient she will do.
2. Empathic observation: Infant feels mother's anxiety in the feeding situation.	Nurse *controls* her own *anxiety* and assists patient toward control of his anxiety (Table 20.2).
3. Input appraisals of defining others: Child hears appraisals. Repeats appraisals verbatim. Internalizing appraisals of others as his or her own views, which are now reflected appraisals.	The *form* and *language* of the nurse's questions and comments are *investigative*, thereby not colliding with or confirming self-views of patient. Nurse inputs are unfamiliar to patient who experiences anxiety. Nurse applies Table 20.2 and then repeats investigative input. Patient hears nurse input. Patient internalizes nurse input as his or her own stimulus to inquire and think about the circumstances. Nurse inputs are reflected back by patient.
4. Actions to go with reflected appraisals (self-views) are acquired.	Patient gradually acts on internalized investigative nurse inputs.
5. Sets up situations to maintain contents of the self-system.	None
6. Supervisory personifications are internalized.	None

Sullivan (1956) claims that the self is an anti-anxiety phenomenon having its earliest roots in mother–infant interaction in the feeding situation early in life. The interactive sequences during the first few weeks in life go like this: The infant cries, signaling an operative need; the mothering one responds, accurately inferring and then meeting the infant's need; mutual satisfaction is *felt* by both infant and mother, both of whom have had their different but complementary needs met. However, at some time during this same time period a change occurs. The sequence now goes like this: The infant cries, signaling an operative need; the mothering one responds as before, except that this time the mothering one is anxious; using an inborn capacity for empathic observation, the infant feels the anxiety as extreme visceral discomfort, stops feeding, and instead cries more; the mother's anxiety increases; the infant now evolves new, unique, adaptive behaviors; the infant cries until exhausted and sleep occurs, or the infant cries, eats, cries, then vomits. In this sequence, both mother and infant are left with their needs unsatisfied.

It is assumed that the infant discriminates the differences in the two sequences, just described, at the level of *feelings*, sorting them in some way into *felt* satisfaction and *felt* discomfort. Thus the infant, perceiving a *felt relation*, "sees" the mothering one in two ways, as "good mother" and as "bad mother," and himself or herself as "good me" and "bad me." The main question, in terms of the developing self-system is: Which sequence becomes the prevailing recurring, expected experience? It can be taken for granted that all mothers will experience anxiety at some point during the feeding experience. The question is how frequently and to what degree?

Infants go through a period of prespeech vocalizations and then the capacity for language development ripens. Most parents are eager for their children to talk. They encourage verbalization, and eventually children say "mama" or "dada." At this point, perhaps more so with firstborn children, most parents respond verbally and with attention, pride, pleasure, and approval. On the basis of a *felt relation* (a connection experienced at a feeling level rather than as a thought) the child recognizes that something important has occurred. In order to call out similar parental responses the child tries harder and more often to hear, form, and say the words that adults in the situation use.

As the child becomes mobile, the adults make more defining statements about the child that are designations of the child, estimates or appraisals of the child's ability or worth. The toddler pays attention to these *input appraisals* of significant others, for otherwise there are no views of the self. These become the initial contents for the self-system. The mode of imitative learning is used along with ability to focus attention as the toddler *hears* and *repeats verbatim* what others say that seemingly refer to him. For example, the parent says, "Johnny is a bad boy." Gradually the toddler *internalizes* the input appraisals. This occurs through revision of the language used, with adult help, in three observable steps: The child will *reflect back* (1) "Johnny is . . . ." (2) "Me is . . . ." and then (3) "I am . . . ." When the personal pronoun *I* is used, the defining input appraisals of others have been *internalized,* have become beginning contents of the self-system, and have been accepted as baseline self-views.

The child now begins to watch in order to notice those behaviors that evoke specific defining appraisals from adults; by watching and by trial-and-error the child connects the actions that go with the appraisals of adults that now are self-views incorporated into the self-system. The tendency thereafter is to set up interactive situations with adults that are more rather than less likely to confirm and maintain the reflected self-appraisals.

Self-system maintenance involves the prevention of anxiety by accepting appraisals into the existing system that are congruent with already-incorporated views. Revision is possible, but anxiety is experienced with it. Important as this early period is in laying down a baseline of self-views, every subsequent major new experience, entering school, various church activities, getting into a peer group, having a chum, being hospitalized, getting into college, various achievements or failures, marriage, and the like, have the potential for forcing changes, constructive or not, in the self-system.

Child rearing and childhood education involve the use of three major patterns in the behavior of adults toward children, namely *approval* (praise, compliment, reward), *disapproval* (blame, punish, rebuke, castigate), and *indifference* (ignore, banish, dismiss, reject, ostracize, expel, abandon). Very young children do those things of which they are capable, the pleasure being in the discovery and use of their capability. In these matters they are often unaware of risks and dangers that may be involved. Parents and teachers, on the other hand, know the possible untoward consequences of some child actions and so they interfere and begin to shape the child's behavior, using one of three patterns. For children, in general, it is more comfortable to be liked, rather than disliked or not noticed. They tend to work for approval, that is, to please parents and to be what parental defining inputs suggest.

Parents and teachers use disapproval to force the child to give up disapproved behavior and behave in ways that adults want, expect, and can approve. Hochschild (1974) has written a poignant biography in which he describes the awesome, lingering effects of parental disapproval experienced in the absence of directly expressed affection and approval. When disapproval becomes the recurring, predominant pattern of the adults, some children lose hope or interest in gaining approval and instead tend to work for disapproval. To be ignored imputes the self-view "I am nobody" on the child, an anxiety-evoking experience; at the least, being punished implies being noticed for something. Very withdrawn psychiatric patients, however, tend to accept indifference and, to make it a mutual pattern integration; they ignore others who ignore them.

Thus approval, disapproval, and indifference by adults upon whom the child is in some way dependent have an impact on the child's evolving self-system. They are in effect input appraisals and they become self-system contents in the same way: They are heard (noticed) internalized, reflected back as self-appraisals, and actions to confirm these self-views are acquired. As a folk saying puts it: "You get the name and then get the game."

The point needs to be emphasized that what reaches the forefront of awareness, as accepted, "owned," self-views, consists of the most frequently recurring appraisals (see Table 20.5). Toddlers and young children think "That's me" in terms of what adults say they are, and in terms of their own experiences. It is in this sense, to the child, an adult verbal appraisal such as, "You are stupid," "You can't do that," "bad," as well as self-appraisals derived from personal failure in efforts toward achievement (as in physical activities and schoolwork) are *perceived* as approved views. The disapproval or indifference of adults and peers becomes approved self-views (as in psychiatric patients) when the evolving individual accepts these appraisals as "That's me—I'm stupid," "I'm a failure," "I can't do anything." It is important to note the distinction between what others, external to the psychiatric patient approved, disapproved, or ignored, and what the patient, earlier in life, perceived, classified and internalized, into his or her self-system.

The destructive effects of input appraisals of adults that have been primarily derogatory in content, incongruent with inborn capacities, with a preponderant use of disapproval or indifference, as patterns used by parents and teachers early in the child's life, can most clearly be seen in psychiatric patients, juvenile offenders, and prisoners.

The significant persons in the life of a growing child are also internalized into the self-system as *supervisory personifications*, a Sullivanian (1956) term. Parents particularly, as well as other adults significant to the growing child, supervise their children by telling, warning, ordering, forbidding, punishing, and by conveying principles or other guidelines for living. Later on, in the absence of these significant others, most children recall both the parental figure and the guidelines, and utilize these internalized inputs in making judgments and decisions particularly in stressful situations. This is useful in that children, some more than others, up to reaching adulthood, became more aware of the risk element in situations they get into. This identification with parents should be transitory, so that when full adulthood is reached the supervisory personifications are edited out. Actions are then based upon self-discipline and responsibility, and not on "my mother told me to . . . ."

Psychiatric patients invariably sustain autistically controlled interpersonal relationships between themselves and their incorporated supervisory personifications. This remnant of earlier self-system development is employed in the production of hallucinations. It is also an anxiety-maintaining phenomenon, especially when the parent (now an illusory supervisory figure) peppered the guidelines given to the patient as a child with *should*s, *ought*s, *must*s, *cannot*s, *don't*s, and the like and without practical instructions to go with these injunctions. These words generally accompany expectations that were and still are unlikely of being met by the individual.

Stability within the self-system also requires a sorting out of incongruent views into separate categories, the figurative boundaries between them being a function of attention and its relation to the overall anti-anxiety performances of the self (see Table 20.5). Those self-views that have been accepted into *awareness*, that is, focal attention, are easily noticed, openly claimed, and comfortably expressed, usually with the use of personal pronouns such as *I, me,* or *mine.* Originally, these were input appraisals, defining statements, which defining others made to the person, which subsequently were accepted and internalized into the person's self-system. These were the *recurring,* frequently repeated, defining statements that adults made about the infant, then-growing child. In this sense they were perceived as approved: What others said the child was. They may have been primarily affirmative *or* destructive inputs to the child's evolving self-system. This distinction is worth noting. Most so-called social rejects—prisoners, juvenile offenders, psychiatric patients—experienced an overload of destructive input appraisals in life; these then tend to be the contents of their self-system that is up front, in awareness.

Although early infancy and childhood are crucial in self-system development, all later experiences also influence the self. The growing child gains self-esteem and many competencies when acceptance by peers is forthcoming. Agemates, especially during the first six years of school, are all seeking to establish their position, their status, among peers and to gain acceptance into the peer group of their own choice. They are usually brutally frank with each other; name-calling is common. For some children, these peer definitions become self-views. Others gain strategies to avoid internalizing peer designations; the phrase "sticks and stones will break my bones but names will never hurt me" represents one such tactic. Children often ignore or are totally indifferent to those children who act helpless and who are unable to compete, compromise, and cooperate in relation to the needs of the evolving peer group. These later "rejects" may have growth-enhancing remedial experiences later on, although some become isolates and vulnerable, at risk for psychiatric problems. In describing his experiences through seventh grade, a scientist says "I was *really* left out" (Wright, 1988, p. 35).

Self-worth is further influenced by success in a chum relationship ("best friend"), achievements in school, sports, and community affairs. However, the contents of self that a child brings into these opportunities, for enlargement and revision, weigh heavily in determining how situations will be set up—in the direction of success or failure, peer acceptance or rejection, or to be a winner or a loser.

Self-views are also sorted into categories called *selectively inattended* and *dissociated*. In order to prevent anxiety, individuals inattend to aspects of what is going on, including not noticing some of the self-system contents. These are generally self-views *perceived* as disapproved. The characteristic of selective inattention is that the degree of anxiety involved is minimal; therefore it is possible for the individual to notice if attention is directed to it by others. Dissociation, the tendency not to notice and to be unable to do so without experiencing severe anxiety or panic, is a more difficult attention problem. The security of the self-system is maintained by not noticing these aspects of self (see Table 20.5).

The contents of the self-system are conveyed, wittingly and unwittingly, in relationships between people, by language usage, actions, body gestures, appearance, and the like. For instance, psychiatric patients most often will say freely, directly, "I am no good, stupid, worthless," and so forth. Some prisoners say, without a trace of anxiety, "I am a killer." These statements to which the personal pronoun *I* is attached, are the operative self-views of the persons involved. For most people, the mere thought about oneself, "I am a killer," is so abhorrent that it raises a touch of uncanny sensation (sometimes experienced as shivering or goose bumps). Because it collides with and is inadmissible to self-views in awareness, it is a dissociated, "not-me" self-view.

Contents of Self-System

The major contents of the self-system include the following: *Self-views* are definitions, conceptions, of oneself, that are comprised of baseline reflected appraisals, inputs originally from caretakers early in life, and incremental additions, elaborations, and revisions resulting from the person's subsequent life experiences. Aims, attitudes, opinions, and goals are among these contents (see Table 20.6).

Self-images are imagined pictures of oneself, drawn from memory or fantasy, which are projected onto or otherwise conveyed to the outside world. Images are generally representations of how one wishes to be seen by others and, therefore, may not always be congruent with self-views and other self-system contents.

Self-worth is originally a by-product of an interpersonally intimate, two-person, same-sex, best-friend, chum relationship, usually experienced around ages 9 to 12, in which validation of personal worth outside of the family, by a peer, occurs (Sullivan, 1956). Self-worth includes the extent of personal liking or valuation of oneself, one's characteristics, talents, abilities, and the like. The ability to evoke meritorious valuations from others, with regard to personal attributes, performance levels, moral or principled actions, or usefulness to others, are also aspects of self-worth. Self-worth judgments are acceptable when they are in accord with the prevailing self views. Self-respect is an ingredient of self-worth.

Self-esteem, which is an internal sense of self-regard, includes confidence in one's abilities and judgments, and serves as a measure of self-praise or the favorableness the person attributes to himself. Estimates of self-esteem tend to be higher when the person has self-reliance, awareness of and confidence in his own powers and resources, and when there is self-determination—inner control, self-regulation, and self-discipline. Self-control over one's actions and feelings requires an awareness of them in current situations, reflection on their consequences for self and others, and self-discipline in subsequent situations. No one, of course, is totally self-sufficient. Interdependence among persons is a condition of social life. However, recognizing one's separateness and independence is an important aspect of self-identity.

The major source of self-esteem is achievement—socially acceptable accomplishments, recognized by oneself and others, which result from using one's capabilities. *Stature,* within a field of endeavor—an occupation, profession, or social group—derives from estimates of achievements, attributed by others and the importance assigned as to their merit or usefulness. Intrinsic and assigned merit are not always identical. *Status* refers to the official and informal position or rank of an individual, in relation to others, in a group such as the family, workplace, social group, and the like.

Official and informal status may not be similar or identical. *Prestige* means having the personal social power to command admiration or esteem of others and thereby to maintain status. Prestige includes one's reputation and ability to influence others, particularly in terms of successful achievements of interest to them.

Nursing Applications

Nurses have the difficult work of aiding psychiatric patients to change their socially dysfunctional self-systems that inherently resist change. The construct presents the structure employed in establishing a self-system and suggests the nursing applications (see Table 20.7) that can be drawn from it. The work of both nurse and patient goes on during verbal interactions in nurse–patient relationships.

In this work, nurses are, in effect, definers of patients. Such definitions are inherent in statements made to, about, or in response to patients. What is being suggested in this paper is that these input appraisals of nurses be oriented primarily to the patients capability rather than being of defining content. When a nurse says: "Describe what happened" or "Illustrate that," the verbalization rests on the assumption but does not say directly that the patient has the necessary capability that the patient's response requires. If the patient does not respond as asked, the nurse then assumes on the basis of Tables 20.5 to 20.7, that the input has not yet been heard, because it is unfamiliar. Later on, as the same messages are posed, the patient will hear, eventually internalize, and make the necessary effort to describe or to illustrate. Timely repetition of such instrumental nurse inputs eventually serves the patient as internalized stimuli for self-change. It is in this sense that *nurses are definers who are significantly different* from the "defining others" who during pre-hospitalization applied content appraisals to the patient. The theoretical construct addressed suggests the design of the nursing intervention most likely to move the patient in a remedial direction.

Verbal statements made to patients can *collide* with, *confirm*, or *stimulate change* in a patient's self-views. Collisions occur when what the nurse says disputes, refutes, or otherwise disconfirms a self-view that is inherent in what a patient says to a nurse. Such collision will evoke anxiety to some degree in the patient. Confirmation of a patient's self-view means that the nurse's response conveyed agreement with what a patient has just said with reference to the self. This is problematic on two counts. Patients become dependent upon the nurse's agreement or praise or approval, rather than developing ability for self-evaluation. Moreover, if the patient's self-reference is derogatory, the nurse has affirmed a dysfunctional self-view. In both cases, collisions and confirmation, constructive change in the patient has not been aided.

An existing self-system is resistant to change; it functions to maintain itself. Therefore, nurse statements in relation to self-views expressed by patients should bypass the operative system. *Instrumental inputs* by nurses are more likely to serve this purpose. Instrumental statements serve as the means by which nurses address the components of the process rather than the contents of a patient's self-system (see Table 20.7). They are designed as verbal contrivances most likely to evoke interest, effort, and eventually use of latent capability for self-change by patients.

Instrumental inputs are *investigative* questions raised when a problematic self-view is being presented by a patient to the nurse. Such inquiries include but are not limited to such queries as: "When did you get that idea?" "What's the source of that notion about you?" "When did you first think of yourself in that way?" "What's the evidence for that self-reference?" "Illustrate that," "Describe one time that view applied to you," "What do you get out of thinking that about yourself?" "What's the point of classifying yourself that way?" Such questions require the patient to work—to recall, to think, to formulate, to express, and to reflect on what prompted the questions.

Investigative questions seek the origins of, evidence for, and purposes of patients' presenting self-views. It is quite likely that the language, form, and intent of these instrumental inputs will at first be quite unfamiliar to psychiatric patients. The prevailing tendency in social situations is to ignore, to agree, or to disagree with the self-views people present to others, rather than to investigate them. Thus, anxiety is likely to occur, as the patients do not expect questions of this type. The patient's awareness and ability to name anxiety (see Table 20.2) therefore are important antecedent tasks to be accomplished. As the nurse's questions become familiar, expected words, the patient will begin to hear, internalizing and then act in terms of these inputs. At first, this remedial effort proceeds quite slowly and consists primarily of attempts on the part of the nurse to guide the patient in a direction toward having within the self the internalized instruments necessary for self-change. In time, as these instruments are internalized, the patient will initiate use of them as more generalized problem-solving tools.

HALLUCINATIONS

Everyone has the human capacities that are employed in the development of hallucinations (see Table 20.9). Only those persons who have need of interpersonal relationships with illusory figures invent and sustain them. In psychiatric nursing practice, hallucinations are most commonly observed in patients diagnosed as having schizophrenia, although they also occur with other diagnoses such as alcoholism. There are several types of hallucinatory experience, all of which involve the senses: visual (seeing invented images), auditory (hearing invented voices), gustatory (taste), olfactory (smelling invented odors), and tactile (invented crawling things such as "bugs," felt on the skin along with uncanny sensations). It is not uncommon for auditory and visual hallucinations to occur simultaneously. Auditory hallucinations are discussed in this chapter.

There are various definitions of hallucinations in the literature. Some authors refer to these phenomena as "inner speech" (Johnson, 1978). Arieti (1959) defines hallucinations as "an inner experience expressed as though it were an external event." Gould's research (1948, 1949, 1950) demonstrated that hallucinations were "automatic speech," which employed the "vocal musculature." Two social workers designed and tested a technique by which several patients were taught to control their "voices" at the point of "hearing them" by employing their vocal cords in activities such as talking or gargling water (Erickson & Gustafson, 1968). The nursing literature generally defines hallucinations as need-based perceptions having no basis in reality (Beck, Rawlings, & Williams,

1988). Nursing texts usually suggest reality testing, decoding the verbalized hallucinatory content, and shedding doubt when patients indicate hearing voices.

Definition

For purposes of this chapter, hallucinations are defined as follows: Visual and auditory hallucinations consist of illusory figures, perceived *as if* they were real persons. Interactions between the individual and autistically invented images or voices serve to maintain the self-system, the precarious stability of which is increasingly threatened by the effects of social isolation. The figures are invented, initially, for purposes of avoiding anxiety-evoking social situations and to mitigate loneliness. The individual attributes human characteristics to figures drawn from data derived from past experience. These characteristics change, over time, from helping, to derogatory, to terrorizing, and then to pleasant but ever-present. The nature of the characteristics is determined by the person's changing circumstances, in particular, regarding competencies the individual loses through disuse or distortion. Due to lack of social checks and validation, the display of this pathology is evident to external observers who intervene. In the absence of professional psychotherapeutic assistance this psychopathological process evolves toward chronicity as its endpoint (see Table 20.8).

TABLE 20.8 The Hallucinatory Process and Nursing Interventions

Phases and steps in the process	Nursing interventions
Phase I: Problem-solving reveries	None
1. An individual who is alone, lonely, undergoes great stress or severe anxiety, and/or feels some large and burdening responsibility.	Be aware of this as a personal experience.
2. Being unable to command attention of a real person in the situation, the individual recalls a helping person, known in the past and thinks about the help this person would give.	

TABLE 20.8 The Hallucinatory Process and Nursing Interventions
(Continued)

Phases and steps in the process	Nursing interventions
3. The memory assists the individual in enduring the stress and in at least partially resolving the stress-producing problem. 4. The foregoing steps lead to a definite experience of felt relief. All steps in this phase are within the awareness of the individual.	*General considerations* 1. Identify the phase of hallucinations. 2. Identify and name anxiety (Table 20.2). 3. Provide opportunities with real people to mitigate loneliness.
Phase II: Courting similar relief 1. In a subsequent experience of stress, whether it be in greater or lesser degree than in the previous phase, the individual recalls that relief followed an autistic reverie about a particular helping person. 2. In stressful and nonstressful periods the individual now sets up the situation to spend more time in private thought of like kind. 3. The increased time spent in isolation from people—particularly in persons who are lacking in social skills—affords additional, though temporary, relief from even minor anxiety. The relief occurs because the interpersonal strains with real people are reduced. As an aspect of courting this considerable relief, however, a "listening state" develops. Anticipatory anxiety arises of the kind: "Will I or won't I be able to think of him today?" The answer hinges on intrusions of daily social life which must be reduced to a minimum. In search of relief from the now added anxiety more time is set aside for autistic reveries. As a result, there is a consequent adaptive beginning loss of ability to control focal attention and the contents of thought, for such abilities are sharpened by use in verbal interactions with real people, rather than by private thought unchecked by others.	Observe tendency toward withdrawal. Provide opportunities for development of social skills. Encourage interactions with family and friends. Observe "listening state" (Patient alerted; face averted slightly—"to hear"). Provide opportunity to talk with a professional. Observe and intervene to avoid increased "moving away" from real people. Intervene to reduce withdrawal time and solitary activities.

TABLE 20.8 The Hallucinatory Process and Nursing Interventions
(Continued)

Phases and steps in the process	Nursing interventions
Phase III: Marked loss of ability to discipline focal awareness 1. The need for the relief afforded by the autistically invented interactions with illusory figures becomes more compelling as the time spent with real people decreases markedly. In one contact with a real person, often a family member, there is a "sudden breakthrough" of the autistic reverie. The individual will "hear" the illusory figure say sor.ething to which the person responds verbally; the family member will notice and question this behavior; the breakthrough signals the individual's loss of control over focal attention and over the person' discrimination of the difference between private and public fields of interactive discourse.	Observe "inappropriate laughter," that is appropriate only to the content of the interaction of patient-and-illusory figure. Ask a neutral question: "What's going on now?" Respond to such breakthroughs in a least threatening manner; provide nonthreatening discussion with a professional. Schedule activities and interactions with real people to provide compelling pulls toward control over focal attention.
2. The individual feels embarrassment and shame for revealing private behavior to another person who has called attention to it, most often in derogatory terms such as "Are you crazy or something?"	Avoid evoking these emotions. If evoked, aid person to recognize and name them, and to connect them to their antecedents. Work on getting anxiety and loneliness named.
3. The individual now becomes more guarded and secretive, using previously acquired techniques of concealment, which every human being has developed to some extent. Concealment is used to prevent the terror of being noticed publicly again and to sustain the hope of relief through continuing use of the autistically invented relationship with illusory figures.	Use of "thereness" instead of prying.
4. More time is spent in isolation from real people. Plausible excuses such as "I'm tired," "I have a virus," "I feel sick" are	Medical assessment of illness complaints is in order.

TABLE 20.8 The Hallucinatory Process and Nursing Interventions
(Continued)

Phases and steps in the process	Nursing interventions
used to ensure maximum time for autistic activity to go on uninterrupted. As a consequence, there is an even greater loss of ability to control thought, that is, to choose what to think about, to audit (notice) and edit (change) the contents of thought, now the "voices" become much more definite and "pop into mind." In the sense that the individual can no longer control thought ("the voices") at will, the so-called voices control the patient (i.e., splitting within the self-system has also occurred).	
5. There is some dim awareness by the individual and perplexity concerning the loss of ability to discipline thought (control the voices); this increases anxiety that is now almost constantly of severe degree. Terror is also felt from noticing the concern shown by others as the excessive withdrawal hallucinating behaviors become more self-evident. (If the techniques of concealment work the process in this phase may go on for years; if they do not the individual may seek therapy and if not treated as subhuman will respond quickly).	If the individual mentions voices, ask for description of "these so-called voices you say you hear" (i.e., linguistically separate the nurse's from the patient's experience).

Phase IV: Failure of concealment techniques

1. Generally, when the efforts at concealment fail, a family member will hospitalize the patient. This procedure adds new stress and may give rise to panic (See Tables 20.3 & 20.4). Hospital admission disrupts the individual's control of his situation and his inept efforts to obtain relief, particularly from loneliness; it also again

(continued)

TABLE 20.8 The Hallucinatory Process and Nursing Interventions
(Continued)

Phases and steps in the process	Nursing interventions
evokes embarrassment and shame and imposes care by strangers in a totally unfamiliar environment. Heroic measures are now needed to obtain relief and for the self-system to survive. 2. The individual has heretofore narrowed his adaptive powers down to one pattern: autistic reveries in isolation from real people. As a next adaptation, under the new circumstances of hospitalization and in the same direction as the previous one, the patient taps aspects of the self-system and experience having to do with failure (rather than helping); the voices now become derogatory, accusatory, and/or persecutory. This shift in content, and the patient's inability to edit it out of his thought, and the further failure to experience relief, is felt as terror, generally projected. The patient will say, "The voices terrorize me." 3. If the process goes on without corrective professional intervention the terror will persist, disturbing eating and sleeping patterns, until the derogatory content attributed to voices becomes familiar and accepted by the patient as his view of self. Before the days of psychotropic drugs, chronic patients in seclusion rooms could be heard, at this point in the process, pleading, negotiating, bargaining while screaming with terror at their voices. Finally, a compromise would be reached: "I won't talk to staff if you don't leave me."	

Human Capacities Employed in Hallucinations

The development of hallucinated figures makes use of capacities developed early in life (See Table 20.9). For instance, it can be observed that children, particularly before age 6, are able to move freely between autistically invented play and interactions with real people. For them, there is no figurative line of demarcation between fantasy and reality, interactions that involve private or public thought. Small children invent playmates, endow them with names, roles, and personal characteristics, share experiences and have conversations with them. In effect, the children thus have control of both sides of these self-and-other interactions in which one is real and the others are illusory. Moreover, there is no observable anxiety-related discomfort as the children move from the imagined to the real world when adults address them and thus distract their attention from the invented to the actual situation. Children often reenact parent–child scenes, taking the role of the parent, for example on beating a child (doll), in order to experience what it feels like to be the beater rather than the beaten one.

Once children begin school their teachers require them, in the classroom, to give full attention to their schoolwork. This work, which is the same subject matter for all pupils, may be said to be in the *public mode*. *Private mode* or autistic thought, such as imaginary play, is more or less discouraged during classroom hours. Some teachers are more lenient, others are more severe and punitive, in their efforts to get children to discipline their attention and to focus their thought on the common subject matter under consideration at a given time.

Teachers use various disciplinary strategies: Calling on a child unexpectedly to read something; using a facial gesture of forbiddance while saying, "Pay attention," or using some form of disapproval. Most children somehow adapt; they voluntarily give up private mode thought while in the classroom and focus on teacher-directed lessons. There may be lapses, but if caught by the teacher the child may be subjected to humiliation and experience shame and embarrassment in front of agemates who have become important. Slowly, a figurative boundary separates fantasy and reality as these

TABLE 20.9 Comparison of Selected Competencies and Purposes of Children, Adults, and Hallucinating Patients

Preschool children	"Normal" adults	Hallucinating patients
Move freely between autistically invented play and interactions with real people. No anxiety.	Maintain an imaginary boundary between fantasy and reality and are aware of fantasizing when it occurs, anxiety if "caught."	Loss of the figurative line between the autistic and public mode. No anxiety until "voices" threaten to leave.
Invent figures, endow them with human characteristics, converse with figures, take role-of-other to test roles in imagination. No anxiety—total control over all components of interaction.	Relationships with real people. Some control of interaction and potential for anxiety.	Invent illusory figures, using data from past experience; figures are given human characteristics; has interactions with figures. No anxiety—unless figures "threaten," since has total control over all components of the interaction.
Purpose: To use evolving capacities, developing ability to focus attention, testing in imagination, learning the dimensions of observed adult roles, exercising developing verbal and social abilities in safe, self-controlled situation.	Purpose: To use competencies to meet personal needs and to establish and maintain social relationships. Some social control.	Purpose: To avoid people as relief behavior; to attenuate loneliness by having invented interactions; to mitigate powerlessness socially by control over autistic invention.
Beginning in school years, shifts interests to interactions with real people—peers, chums, adults.	Interactions with real people, in homework, and in social situations.	Isolate: Invents relationships based upon need: (1) for help—invents "helping figures;" (2) derogations as a failure, shame, embarrassment, occur—invents "derogatory figures."

powerful emotions spur the child toward more actively policing attention. Or the shame and embarrassment may increase feelings of inferiority, distance from peers, and new ways to act as if attending when the child is all the while daydreaming.

Failure to gain acceptance into a peer group of agemates, or to successfully have a chum relationship, a best friend as noted earlier, or to achieve something of interest in an enduring way, make private thought much more enticing than discussions with others of one's generation. By the time of adolescence, some of these individuals are loners. Some isolates may eventually have corrective experiences with people, find satisfaction in solitary pursuits, or otherwise be successful. Still others become experts in private thought. They experience anxiety and loneliness (Peplau, 1955; Peplau & Perlman, 1982). They are labeled as isolates, rejects, or loners.

As described previously, individuals who experience high anxiety in recurring situations tend toward *avoidance* of such anxiety-evoking situations. Loneliness, an intense, unpleasant, affective, emotional experience, tends to drive the lonely person *toward* people, at any price, as observable in public places such as bars, brothels, clubs, and gangs. Persons who exhibit both these powerful affects and have a history of spending much time in private thought, are at risk for hallucinatory experience. They are, in effect, pulled away from and toward people simultaneously, a circumstance initially attenuated by withdrawal and by hallucinating "helping figures," a safe way to relieve both anxiety and loneliness.

Clinical Examples of Phases of Hallucinations

Hallucination is an interpersonal process having four phases (Peplau, 1963b). Each phase has its own characteristics. Each succeeding phase in the evolving process is heralded by new interpersonal circumstances that intrude and change the hallucinating person's patterns of trying to meet his needs. Those needs include avoiding anxiety, relieving loneliness, and maintaining a precariously integrated self-system. The intrusions are experienced as failure of previously effective, relief-giving concealment and autistic resolution of personal need. As with all psychopathological processes the patient cannot extricate himself or herself from the hallucinatory experience without effective psychotherapeutic help. Therefore, in each subsequent phase in the process, the hallucinating person employs more drastic measures to obtain more desperately needed relief, but to no avail. Without psychotherapeutic intervention the process moves inexorably toward its inevitable end in chronicity.

Phase I of the process of hallucinating is illustrated in the following vignette. Here, an operative need for help was relieved and met by an autistic reverie:

> The wife of a farmer became critically ill in the middle of the night. Her husband and their three children drove her to the hospital, quite a distance from their farm. At the hospital, the husband attended to the arrangements for his wife's care, with staff, the physicians, and nurses. He left his 9-year-old daughter in charge of her siblings, ages 4 and 1 year, in the waiting room alone. The two younger children were very irritable and crying, and the 9-year-old felt her great burden of responsibility and was very worried about what might happen to the children and her mother. Then she remembered a girl she knew at church; they used to talk amiably together when she went to Sunday school. She invented a conversation with her "remembered friend," consulted her on what to do to comfort her small siblings, and sought her approval for actions taken. All went well. At daylight the father returned and was pleased that the children were all right.

An 11-year-old school girl's experience illustrates phase II in the hallucinatory process. Her need evolved out of her failures in earlier developmental events and a very deprived socioeconomic home situation.

> On arrival in the office of the school nurse, Mary asked: "May I talk with you about something that's been bothering me?" Mary then told the school nurse, "There is this other girl who goes everywhere with me. She's a real friend. But now she's telling me what to do and says if I don't do it she'll go away and never come back."

Intervention at the phase II point in the hallucinatory process is most likely to be effective. In the case cited, the school nurse arranged ten "talking sessions" with Mary, during which she discussed her need for real friends, her difficulties in making them, and the way in which she recalled and courted an illusory make-believe friend. The school nurse also talked with the school teachers and the child's mother, and without revealing to them the confidential data obtained in her talks with Mary, she made suggestions to them about including Mary in school group activities, and for talks between Mary and her mother during shared activities at home.

Phase III of the hallucinatory process evolves when interventions into phase II have not been carried out, or have not been effective, or when the occurrence of phase II behavior has not been recognized as such by persons who could be helpful. It is at this point that withdrawal behavior becomes most prominent. It is not the withdrawal behavior per se that is problematic, rather it is what goes on during such retreats from the social scene. Because the individual has felt helpless in regard to having some felt power and control in social situations, with real people, interactions with autistically invented figures become more attractive. The person exercises much ingenuity in finding time, places, and excuses that seem plausible to others, in order to be alone. In other words, he or she sets up situations to court and to have extensive interpersonal interactions with one or more illusory figures. In so doing, what is missing (that would ordinarily be provided by real people) is checking, challenging, validating, or invalidating the highly private thought the person is using exclusively, thereby having total power and control over self and invented others. This experience relieves the previously felt helplessness and powerlessness.

A major problem that arises as a consequence of disuse is the loss of control over the contents of awareness. This is manifested when so-called voices arrive uninvited by the person, "pop into mind," and conversations with them are held so as to be heard; often this occurs in the presence of other people. As one patient put it, "I was out-blued." The nurse, at first, mentally spelled this verbalization as *outblewed*, and decoded it as a blowout. But then she asked the patient to spell the word, at which point the patient also told her that the "voice came in out of the blue."

Whereas previously the patient was able to conceal interactions with figures when real people entered the situation, with a beginning loss of control over focal attention, efforts at such concealment fail to work. Anxiety, shame, and embarrassment rather than relief are felt when a real person observes the individual's hallucinatory behavior. These powerful emotions call out an even greater need for relief from such overwhelming discomfort. Relief is achieved by almost complete withdrawal from real life situations.

Phase III is a very good time for interpersonal intervention, particularly by a professional who is thoroughly knowledgeable about the three constructs presented in this paper, one who uses an investigative psychotherapeutic technique (Field, 1979). Great increases in shame and embarrassment, the escalation of anxiety into panic and enormous fear, generally occur when hospitalization occurs at this point, making the relief-giving symptoms even more important to the survival of the person as he or she perceives it. The careful use of psychotropic drugs to take the edge off anxiety is helpful. Long-term help, however, requires psychotherapeutic work and social interaction by persons sensitive to what is going on in the thought processes of a very troubled person.

Without effective intervention, psychopathologic processes continue to evolve toward an endpoint of chronicity. Phase IV, in which the person's loss of control over focal awareness is almost complete, means that inappropriate behavior, such as talking to so-called voices, becomes quite obvious to all observers. With increasing anxiety, more felt shame and embarrassment, and a dimly perceived sense of patterns of relief behavior that had previously worked, derogatory elements of the self-system come into play. The so-called voices, previously helpful and friendly, now become angry, threatening, and derogatory. The voices threaten to go away, make demands, or terrorize the individual, who now becomes quite confused. Survival looms as the major goal. Hospitalization generally occurs at this point. The people who observe such irrational behavior usually become very anxious and fearful; their expectation to maintain the figurative boundary between public mode and private mode thought and behavior is being threatened. Hallucinatory individuals empathize with the anxiety of others, which tends to increase their own anxiety, and quite frequently panic ensues. All too often the hallucinating individual at this point converts the escalating anxiety into enormous rage, acted out as violence and requiring physical restraints applied by others. The endpoint of phase IV generally is reached during hospitalization. Ineffective available treatments, insufficient knowledge, insufficient or unqualified staff able to use current knowledge fully, and unwitting symptom reinforcement (illness maintenance) by persons in the patient's environment—all are aspects in the production of the patient's chronicity. For the patient, the need for relief from terror is very great. This is achieved by the patient reaching compromises with his so-called voices. These compromises or negotiations are along the lines of "I won't . . . if you won't." Most frequently, the patient promises not to talk with or obey the hospital staff if the so-called voices do not derogate, threaten to leave, or make demands. Because the patient is in charge of his or her part as well as that of the autistically invented figures in this interpersonal transaction, it could be said that the patient achieves peace within—but forever remains mentally ill.

Nursing Interventions

There are some general guidelines for working interpersonally with patients who hallucinate (see Table 20.8). For the patient, the experience of hearing voices or, less frequently also seeing illusory figures, seems real; however, the nurse knows from the theoretical construct that they are illusory figures autistically invented for the twin purposes of avoiding anxiety and mitigating loneliness. This distinction between the patient's and nurse's perceptions should be clearly emphasized in what the nurse says to the patient. For example, when a nurse says, "Tell me about the voices," she has, in effect, linguistically accepted the voices as real. It is possible to maintain the distinction when the nurse says, "Tell me about these *so-called voices* of yours," or "Talk about the *voices you say you hear*," or "When did you first notice these so-called voices of yours?" These verbalizations are cumbersome. Their merit is threefold: (1) It lies in shedding doubt on the reality of the hallucinatory figures. (2) In attributing them solely to the patient, the nurse does not confirm or deny them, and therefore does not agree to their reality. And finally,

Concepts

(3) the perceptions of nurse and patient distinguished one from the other, are kept completely separate. If the nurse uses verbal inputs such as those suggested, sustaining the message but varying the language, eventually the patient will hear, internalize and act on— that is, begin to question or doubt—the reality of his or her so-called voices.

Sometimes, particularly with patients in phase IV, the so-called voices interfere with and tell the patient not to talk to the nurse; patients tend to convey that message. A useful nurse response is some variant of: "You tell your so-called voices they have twenty-three hours of your time, while I have only this hour with you; so the least your so-called voices could do would be to go away while you and I talk."

Eventually patients must dismiss their voices, which they can and will do only *after* they have generated awareness of their anxiety and loneliness, and of their behavioral responses to these powerful energizers. Usually many hours of therapeutic work precede dismissal of voices in phases III and IV. In the meantime, along with and not as a substitute for therapy, engaging patients in physical activities with staff and with other patients, such as throwing a ball, is remedial, because watching for the ball in play engages their attention. Talking about anything helps, because it is almost impossible to hallucinate while talking with another person. The way out of their "trapadaptation" is long, and the work is difficult and can only be accomplished when knowledgeable, sustained professional assistance is provided for hallucinating patients.

REFERENCES

American Nurses Association (1989). *Classification systems for describing nursing practice.* Kansas City, MO: Author.
American Nurses Association (1980). *Nursing: A social policy statement.* Kansas City, MO: Author.
Arieti, S. (1959). Schizophrenia: The manifest symptomology, the psychodynamic and formal mechanism. In S. Arieti (Ed.), *American handbook of psychiatry* (Vol. 1) (pp. 455–484). New York: Basic Books.
Beck, C. K., Rawlings, R. P., & Williams, S. R. (1988). *Mental health — Psychiatric nursing.* St. Louis: Mosby.

Bouwsma, W. J. (1988). *John Calvin: A sixteenth century portrait*. New York: Oxford.

Cooley, C. H. (1902). *Human nature and the social order*. New York: Scribners. (Reprinted in 1964 by Schocken Books)

Erickson, G. D., & Gustafson, G. (1968). Controlling auditory hallucinations. *Hospital and Community Psychiatry, 19*(10), 327–329.

Field, W. E., Jr. (1979). *The psychotherapy of Hildegard E. Peplau.* New Braunfels, TX: PSF Productions.

Gecas, V. (1982). The self-concept. *Annual Review of Sociology, 8,* 1–33.

Gordon, M. (1985). *Manual of nursing diagnosis.* New York: McGraw-Hill.

Gould, L. N. (1948). Verbal hallucinations and activity of vocal musculature. *American Journal of Psychiatry, 105,* 367–372.

Gould, L. N. (1949). Auditory hallucinations and subvocal speech: Objective study in a case of schizophrenia. *Journal of Nervous and Mental Disease, 109,* 418–427.

Gould, L. N. (1950). Verbal hallucinations as automatic speech: The reactivation of dormant speech habit. *American Journal of Psychiatry, 107,* 110–119.

Hochschild, A. (1974). *Half the way home.* New York: Viking-Penguin.

Johnson, F. H. (1978). *The anatomy of hallucinations* (pp. 1–40). Chicago: Nelson-Hall.

Kim, M. J., McFarland, G. K., & McLane, A. M. (Eds.). (1987). *Pocket guide to nursing diagnosis* (2nd ed.). St. Louis: Mosby.

King, I. M. (1981). *A theory for nursing.* New York: Wiley.

McLane, A. M. (Ed.). (1987). *Classification of nursing diagnosis: Proceedings of the seventh national conference.* St. Louis: Mosby.

Mead, G. H. (1934). *Mind, self, and society.* Chicago: University of Chicago Press.

Parsons, T. (1961). *Theories of society* (Vol. 1). New York: Macmillan.

Peplau, H. E. (1955). Loneliness. *American Journal of Nursing, 55*(12), 244–248.

Peplau, H. E. (1963a). A working definition of anxiety. In S. Burd & M. Marshall (Eds.), *Some clinical approaches to psychiatric nursing* (pp. 323–327). New York: Macmillan.

Peplau, H. E. (1963b, October/November). Interpersonal relations and the process of adaptation. *Nursing Science,* pp. 272–279.

Peplau, H. E. (1964). Professional and social behavior: Some difference worth the notice of professional nurses. *Quarterly* (published by the Columbia University Presbyterian Hospital School of Nursing Alumni Association, NYC), *50*(4), 23–33.

Peplau, H. E. (1978). Psychiatric nursing: Role of nurses and psychiatric nurses. *International Nursing Review, 25,* 41–47.

Peplau, H. E. (1987). Interpersonal constructs for nursing practice. *Nurse Education Today, 7*(5), 201–208.

Peplau, H. E. (1988). *Interpersonal relations in nursing.* London: Macmillan. (Reissue of 1952 book)

Peplau, L. A., & Perlman, D. (1982). *Loneliness: A sourcebook of current theory, research and therapy.* New York: Wiley.

Roy, C. (1984). *Introduction to nursing: An adaptation model* (2nd ed.). Englewood Cliffs, NJ: Prentice-Hall.

Sears, D. O., Peplau, L. A., Freedman, J. L., & Taylor, S. E. (1988). *Social psychology* (6th ed.). Englewood Cliffs, NJ: Prentice-Hall.

Sullivan, H. S. (1956). The interpersonal theory of mental disorder. In H. S. Perry, M. L. Gawel, & M. Gibbon (Eds.), *Clinical studies in psychiatry* (pp. 3–11). New York: Norton.

Tuma, H., & Maser, J. D. (Eds.). (1985). *Anxiety and the anxiety disorders.* Hillsdale, NJ: Erlbaum.

Wright, R. (1988). Did the universe just happen? *The Atlantic Monthly, 261*(4), 29–44.

Wylie, R. (1974). *The self concept* (revised ed., Vol. 1). Lincoln, NE: University of Nebraska Press.

CHAPTER 21

Thought Disorder in Schizophrenia: Corrective Influence of Nursing Behavior on Language of Patients

The language behavior of the schizophrenic patient reflects, and unless disrupted, perpetuates and worsens the thought disorder connected with this form of mental illness. Moreover, the language behavior of the nursing staff, in nurse–patient relationships, tends toward correction or reinforcement of such thought disorders. In this paper, these two ideas will be amplified and discussed.

It was Whorf (1956) who first recognized that language influenced thought, rather than the other way around. Moreover, he hypothesized that language, used habitually, also influenced subsequent perception and understanding of the environment. Language, then, is an important human instrument for representing

Paper originally presented at Bellevue Hospital, Psychiatric Unit Nursing Staff, New York, NY, May, 1966. Schlesinger Library, Radcliffe College, Cambridge, MA. No. 84-M107 Hildegard E. Peplau Archives, carton 40, volume 1456. Copyright 1986 by Schlesinger Library. Adapted and edited by permission.

experience, for looking at the environment, as well as for communicating these matters with other people, either in such a way as to be understood or to maintain mental illness.

The language behavior of schizophrenic patients should be of considerable interest to professional nurses because it reflects what is going on with the patient. Nurses are required by their work to observe the verbal exchanges that go on between themselves and patients. Their aim is to correct the thought disorder by influencing the language of the patient.

It is essential to point out that the verbal behavior of the schizophrenic patient is not the only concern of the nurse. Nonverbal behavior, including muteness, as well as disturbances of affect and action, are of equal concern in the total nursing care of these patients. However, the focus of this paper is on language patterns of patients that indicate particular difficulties in the use of the thought process, and tactics nursing personnel can use to correct these problematic language patterns.

WIPING OUT THOUGHT DUE TO SUDDEN INCREASE OF ANXIETY

Schizophrenic patients wipe out thought by actively courting dissociative tactics for dealing with experience. In order to relieve or prevent anxiety, the patient initially tried to block out what could be observed, and the relief obtained led to the habit of not noticing. However, because each next anxiety-producing idea or observation required similar relief, the aim being comfort rather than grasp of what was going on, the patient acquired a large repertoire of dissociative tendencies. Some of these are reflected in the language of the patient.

Some clinical variants of this pattern would include the following phrases, used recurringly by a particular patient: "I can't remember," "That's all," "I told you all," "My mind is a blank," "I don't remember," "I forget," "Nothing," "I don't really recall," and so on. The patient uses these phrases automatically. The patient has long since given up the effort required to try to remember, and this would continue to be the case long after these language patterns no longer provided the relief they afforded the patient through their initial usage.

There are two nursing tactics that would help undermine this language behavior of the patient in the direction of new and more useful behavior: (1) The nurse can aid the patient to identify the underlying anxiety by using such phrases as: "Are you anxious?" "Are you upset right now?" "Are you nervous?" or "What prevents you from remembering?" Recognizing anxiety is a first step in controlling and using it to advantage. [Editor's Note: See Chapter 20, pp. 278–294 of this volume, for a complete discussion of the concept of anxiety.] (2) The nurse can suggest a topic or area for discussion that might help the patient to get started talking. Useful phrases would include: "Tell me about coming to the hospital," "What was it like in your neighborhood at home," or "Talk about when you were in school."

AUTOMATIC KNOWING

In this pattern, the language of the patient conveys the idea that either the patient or the nurse knows something without any data being presented by either party. The patient "knows" without asking or telling. Often, very young children recognize and report meaning of an experience, without giving details, on the basis of "empathic observation" or by taking in rapidly a great many details and then generalizing with equal rapidity and, coincidentally, correctly in some instances. One root of this form of language and thought disturbance is the "forbidden gesture" (Sullivan, 1953, p. 86)—the common experience of children in which the parent or teacher has used the "dirty look" to convey annoyance and evoke obedience. The child, without asking, reads meaning into the data and fails to check with the adults as to accuracy. Automatic knowing has this "mind-reading" quality to it also.

The most common phrase that illustrates this language problem and its accompanying thought disorder is "you know." It is not difficult to find psychiatric patients who use this phrase up to ten times in as many minutes of discussion. The corrective tactic of the nurse is to say, "No, I don't know; tell me," or "What is it I am supposed to know?" or "On what basis am I to know what?" The contagion of the phrase "you know" requires the nurse to alert herself to hear it, then to respond with awareness of its use.

Sometimes this language pattern is also coupled with dependency, and the combined problem is then reflected in the phrases used. The patient might say: "I think I told you. . . ." or "I told you about. . . ." Often the nurse has no recall of such a discussion. In these instances, the nurse might say simply: "Tell me again" or "What was it you told me?" It is important that the nurse avoid participating in the dependency by reinforcing the patient's habit of assuming that others have already been told something.

Another variant of automatic knowing may have to do with statements about other people rather than about the nurse. For example, a patient might say "My wife thinks. . . ." or "My wife feels. . . ." In everyday language this same communication difficulty is common. However, when this phrase is used socially and the hearer says, "On what basis do you know that is what your wife thinks or feels?" the speaker would no doubt be able to describe the wife's behavior or repeat statements from which the inferences were drawn. The patient, however, cannot supply the missing data. The habit of knowing automatically is pathological for the patient who is unable to provide the data from which the inference is made. The nurse tactic with patients aims to influence the language difficulty; it is, therefore, based on the assumption that the patient can only know what the patient has observed. The nurse's tactic, therefore, is to aid recall of these data. In most instances the patient will have difficulty in recalling most or all of the wife's actions or statements to which he now refers. The patient cannot know (except on an automatic basis) what his wife thinks or feels, only what she says and does—which the patient can hear and observe. The nursing staff can help the patient to find out.

Still another variant is the patient who says, "They understand," assuming that others (perhaps patients in the ward or staff) know his or her predicament without any further data. Or the phrase might be, "They don't like the way I look"; that is, the patient has automatically drawn an inference about others. In order to undermine these tendencies toward "mind reading," the nursing personnel need to ask for the data from which these conclusions have been drawn.

TENDENCIES TOWARD
OVERGENERALIZATION

The mentally ill are noteworthy for their inability to describe the raw data of experiences that have been problematic for them. However, this incompetence can be successfully masked in a number of language patterns, of which overgeneralization is but one. The tendency toward global vagueness, sweeping assertion, or large overgeneralization is inherent in such phrases, used recurringly by patients, as the following: "Everything happened today," "Lots of things go on!" or "The whole world is a mess." Similarly, the problem may be reflected by the use of stereotyped phrases such as proverbs or cliches, which show use of "packaged" generalizations and the unwillingness of the patient to risk generalization on his own. These phrases might include the following: "Time will tell," "Still water runs deep," "That's fine," or "That's nice."

Nursing intervention directed toward this thought disorder is based on recognition that patients need to be helped to reproduce some raw data from their own experience by describing events. The nurse might say: "Give me an example of something you see as nice!" or "Describe one thing that happened today," or "Tell me the details of one piece of the worldly mess you are talking about." The nurse might also say: "Put the proverb into words of your own," or "What is the main point of that phrase (or proverb, or cliche)?" These tactics of the nurse, if used with persistence, will aid the patient to move toward some greater flexibility in language usage, which will in turn influence thought. Also, the nurse's encouragement to describe events will aid the patient in learning how to abstract more useful meaning from problematic experiences.

INADEQUATE CLASSIFICATION
OF EXPERIENCE

Language used habitually influences observation of subsequent experiences. Hence, when a patient classifies his perception of his wife as "jealous," despite the fact that this classification may be inadequate, subsequent interactions with her occur in light of this categorization. Erroneous or inadequate classifications may include such phrases as: "My wife blocks everything I do," or "My wife traps me," or "My sister was the favorite of my mother," and the like. In using these classifications, the patient who is mentally ill is losing or has lost connecting links between these categories and the raw data of experiences. Again, the nurse elicits examples, instances, or descriptions of particular events to which the "favorite" or "trap" categories were first applied. As the patient recovers and reviews these data, now described to another person, the classification can be rechecked and revised. The nurse could say, "Tell me the details of one particular time your mother showed that your sister was a favorite."

PROBLEMATIC USAGE OF PRONOUNS

Pronouns are used in place of names in situations in which the referents are known to the participants or can be readily identified on request. The mentally ill, however, use pronouns for quite other purposes. The identity problem of nonseparateness of self is seen commonly in schizophrenic patients who use *we* to refer to the self plus some vague incorporated illusory other. This tendency to refer to oneself and the incorporated other person as a unit is inherent in the recurring use of *we, let's,* or *us.* The nurse who does not ask, "Who is *we?* You and who else?" or otherwise disrupt this language pattern helps to perpetuate the nonseparation problem reflected in this language. Similarly, the lack of self-awareness, almost dissociation of the self, is implicit in such patient phrases as "You can tell" (when referring to self) or "One gets paranoid feelings because they want you to stop gambling." In these instances the nurse needs to ask: "Who can tell?" or "Who gets these so-called paranoid feelings?" Another variant of problematic pronoun usage is coupled with "automatic knowing"—the use of *they.* The patient might say, "They are out to get us" and be unable to identify either the *they,* or *us.* That is a problem with which the patient needs help.

It is helpful to aid the patient to name the real people hidden in the pronoun by asking, "Who are they?" In using this tactic, with persistence, every time that the patient uses *they,* the nurse will find that the patient's language behavior follows a predictable sequence: (1) *they;* (2) *the people, everyone;* (3) a class of people such as *the doctors, the nurses, my family;* and, finally, (4) names of people to whom the pronoun refers. Persistence in the language behavior of the nurse is the key that aids the patient to reach step 4 in time.

On the other hand, the nurse might find the patient who combines step 2, *the people* as indicated above with a tendency toward over-generalization. For example, one patient said: "People here have to understand that people outside are cruel to people with mental illness." Thus, the patient uses *people* as one classification to refer to different categories—*people here, people outside,* and *people with mental illness,* qualifying each by one small unique characteristic. Unless someone asks: "Who are the people outside that you are referring to?" or "What are the names of the people that you have in mind?" this habit of thought will continue and get worse. Moreover, other patients reinforce the thought disorder when they merely nod their heads or verbally agree with the patient. The patients, then, more and more share such generalities and incorrect language usage, and thereby continue to lose more and more ability to get the raw data to which these generalizations refer. If this situation goes on, as it does in large public mental hospitals every day, chronicity is produced. The problems then become less and less amenable to verbal intervention by anyone except over years and years of patient psychotherapeutic work. Prevention and early intervention in the language usage of first admissions are indicated.

There are other incorrect usages of pronouns that reflect thought distortion. For example, the patient can use a plural pronoun but be talking about one person. One patient who had been using *they* recurringly finally reached the point where he said, "They, I mean my sister-in-law." This too is characteristic and to be expected—that the old language habit persists side-by-side with the new language behavior until finally the latter becomes the modus operandi.

Mentally ill people tend to lose connections of all kinds with reference to their experiences. Nurses deal with aspects of these experiences reflected in language such as the pronouns the patient uses. The nurse can help patients to recapture the names of the real people they have in mind when using these pronouns. As has been suggested above, this effort on the part of the nurse also influences other aspects of pathology such as concealment, nonseparateness, dissociation of experience, and the general disconnectedness with which the patient treats experiences.

FOCUSING ON NONOCCURRING EXPERIENCE

Many textbooks suggest that nursing staff should help patients to face reality. One of the concrete ways to do this is through the verbal response of the nurse when the patient uses language to refer to things, events, or people that are not aspects of reality. There are several different varieties of this problem. The patient might talk only in future-oriented terms. The future, especially for mentally ill persons, is not something the nurse can discuss with the patient with any useful purpose until and unless the nurse knows a good deal about the past and present experience and behavior of the patient. Future-oriented language is like fantasy; it deals with things that have not yet happened. Consequently, the patient can invent all of the data and thus control it. For example, if a nurse says to a patient who has been hospitalized for ten years, "Tell me what has gone on since I saw you yesterday" and the patient responds, "Well, I'm fine; I'm planning to go home and be with my family and keep my house clean and take care of my husband and my children," it is obvious that the patient is future-oriented. But, for this patient, the chances of any of these ideas being realized are slim. So, the nurse needs to say, "Tell me about the last day that you were home" or "Tell me about the last time you visited with your husband (or children)." The aim is to aid the patient to talk about real experience—about something that did happen.

In a similar vein, some patients are primarily *if-* oriented; these patients will use such recurring phrases as "If I did. . . ." or "I wonder what. . . ." Again, it is more useful for the nurse to seek examples of actual, direct, past, or present experience than to participate in the autistic invention and thereby to make it mutual. In this same category are the negative oriented communications in which patients talk about what did not happen—what was not thought, felt, or done. The patient might say: "I don't suppose. . . ." or "I didn't have. . . ." or "I don't think. . . ." or "I don't feel good," or "I'm not here for good," and so on. The nurse ought to seek what did happen—what the patient does think, did feel, is in the hospital for, and the like. The nurse can do this by saying, "Name the feeling you do have," or "What are you thinking now?"

There is another category of nonoccurring experience that includes such phrases as "I should. . . ." "I must. . . ." "I ought. . . ." and the negative of these such as "I shouldn't. . . ." "I can't. . . ." and the like. In these phrases the nurse seeks what did actually happen—what the patient did do in particular experiences which can be described.

INADEQUATE RELATIONS AMONG SEVERAL MEANINGS OF EXPERIENCE

There are several variants of language usage that reflect the difficulty of the patient in focusing, policing, or controlling the contents of his attention. This ability to control focal attention develops slowly, in the family and in school. Both child rearing and teacher discipline of pupils include particular tactics, which more or less force the growing child to gain some control of what is up front in the mind. With the mentally ill, because of anxiety and disuse of the ability to exert such control, there is increasing loss of control over focal attention. This problem is reflected in the language behavior as well as in the actions of the patient. It is reflected in various forms: Prototaxis, the tendency to treat each moment of experience as if it were unconnected to prior or subsequent experience, is seen in chronic mentally ill patients, in severely brain damaged, as well as in patients in acute panic. The tendency is toward concreteness, repetitiveness, focusing on a detail, and the general absence of any associations between ideas. The nurse needs to recognize prototaxis. If it is due to anxiety, the tactic is to aid in anxiety reduction; if due to chronic disuse, the tactic is to stay with the concrete detail and work for its enlargement; if due to brain damage, the tactic is to treat the patient prototaxically, recognizing that ability to make connections may be temporarily or permanently lost.

One chronic patient illustrated this juxtaposition of three unrelated ideas: "I want to go home because my brother is 16 and my sister is married." The connections here are *because* and *and;* the ideas that connect these three facts are lost—the patient has not presented them. Another patient said: "I'm enjoying it here; that's why I want to go home." There are many different types of such juxtaposition. Two common types are inadequate cause–effect relations where neither the suggested cause nor effect are clear and may not be related, and temporal sequence disorientation, where ideas are not put in relevant serial order.

Another type of statement indicates more or less complete loss of control of the contents of focal awareness. Some examples would include: "The thought hit me," "Sleep hits me all of a sudden when I get up," "The idea struck me," "I picked up his thought without his knowing it," and so on. These kinds of statements should alert the nurse to what is going on—the patient is losing more and more control. Instead of deciding what to think and what not to think, at any given moment the patient's "thoughts think the patient." Thoughts "pop into his mind" without any choice on his part. The next step in this process is hallucination or delusional thinking.

The main problem of psychiatric patients is anxiety. It influences language and thought. It has the effect of a "blow on the head"—wiping out details of experience and therefore leading to language usage based upon inadequately seen or recalled data. Not all such data can be fully recalled by the patient, but there should be effort in that direction. It is not necessary, either, that the patient recall every detail of every experience that has been undergone—even if this were possible, which it is not. What is necessary is for all people to have gradually enlarging ability to describe experiences in which they are participants, to talk these over with at least one other person and therefore to check their observations and conclusions as to accuracy and relevance. This is the way to mental health. Nursing is a way of helping patients to do this. In the psychiatric setting, the language of the patient presents the most useful data concerning many of the difficulties that need correcting. In this kind of corrective work, the effects of the language and language tactics of the nursing staff are of paramount importance. The nurse's language influences the patient's language and that, in turn, influences the patient's thought; and the patient's thought in turn guides his or her actions and is required to formulate the patient's feelings, the relevance between thought, feeling, and actions, and the relationship among events and people with whom the patient interacts as a social being.

In this chapter I suggest seven categories of language disturbance seen in psychiatric patients, about which nursing personnel can do something constructive in their verbal interchanges with patients—however long these may be. This discussion, however, is not intended to be a comprehensive statement on each of these categories or to constitute the sum of language difficulties seen in the mentally ill (see Chapter 22, this volume).

REFERENCES

Sullivan, H.S. (1953). *The interpersonal theory of psychiatry.* New York: Norton.
Whorf, B. (1956). *Language, thought, and reality.* New York: Wiley.

CHAPTER 22

An Explanatory Theory of the Process of Focal Attention

Professional nurses are constantly searching for theoretical concepts and processes that will elucidate or explain the meaning of
their observations of patients and prove useful for deriving
theory-based nursing practice. One such process Schachtel (1959)
calls *focal attention*. This theory clarifies observable behaviors
connected with the selection of a focus of attention and ability to
sustain interest in and derive meaning from it. This human function sometimes does not develop, or evolves incompletely, or the
ability is lost for organic or functional reasons. Strategies used by
professional nurses can help develop or restore focal attention
ability. Such nursing interventions, essential for health promotion,
are important practices during psychotherapeutic work and for
use in nurse–patient interactions in any clinical milieu.

Original paper, 1983. Schlesinger Library, Radcliffe College, Cambridge, MA.
No. 84-M107, Hildegard E. Peplau Archives, carton 32, volume 1163. Copyright
1986 by Schlesinger Library. Adapted and edited by permission.

DEFINITION

Focal attention has specific characteristics differentiating it from *focal awareness*, which refers to a more global recognition of an impinging environment. Focal attention includes: (1) observing in a particular direction; (2) noticing an external or internal object, such as a thing, idea or feeling; (3) making an active effort to grasp the object intellectually; and (4) using not only a sustained approach but also subsequent efforts to explore the object's various aspects and relations. Acts of focal attention, therefore, are governed by curiosity and intense interest in an aspect of a larger field. As can be inferred from the description of steps in evolution of focal attention that follows, the use of each step forces development of subsequent ones, and ultimately of related competencies required for the highly disciplined use of this ability as seen in professionals, eminent scholars, or scientists.

PHASES AND STEPS IN THE EVOLUTION OF FOCAL ATTENTION

Phase one might be entitled *evolution of the capacity*. It can be assumed that in utero all of the physiochemical conditions will be available to the growing fetus, and that no specific need differentiation by the infant occurs. A first step in developing the capacity for focal attention occurs when the infant takes notice, perhaps as a "felt relation," (Peplau, 1952) that the mother's breast is apart from the self. Later, this "vaguely directional" or not wholly global observation is elaborated as the infant notes that his or her need and the mother-as-the-source-of-need-satisfaction are not merged. The infant's tentative awareness of this separateness results from two major aspects of experience: (1) object constancy, that is, the internalization of mothering experiences as a ready source of response to personal need; and (2) the reliability of crying as the tool that calls for the source of need satisfaction when required. Obviously, then, the alert, caring, constant response of the mother (or parenting person) to the infant, in the first month of life, has much to do with satisfactory development in this phase in the earliest functioning of the capacity for focal attention.

Phase two might be called *reactive attending*. After birth, the newborn infant begins, gradually, to differentiate need tensions from the sources of need satisfaction. Here the infant's beginning differentiation from mother continues in two substeps. (1) At first, there is vaguely directional staring at large objects. At about the 5th week, the infant will focus briefly on most large objects that happen to come into the range of vision. By the tenth week, the focus is more prolonged. However, although the infant notices the object, the interest that is manifested does not persist, so shortly, from the infant's standpoint, the object ceases to exist. (2) In the next few weeks, the infant begins to follow a moving object and begins to retain longer interest in it. This development heralds the next phase.

Phase three marks the further development of *selective attending*. By the 9th to 12th months, there is observable evidence of ability to focus on small objects. If the object disappears, the infant will begin to look for it. The *idea* of object as contrasted to object per se now engages the attention of the infant. This is also a time when speech begins to emerge; therefore, the thought process can now evolve beyond an extremely primitive stage, and ideas begin to generate. Similarly, the developing self-system begins now to include a baseline of reflected appraisals, inputs to the infant from significant persons. Later, with the use of the personal pronoun *I*, there is further development of relational thought, and therefore more connections between self-other and self-objects are noticed (Sullivan, 1953).

With most children, by age 2, the foregoing phases and steps in focal attention are complete. Nevertheless, between age 2 and the beginning of school at age 6, depending upon the child-rearing tactics of parents, most children can and still do move quite freely between the private mode of thought (autistic, highly individual, fantastic) and the public mode (reality-oriented ideas held in common and shared with others).

Phase four represents a period of testing and further development of ability to focus attention. In the first three grades of school the child is required to police his or her attention to maintain the focus designated by the teacher. Thought is now in the public mode. Thus, the child learns to (1) inattend fantasy (the private mode); (2) to shift attention voluntarily from person thought to the teacher-designated focus; (3) to audit (that is, to hear and notice his or her own speech and behavior), and (4) to edit or change personal behavior in conformity with requirements of school. These four complex tasks evolve or fail to do so as a consequence of the child's interactions.

Traditionally, teachers have used tactics to force children to refine their ability to focus attention. The teacher reminds the child periodically by saying, "You are not paying attention." The teacher might warn, punish, humiliate, belittle, or even abandon the child. Many children have reading disabilities or other problems in focal attention for which remedial help is needed and for which specialized, theory-based modern strategies are required by teachers and school nurses.

IMPLICATIONS

Persistent inability to focus attention in phase four is an early sign that should be heeded, because early attention to it might prevent mental disorder. Reparative experiences related to phases two and three might be required if the difficulty can be pinpointed as stemming from early childhood experience in the home situation. Other causes of disability, however, may be directly related to the current schoolroom experience. For instance, anxiety prevents the child from using inherent ability if, for example, he or she observes destructive fights between parents before coming to school. More compelling needs then compete with the teacher-directed ideas for the focus of a child's attention. Suppose the child has come to school hungry or cold, or has a great longing for but does not have the social skills to gain interest from peers rather than the adults. That child may be distracted from a teacher-directed focus. In addition, fear of being different from his or her family, especially when at home there is scattered thought and disorganization, may compound the difficulties inherent in the child's efforts to focus attention on learning. A significant problem occurs when there are gross discrepancies between appraisals within the child's self-system and the actual capacities available for further development. School nurses and teachers need strategies to counteract habit and, especially, tendencies toward disuse of capacity for focal attention.

Although teachers in the first three grades focus on teaching beginning skills in reading, writing, and arithmetic, from a developmental point of view, the main interest and curiosity of the child tends to be focused on making way with his or her agemates. Moreover, simultaneously, in the ages 6 to 9 juvenile era, the child has perhaps the most complicated social learning at the forefront. At that time, the child must learn how to make smooth transitions from home, to school, to peer group, and perhaps to religious group situations. Each of these four situations has requirements of its own. Ability to focus attention must be enlarged quickly because the child must now, voluntarily, discipline thought, to please in turn members of the family, the teacher, peers, and religious teachers. There are similarities and differences among these four social situations that need to be perceived and kept in mind if success is to be had and humiliation and failure are to be prevented.

The juvenile-era child operates primarily in the parataxic mode, that is, he or she searches for the familiar, relating to new situations in the present in terms of familiar elements known from similar situations experienced in the past. The child must now focus on, notice, and take into account differences in these situations. The child who does not develop this shift in ability to focus attention may suffer shame and embarrassment. Or the child may feel envy for children who somehow can make smooth transitions, can manage with a modicum of success in all four situations, and therefore are liked, gaining much approval. Such powerful emotions then contribute to and compound any earlier difficulty in focal attention. Withdrawal, apathy, distractibility and other early signs of difficulty are seen in children called "misfits," the children who do not make satisfactory developmental progress in the first three grades of school. Not all these children, but altogether too many, may later be diagnosed as having psychiatric disabilities. In later eras of development new and more complex intellectual and interpersonal competencies built on earlier ones are required by increasingly adult, complex, life situations. It is these requirements, which compound the dysfunctions, that perhaps result in mental illness.

DYSFUNCTIONS OF FOCAL ATTENTION

There are many kinds of dysfunction directly related to focal attention, variations of which professional nurses observe in the behavior of patients, especially the mentally ill. Although other explanatory concepts suggest some guides for intervention, the process of focal attention provides others. The following are some of these dysfunctions and recommended intervention strategies.

Prototaxis

Some patients focus more or less exclusively upon the "now" moment. Such behavior is similar to that seen in phase two described above. It is characterized by the absence of relational thought, namely, the ability to notice, formulate and act in light of connections, such as before and after (then and now) or between the present and future (actions and their effects). Prototaxis is seen in patients having severe anxiety or panic, in brain-damaged patients, and for reasons as yet unexplained in "psychopaths." The aim of the nurse is to enlarge the focus on the "now" moment (that is, the present, presenting item) in the hope of evoking some connecting link to a "then" moment (that is, the previously experienced item). The nurse would say, "Talk about that," "Say some more about that idea," "Describe further what you just said." In patients who are severely anxious, the nurse also has the useful option of having the anxiety named.

In brain-damaged patients, the nurse might seek other laboratory and professional reports so as to establish a basis for judging whether seeing, stating, retaining, and acting on connections between past and present are possible for a particular patient. If they are not, the nurse would merely react to the immediate demand, acceding to it or not, but recognizing that connections between the immediate demand and previous similar demands from the patient cannot be forced. The nurse who becomes annoyed when a brain-damaged patient repetitively asks the same question does not know the concept of prototaxis—nor does the nurse apply it in nursing practice.

Scattering of Thought

Patients sometimes use what is called *flight of ideas,* a long chain of ideas presented, one in juxtaposition to the other, with little if any association or connection between them. The inability of the patient to focus on one of these ideas, sustain interest, develop and state the idea clearly and fully to a hearer, is most noticeable. Consequently, the nurse tactic is to aid the patient to maintain a point and elaborate it. Sometimes this is easier for the patient to follow if the nurse asks about the very last idea presented. Frequently in scattering there is also severe anxiety, and the nurse has a theory-based intervention for this difficulty.

Circumstantiality

Some patients are unable to come to a point directly. They either lose the point in tangential verbiage or delay getting to it, thereby taxing the comprehension and interest of the hearer. Having and using a power tactic that evokes helplessness and felt loss of control in the hearer may not have been an ingredient in the early evolution of this language–thought difficulty, but in the mentally ill what is seen is an automatic, habitually used pattern of language behavior. The aim of the nurse is not to get lost in the patient's verbalization, but instead to attempt to grasp the point, and to ask about that point, repeatedly!

Elusive Marginal Thought

Everyone has difficulty at some time or other pulling in ideas (names of people, for example) that are on the "edge of mind" or "on the tip of the tongue," as the folk saying has it. The mentally ill, however, tend to court unawareness and have more frequent difficulty along this line. The aim of the nurse is to encourage the patient to police attention and to bring the elusive idea within the focus of attention. Verbal tactics, such as "Say immediately what comes into your mind," "When an idea occurs to you, say it," or "Give it a try, say what you think" are useful.

Ruminative Thought

The patient who ruminates has an idea in the focus of attention, is unable to push the idea out of mind, and in essence maintains a nonproductive overfocus on one detail of that idea or a symbolically related idea. The patient is unable to examine the "worrying idea" in all aspects, considering or weighing their respective merits in order to reach a resolution and then dismiss the idea so the focus of attention could shift to another subject. Such patients will say, repetitively, "I can't stop worrying." A useful intervention is, "Say the worrying idea out loud now; talk to me about it." Verbal maneuvers in a similar vein that encourage the patient to examine the ideas that go "around and around," in time disrupt the difficulty. The patient who says, "I can't get my mind off my father" often responds in a manner that helps when the nurse says, "Talk about you and your father."

Almost Complete Loss of Control

Chronic patients in mental hospitals often manifest almost complete loss over focal attention, in part due to disuse of the ability. These are patients who find it difficult, if not impossible, to harness their ideas and state them, to hang onto ideas and consider them, or even to recognize the source of ideas that are heard. To assist patients to exercise these functions in daily nurse–patient verbal encounters is an important nursing practice that helps patients to regain ability for focal attention. These are the patients who say, "My mind is a blank," "I don't think of anything," "I thought of something a minute ago but not now," or "The voices just pop into my mind and I can't stop them from calling me names" (Peplau, 1963). Obviously, these are not simple nursing problems. They are problems to be corrected or prevented in all patients by theory-derived verbal strategies of nursing personnel from the very first day of admission. An optimistic bias ought to guide work with these patients as general principles are applied in order to bring about some return or further development of ability to focus attention.

GENERAL PRINCIPLES

One aim of nursing actions with all psychiatric patients is the development or restoration and further refinement of ability to focus attention. The concept of focal attention defined in this paper suggests various dimensions of the problem. Ten principles, derived from the concept, are presented below. The relation of these principles to the phases in development of focal attention, and the inherent quality of corrective experience for patients in the suggested nursing practices can be inferred easily by the reader. When these principles guide the sustained, concerted actions of professional nurses, favorable improvement in focal attention can be anticipated. However, because there is no magic in such actions, it goes without saying that the nurse must sustain the actions over time, varying the language but not the message.

1. When the nurse maintains an identity separate from that of patients, reflecting this separation in his or her language and gestures, this stimulus may evoke in patients differentiation of self from significant others.
2. When one set of knowledgeable nursing personnel is assigned around-the-clock to each patient, and these nurses apply theory to understand the patients' difficulties, and use that theory in their daily practices, object constancy becomes a possibility in that dependable resources for meeting and formulating needs become internalized, later to be used in the nurses' absence.
3. Inasmuch as psychiatric patients use only the tools for communication and social interaction they have, respect for these tools, coupled with concerned effort at developing a next step in evolution of higher-level social approaches, is a main aim of the professional nurse and those she or he supervises.
4. When patients experience the genuine interest of the same, consistent staff, they are aided in the development of initial phases of selective attending. The use of remotivation, TV discussions, group discussion, ward-group teaching of specific concepts in simplified, visual form, are among the foci nurses could develop.
5. Because most psychiatric patients operate from a self-system overloaded with ideas of derogation, worthlessness, and

hopelessness, it is incumbent upon nursing personnel neither to collide with nor confirm such operating self-views of patients, because these approaches require the patients to redouble efforts to sustain and make more concrete the views currently held.

6. The professional nurse who evaluates her or his own ability to select a focus, sustain interest in and derive meaning from it, is more likely to be able to aid patients to gain competencies along similar lines. Tactics to force attention on one thing, and therefore to develop ability through use of focal attention include such verbal tactics as "Tell about one time," "Describe one event," "Talk about one problem," and "Say one thing that worries you."

7. Anxiety underlies focal attention problems and perpetuates the difficulty until the anxiety is named and otherwise recognized, understood, and to some extent controlled by the patient.

8. More compelling needs—for respect, privacy, interest—preclude development of ability to focus attention and should be given first priority.

9. All nursing personnel can promote such competencies as self-expression, stating thoughts, describing actions, and naming feelings in all patients, thereby encouraging development of abilities closely related to resolution of focal attention dysfunctions.

10. Every ward provides opportunity for corrective peer-group experiences when the nursing personnel take seriously the theories related to this developmental need and its relation to focal attention problems of the mentally ill.

REFERENCES

Peplau, H. E. (1952). *Interpersonal relations in nursing.* New York: Putnam.
Peplau, H. E. (1963). Interpersonal relations and the process of adaptation. *Nursing Science, 1,* 272–279.
Schachtel, E. G. (1959). *Metamorphosis.* New York: Basic Books.
Sullivan, H. S. (1953). *Conceptions of modern psychiatry.* New York: Norton.

CHAPTER 23

Process and Concept of Learning

Learning is an active process which utilizes the thinking and perceiving abilities and knowledge previously acquired for three major purposes: (1) acquiring new knowledge to explain events, (2) facilitating change, and (3) solving problems.

Steps in learning as a concept and as a process	Operations, performances, behaviors, separate skills, associated with each step in learning. (Major use of the perceptual processes—see, hear, smell, touch, etc.)	Examples of statements by the nurse to facilitate development of each step in a patient, in the total sequence of the process of learning
1. To observe: The ability to notice what went on or what goes on now	To see with one's eyes To hear To feel using empathic observation To feel using tactile senses	What do you see? What is that noise? Are you uncomfortable? Do you have something to say to me? Could I share the thought with you or is it private? Tell me about yourself. What happened? I don't follow. Tell me, what did you notice? You noticed what? Did you see this happen? Who was with you? When did this occur? What is the color? Where were you? Tell me. Then what? Go on. Give me a blow-by-blow description. Tell me every detail from the beginning.

Assumption: The patient can describe the situation as he or she viewed it with encouragement and assistance from a person who can focus exclusively on the situation of the patient.

Learning	Operations	Nurse statements: Who, what, when, which, where
2. To describe: The ability to recall and tell the details and circumstances of a particular event or experience.	Increased verbalization Greater recall Enumeration of details Focus on details of one event	Tell me about the feeling. What name would you give to your feeling? Tell me more. Then what?

Learning	Operations	Nurse statements: Who, what, when, which, where
	Movement of patient's general and ambiguous terms for person(s) and nurse's question words assisting patient to be specific	Go on,— Give me an example. Who are they? What about that? For instance? Describe that further. Give me a blow-by-blow account of that. What did you feel at the time? What happened just before? Which was it? Who was the person? What did you say? What did your comment evoke in the other?

Patient's terms	Nurse's question words
1. Everybody They Them Technicians	Who?
2. The nurses The doctors	Which?
3. The ones who work from 8 to 4 (narrowing)	What are their names?
4. Miss Jones (specific name)	

Use nurse statements of observation step, as well.

Explain.
Help me to understand that!
What do you mean?

Learning	Operations	
3. To analyze: The ability to review and to work over the raw data with another person	Examples of the kinds of analysis used by the nurse	What do you see as the reason? What was the significance of that event? What are the common elements in these two situations? What is the connection? Boil this down to the one important aspect. What caused this? What was your part in it? In what way did you participate? In what way did you reach this decision? What caused this feeling? (I expected you at 8:30; you were late; that caused my anger.) Have you had this feeling before? Is there anything similar in this situation to your previous experience?
	Identify needs Decode key symbols Distinguish literal and figurative Sort and classify 1. Impressions 2. Speculations 3. Thematic abstractions 4. Hypotheses 5. Generalizing Compare Summarize Sequence Application of concepts Application of personality theory as a frame of reference *Formulating relations* resulting from the foregoing: 1. Cause and effect 2. Temporal 3. Thematic 4. Spatial	
Step 3 may occur simultaneously with Step 4.		

Learning	Operations	Nurse statements: Who, what, when, which, where
4. To formulate: The ability to give form and structure, to restate in a clear, direct way, the connections resulting from Step 3 (analysis)	Restatement of data in light of Step 3 Verbal or written result of analysis of data	State the essence of this situation in a sentence or so. What did you feel? What did you think? What did you do? Tell it to me in a sentence or so. Tell me again. Was there a discrepancy between what you felt, thought, and did? What would you say was the problem? What name would you give to the patterns of your behavior as you interacted with another person?
5. To validate (by consensus): The ability to check with another person and to reach agreement as to the result of Step 4 (formulation), or to state clearly the issue if there is divergence in the formulations of the two persons	Checking with, comparing notes of two or more people Pt: Are you anxious? (Pt trying to validate.) N: (Is anxious.) No, I'm not Yes, I could say I am. What called my anxiety to your attention?	Is this what you mean? Let me restate. Is this what you were saying? Do you go along with this? Is this what you believe? It seems that—Is this the way it appears to you? Is it that you feel angry when people tell you what to do? Am I correct in concluding that ___? Are you saying ___?
6. To test: The ability to try out the result of Step 4 (formulation) in situations with people, things, etc., for utility, completeness		(Set up situations where patient can try out new behavior patterns.) Now that you have thought about this and come to this conclusion, why don't you try it out? What would you do if a situation like this came up again? In what way can you use this conclusion to prevent repeating this mistake?

Learning	Operations	Nurse statements: Who, what, when, which, where
		In what way will this conclusion help you in the future? What difference will it make now that you know this?
7. To integrate: The ability to see the new in relation to or as an integral part of the old; to add to previously acquired usable knowledge for active use by the person	Enmeshing the new with the old	
8. To utilize: The ability to use the result of Step 4, (formulation) as foresight		(Set up situations where patient can use new behavior patterns.)

Editors' Summary

CONTRIBUTION TO THE DEVELOPMENT OF NURSING THEORY

Hildegard E. Peplau based her interpersonal theory of nursing primarily on the work of Harry Stack Sullivan. Her theory was the first conceptualization of nursing to emphasize interpersonal relations between the nurse and the patient, and to focus on the analysis of the interpersonal processes central to that interaction (Meleis, 1985). She observed that the crucial elements in nursing situations are the nurse, the patient, and what goes on between them (Peplau, 1954). This interactional or interpersonal point of view was in sharp contrast to the prevailing notion that a pathological condition resided within the patient, and the nurse's role was to assist the physician to fix that condition without consideration of the interpersonal elements—not to mention the nurse's autonomy. So Peplau directed nursing's attention to the need to develop a consciousness, that is, a theory, about what the nurse and patient did together. Her theory also provided the knowledge to turn nursing in the direction of autonomous practice during an era when nursing was dominated by medicine (Fitzpatrick & Whall, 1983).

Peplau's contributions to nursing theory are placed historically, after those of Florence Nightingale who, in the late 1800s, addressed the need for nurses to be educated and to conduct research regarding the effect of hygiene and the environment on patient's welfare (Meleis, 1985). Peplau's 1952 book is an application of interpersonal theory to nursing and became the first modern nursing theory.

By introducing interpersonal relations theory into nursing she addressed what she saw as an identity crisis for nursing. Traditional bedside nursing with intensive hands-on care was gradually being phased out at that time, as early ambulation, increase in medical science, and development of medical technology were being introduced. What was the nurse to do if she could not be a traditional bedside nurse and give physical care? This identity crisis required a major change in nursing, and Peplau provided the direction for that change (Peplau, 1983). Nurses would learn to nurse through interpersonal relations.

In addition to the identity crisis in nursing, a second social trend influenced Peplau to develop theory in nursing. Nurses were portrayed by the popular press as "airheads": kind, friendly, but certainly not thinking professionals. To a large extent, nursing itself accepted this view of its members. Peplau (1987) states, "Well into the 1940's, many textbooks for nurses, often written by physicians, clergy, or psychologists, reminded nurses that theory was too much for them, that nurses did not need to think but rather merely to follow rules, be obedient, be compassionate, do their 'duty,' and carry out medical orders" (p. 18). Peplau recognized that in order for nurses to be effective in their work, they must be professional; and in order to be professional they must know and use a body of knowledge. She set out to provide that knowledge.

Characteristics of Peplau's Theory

Peplau's theory may be characterized as *middle range*, a term coined by Merton (1957) to describe theories that fall between the all-inclusive, abstract, grand theories on the one hand and the very specific collection of empirical facts on the other. Merton wrote about the need for middle-range theories when theory development in sociology was focused on grand theory that attempted to explain all social behavior and to provide an integrated conceptual structure from which all theories could be derived. Middle-range theories focus on a limited aspect of reality and provide "clear, verifiable statements of relationships between specified variables" (p. 9). Grand theory in nursing attempts to explain mankind or the human condition. Middle-range theories, such as Peplau's, explain manageable aspects of the universe, for example, the relationship between nurse and patient, or the development of an individual's self-concept. Identification and explanation of phenomena such as anxiety, conflict, and hallucinations are examples of middle-range theories developed by Peplau. The aim of middle-range theories in nursing is to provide empirically verifiable concepts and propositions where the applicability to practice is made explicit.

Peplau's method of theory development is both inductive and deductive. She used her own clinical practice and the practice of students to inductively derive theories that she subsequently tested in clinical settings. She also applied existing social science theory, notably the interpersonal theory of Sullivan, to nursing data. The process of combining induction (observation and classification) with deduction (the application of known concepts and processes to data) provides a creative nonlinear approach to the formation of ideas: one that uses the data of practice, as well as extant theories, as the basis of those formulations.

Peplau described this process of practice-based theory development in her address at the First Nursing Theory Conference in 1969 (Peplau, 1969). The nurse first observes a phenomenon in practice, then applies a name to the phenomenon, selecting that name from available concepts. The concept provides an explanation and a structure to obtain more data, for the professional goes beyond mere naming. Data collection provides a broader base of information and may lead to discarding the initial concept and selecting or inventing another one. Finally, the concept or name suggests intervention for the phenomenon. In short, the nurse observes, interprets, and then intervenes, a process that has relevance for both practice and for practice-based research.

Elaboration of the interpretation phase of the three-step process as it applies to clinical research may clarify the way Peplau approached analysis of clinical data. The data she used were verbatim recordings of her own interactions with patients and those of her students. She examined those data looking for regularities, and began by transcribing similar looking data to 3 × 5 cards, which allowed her to sort, classify, and count. For example, when she first began to teach psychiatric nursing at Teachers College in 1948, she asked the students to make carbon copies of their nurse–patient interactions. She took

these home and studied them and noticed that all the students absolutely could not talk in a friendly way to the patient until the patient
had said, "I need you" or "I like you." Her theory of anxiety came from
the analysis of nurse–patient data such as these. She collected all
examples of anxiety and analyzed them to locate the serial order of
the occurrence of the operations (Peplau, 1981).

Definition of Nursing

Peplau (1952) defined nursing as follows:

> Nursing is a significant, therapeutic, interpersonal process. It functions
> co-operatively with other human processes that make health possible
> for individuals in communities. . . . Nursing is an educative instru-
> ment, a maturing force, that aims to promote forward movement of
> personality in the direction of creative, constructive, productive, per-
> sonal and community living. (p. 16)

This early definition of nursing focused on nursing as a process that
is goal directed, with serially ordered operations. The operations
involved are interpersonal and technical in nature. She defined the
nursing process as "educative and therapeutic when nurse and patient can come to know and to respect each other, as persons who
are alike, and yet, different, as persons who share in the solution of
problems" (p. 9).

An elaboration of the definition of nursing was published in 1969[1]
in a discussion of the need to delineate the parameters or boundaries
of nursing's unique focus. "Nursing can take as its unique focus the
reactions of the patient or client to the circumstances of his illness or
health problem thus overlapping medicine only when dealing with
disease processes more directly" (Peplau, 1969, p. 37). Identification of nursing's unique focus as the reactions to illness or health

---

[1]An earlier discussion of the unique focus of nursing can be found in a 1965 unpublished paper: "The purpose of the practice of a professional nurse revolves around
more than merely helping to heal the physical ailments of the patient, although of
course, this is one important activity of the nurse. The nurse . . . must relate herself meaningfully to the reaction of the patient to his illness, the psychological and
social changes which his illness in effect forces upon him" (Peplau, 1965, p. 2).

problems is important historically, for it became a central element of the definition of nursing in *Nursing: A Social Policy Statement* (American Nurses Association, 1980). Peplau participated on the Social Policy Statement committee and was obviously influential in forming the currently accepted definition of nursing: "Nursing is the diagnosis and treatment of *human responses* to actual or potential health problems" (p. 9).

The human responses that nurses diagnose and treat are phenomena that are observed, for the most part, within an interpersonal context. The professional dimension of nursing demands that the nurse do more than diagnose the human response. "Diagnosing is not the same as understanding a particular phenomenon" (Peplau, 1985a, p. 10). Understanding a phenomenon requires explanations of its etiology, its course, its meaning, and clues to intervention. Often phenomena are conceptualized by Peplau as processes with sequential steps that provide a structure for obtaining more information and also provide a framework within which to formulate strategies for intervention.

Concept Clarification

It was apparent to Peplau early in her career that the first step in developing a theory of nursing was to delineate the phenomena that were of concern to nurses. Operationalizing concepts was one way to make clear the sequential steps in the formation of a particular phenomenon. "When the sequential nature of behavior is clarified, it can be said to be understood" (Peplau, 1951, p. 1). Three of these concepts, anxiety, learning, and loneliness, illustrate the substantive nature of her theory.

Anxiety

Peplau (1982) defined anxiety as an energizer of behavior produced in response to stress. Because it is an energy, it cannot be observed directly, although "its subjective experience of discomfort can be *felt* and its transformation into relief behaviors can be observed" (p. 10). Only the behavioral manifestations of anxiety can be observed and the concept of anxiety inferred from those behaviors. Anxiety is caused by any threat to personal security, such as threats to biological integrity or threats to the self-system (Peplau, 1963a). "Anxiety is always communicated interpersonally. One anxious person communicates it to another person or persons in a situation; the latter empathically observe the anxiety" (Peplau, 1963a, p. 325). Peplau considered any threats to security, particularly the experience of unrealized or unmet expectations, as central etiological factors in causing anxiety. "Any expectation that is held, and is related to the security of the self-system [and is not met], is a threat. Any threat to existence, of non-being, of non-belonging, of psychological or physical impotence, to closely held values . . . involves expectations that are actually or potentially not met; and will evoke anxiety in the person involved" (Peplau, 1982, p. 5).

Peplau (1963a) developed the concept of anxiety on a four-point continuum including mild, moderate, severe, and panic. She elaborated this scale in relation to the effects of varying levels of anxiety on the individual's perceptual capacity, focal attention, and capacity to learn or adapt.

Peplau (1963, 1982) categorized the relief behavior that results from anxiety into four major patterns of behavior: (1) acting-out behavior, including both overt responses, such as anger, and covert responses, such as resentment; (2) withdrawal; (3) somatization; and (4) learning. Only the last pattern, using anxiety to motivate learning, results in movement of the individual toward health. She defined anxiety operationally by providing a serially ordered explanation of its occurrence:

1. Expectations that are held become operative (active).
2. Those expectations are not met (something opposite, unexpected, happens).
3. The extreme discomfort called anxiety is experienced.
4. Relief behaviors are called out and used. Relief behaviors used recurringly become habits—some as automatic anxiety relief behaviors, others (hopefully) as ways of using anxiety to energize investigation and learning.
5. Justification of the relief behaviors (Peplau, 1982, p. 3).

Because Peplau's theory was grounded in practice and was therefore intended to inform practice, her conceptualization of anxiety was developed to provide a theoretical structure for the application of the steps in the development of anxiety to nursing action. The intervention starts with step 3, where the discomfort of anxiety is felt subjectively. The intervention is to assist the patient to name the anxiety by asking, "Are you anxious, nervous?" and so forth. Secondly, relief behaviors, step four, are addressed by assisting the patient to connect the subjective feeling of anxiety which he or she has now named to the behavior that brings relief. Next, the nurse goes to step one in the process, expectations are held, and assists the patient to identify expectations that may have been operating immediately before he or she felt anxious. And last, the reasons for the expectations' not being met are addressed by identifying why (Peplau, 1982).

The rationale for the sequence of these interventions is based on the assumption that you begin with the simplest competency. Naming is easier than making connections between two behaviors, which is easier than identifying and analyzing expectations (Peplau, 1982).

Peplau defined the abstraction *anxiety* in order to make the steps in development and intervention clear. It is not that she discovered anxiety. She made it usable so that even a beginning clinician could spot it and know how to proceed to intervene.

Learning

The concept of learning (Peplau, 1963b), defined in sequential steps as a process, is an elaboration of the three-step process mentioned earlier (observation, interpretation, and intervention). Although the process of learning could be applied to both the nurse and the patient, it was generally viewed as a guide for work with patients. In other words, it was the patient who was viewed as the learner; the steps were used by the nurse as a structure to suggest intervention. The steps in learning are: (1) to observe; (2) to describe; (3) to analyze; (4) to formulate (may occur simultaneously with step 3); (5) to validate; (6) to test; (7) to integrate; and (8) to use.

Interventions, for example, to assist patients in progressing through steps 1 and 2 of the process, observation and description, would involve strategies to increase the patient's capacity to notice aspects of his or her life and to learn to describe these in detail. Analysis involves interpretation of the described data. Peplau detailed ways that the nurse could analyze data: Decode symbolic material, sort and classify, compare, generalize, and apply theory. Formulation is a precise statement of the analysis. Validation requires checking the results with at least one other person. Testing requires trying out the new learning, which is then integrated with previous knowledge and used in similar situations.

Loneliness

Peplau's paper on loneliness (1955) was one of the earliest presentations of the concept from an interpersonal framework. She defined loneliness as "an unnoticed inability to do anything while alone" (p. 1476). It is experienced as a "feeling of unexplained dread, of desperation, or of extreme restlessness. These feelings are so intense, so unbearable, that automatic actions are precipitated" (p. 1476). She differentiated lonesomeness, aloneness, and loneliness. The roots of loneliness were described and linked to "early life experiences in which remoteness, indifference, and emptiness were the principal themes that characterized the child's relationships with others" (p. 1476). Drawing upon her private practice, she presented clinical examples of patients who were lonely with the defenses they used to protect themselves from awareness of the dreaded experience.

Theories of Intervention

Modern psychiatric nursing theories that are used to guide intervention were formulated by Peplau. She defined psychiatric nursing as "the diagnosis of those human responses of clients, in relation to psychosocial or psychiatric problems, that detract from and prevent healthy living in the community, which nurses treat in the course of nurse-patient relationships" (Peplau, 1984, p. 2). She is best known for her introduction of psychotherapy with individual patients into psychiatric nursing, although this was not her original intention. She has also contributed to our understanding of intervention in the therapeutic milieu.

Psychotherapy

The use of the term *psychotherapy* in nursing is a recent development. When Peplau first wrote about psychiatric nursing, she termed interventions with individual patients *nurse–patient relationships.* Later it was called *one-to-one* relationship, then *counseling,* and finally *psychotherapy.* Later definitions of the work emphasized the difference between specialists and generalists in the field; that is, specialists were able to conduct psychotherapy, generalists counseled and conducted nurse–patient relationships. Resistance of other mental health professionals, as well as other psychiatric nurses, to nurse psychotherapists contributed to the use of euphemisms for psychotherapy because other terms were less threatening and more acceptable.

Peplau (1965) viewed the nurse–patient relationship as a way to implement the purpose of nursing which she described as "to find ways to come to know a person as a human being in difficulty and to help that person to stretch his capabilities and exercise innate capacities if only one-quarter of an inch" (p. 4). She later (1969) clarified this purpose by promoting the idea that nursing could claim a focus that assisted patients in gaining interpersonal and intellectual competencies beyond those they had at the time of illness, and that such competencies could be evolved through the nurse–patient relationship. Further, she believed it was necessary for nurses in general practice to have formal knowledge of counseling procedures in order to be effective in brief relationships they would encounter in any setting (Peplau, 1962).

The assumptions underlying Peplau's theory of psychotherapy provide clues to the philosophical basis of her ideas. She viewed humans as essentially rational, cognitive, and goal-directed beings who are capable of exercising self-control to achieve desired goals. People are primarily relational, that is, they develop and express themselves within a context of relationships with others. Behavior is motivated by a desire both to relieve the discomfort of anxiety as well as to move toward positive growth and a state of health. It is the dynamic tension between the need for relief from anxiety and the need to grow and develop—that is, to learn—that provides the focus for the work of the nurse psychotherapist. That work is devoted to assisting the patient give up relief behaviors enough to realize his or her innate need to develop capacities. The following major assumptions guide the work.

1. "Every human being needs to explain to himself what is happening to him and why" (Peplau, 1965. p. 20).

2. "Difficulties in living which lead . . . to mental illness . . . are subject to investigation and control by the patient with professional counseling assistance" (Peplau, 1962, p. 52).
3. "Illness provides an opportunity for learning and growth" (Peplau, 1969, p. 37).
4. "Mental illness is a product of relationships that go on in systems" (Peplau, 1984, p. 3).
5. Psychotherapeutic work of the nurse is based on an extension of the Whorfian hypothesis: "Language influences thought; thought then influences action; thought and action taken together evoke feelings in relation to a situation or context" (Peplau, 1969, p. 35).

Peplau proposed that nurses use an investigative approach, which she defined as the "art and science of stimulating patients to change themselves" (1975, p. 2). Investigative counseling is primarily verbal; only that which gets talked about can be understood and changed. Peplau acknowledged the importance of the nurse's attitude, which is often displayed nonverbally. However, she concentrated on the language behavior of the counselor consistent with her belief that language influences thought. Therefore, the language of the nurse becomes crucial in providing prompters for the work of the patient; the corrective effort of the nurse is directed at the language the patient uses (Peplau, 1984). Nurses also serve as models of healthy behavior through their language and actions.

The focus of the interview is on the patient. Nurses were cautioned to avoid socializing with patients in therapy sessions. If friendship could help patients, they would not need professional therapy. Although the primary focus is on the patient and his or her difficulties, nurses learned to be participant observers in their interactions; they observed their own behavior and that of the patient and altered their behavior in an effort to effect change in the patient's behavior. Such an approach requires a heightened awareness of the therapist's verbal behavior, including thoughts and feelings that prompt it.

Even though the effort is to induce change in the patient, nurses cannot control the patient's responses. They can only control their own behavior, and are obligated to do so out of respect for the patient. Patients are accorded unconditional respect; they do not need to earn respect.

Structure is an important characteristic of Peplau's psychotherapy method. Interviews are structured in regard to time, place, and purpose (one-way focus on the difficulties of the patient), so that the patient is clear about what the nurse intends (Peplau, 1965). Although the interview is externally structured, internally the patient takes the lead for the direction and focus. Trust develops when nurses are clear about the structure and do what they say they will do.

The nurse is an active listener in the therapy situation. The focus is on the patient with the "aim to get to see the patient's view of himself and his predicament the way it looks to him—so that he can see it too" (Peplau, 1965, p. 6). Nurses use theory to structure their observations and to guide interventions to elicit more detailed description and validated analyses of the patient's situation. Peplau (1964) emphasized the importance of eliciting description about the structural elements of an experience first. "Who was there?" "What went on?" "Where did it happen?" The assumption is that such details help to reduce the patient's anxiety, thereby increasing perception, ultimately bringing clarity to the experience. This tactic also mitigates the general tendency among those who are mentally ill to remember and describe experiences in terms of vague and overly abstract generalizations. "The corrective experience is to ask for the opposite [of an overly abstract generalization]—instances of experience given in verbatim fashion" (p. 11).

Peplau advised nurses to keep their theoretical interpretations to themselves, but to use them to lead patients to discover their own meanings from a validated review of their experiences. Inductively derived interpretations, such as themes abstracted in the interview or decoded symbolic material, formed the basis for guiding the patient to a greater understanding of the meaning of the behavior.

Therapeutic Milieu

Although Peplau is best known for her work in developing a theory of intervention with individuals, she also wrote about the problems of psychiatric nursing in the therapeutic milieu. Early in her career she asked students to conduct ward studies: analysis of observations of behavior on units. Interpersonal theory and systems theory were applied to analyze these studies and suggest corrective action. A central concern that grew out of this work was a recurring observation that staff unwittingly participated in the perpetuation of chronicity.

Ways staff perpetuate chronicity are to: (1) exploit patients by using them for work that has no training or monetary benefit; (2) burden them with their own problems; (3) make pets of certain patients; (4) take sides in patient disputes so one wins and the other loses; (5) reconfirm a patient's self-view as helpless by responding to dependency bids; (6) derogate or punish patients; (7) encourage patients to tattle on each other; and (8) participate in efforts of patients to split staff (Peplau, 1978). These patterns of chronicity perpetuation can be avoided by developing awareness of pattern integrations that occur between staff and patients.

Peplau (1985b) defined pattern integration as the merging of patterns of need of one person with those of another or others so that there is a fit. The merging of needs forms a separate entity so that the part of each incorporated into the whole becomes necessary for the unit to be complete. "Many of the expectations and functions associated with problematic need-pattern integrations tend to become automatic, that is, they transpire without thought" (p. 3).

Intervention in problematic patterns of patients on a psychiatric unit requires an admission assessment that elicits data about patterns. One way to obtain that data is to request "critical incidents that occurred in various phases of life, in which the patient's interactions with others are described in sufficient detail to infer problematic patterns" (p. 8). Once patterns are identified, nurses can plan nursing actions which address a few problematic patterns of each patient. More importantly, they can avoid participating unwittingly in the perpetuation of a given problematic pattern.

CONCLUDING REMARKS

We have presented a brief discussion of Hildegard E. Peplau's contributions to nursing and to the specialty of psychiatric nursing through the development of her theory of interpersonal relations.

We have focused primarily on her contributions to nursing theory
by describing the characteristics of her theory, definition of nursing, illustrative concepts, and her theories of intervention in psychotherapy and therapeutic milieu. Peplau also contributed an
extensive body of work on professional issues.

Peplau's theoretical ideas, particularly her definition of nursing
and nursing process, elaboration of anxiety and learning, and her
psychotherapeutic methods, have become a part of the collective
culture of the discipline of nursing. Many commonly understood
and assumed ideas basic to nursing stem from her work. As we
accumulate knowledge, we tend to lose sight of the individual contributions of the originators of that knowledge. In other words, it
becomes knowledge in the public domain. For historical and intellectual reasons, it is extremely important to credit and evaluate
those early contributions in light of their relevance to our discipline
today. It is apparent from this brief review that Peplau's theories
continue to be germane to our research and practice.

REFERENCES

American Nurses Association. (1980). *Nursing: A social policy statement.*
  Kansas City, MO: Author.
Fitzpatrick, J. J., & Whall, A. L. (1983). *Conceptual models of nursing
  analysis and application.* Bowie, MD: Brady.
Meleis, A. I. (1985). *Theoretical nursing: Development and progress.* Philadel-
  phia: Lippincott.
Merton, R. K. (1957). *Social theory and social structure.* New York: Free
  Press.
Peplau, H. E. (1951). *Class syllabus.* New York: Teachers College, Colum-
  bia. Schlesinger Library, Radcliffe College, Cambridge, MA. No. 84-
  M107, Hildegard E. Peplau Archives, carton 11, volume 33.
Peplau, H. E. (1952). *Interpersonal relations in nursing.* New York: Putman.
  (Reissued 1988; London: Macmillan)
Peplau, H. E. (1954, November). *Interpersonal relationships in psychiatric
  nursing.* Paper presented at the Annual Institute, Psychiatric and
  Mental Health Section, Illinois State Nurses Association, Chicago,
  IL. Schlesinger Library, Radcliffe College, Cambridge, MA. No. 84-
  M107, Hildegard E. Peplau Archives, carton 20, volume 675.
Peplau, H. E. (1955). Loneliness. *American Journal of Nursing 55,* 1476–
  1481.
Peplau, H. E. (1962). Interpersonal techniques: The crux of psychiatric
  nursing. *American Journal of Nursing 62,* 50–54.

Peplau, H. E. (1963a). A working definition of anxiety. In S. F. Burd &
    M. A. Marshall (Eds.), *Some clinical approaches to psychiatric nursing*
    (pp. 323–327). New York: Macmillan.
Peplau, H. E. (1963b). Process and concept of learning. In S. F. Burd &
    M. A. Marshall (Eds.), *Some clinical approaches to psychiatric nursing*
    (pp. 333–336). New York: Macmillan.
Peplau, H. E. (1964, July). *General application of theory and techniques
    of psychotherapy in nursing situations.* Paper presented at Cedars of
    Lebanon–Mount Sinai Hospitals, Los Angeles, CA. Schlesinger Li-
    brary, Radcliffe College, Cambridge, MA. No. 84-M107, Hildegard
    E. Peplau Archives, carton 39, volume 1451.
Peplau, H. E. (1965, February). *Interpersonal relationships in nursing.*
    Paper presented at Council on Hospital Services Institute, District
    of Columbia–Delaware Hospital Association, Washington, DC.
    Schlesinger Library, Radcliffe College, Cambridge, MA. No. 84-
    M107, Hildegard E. Peplau Archives, carton 24, volume 834.
Peplau, H. E. (1969). Theory: The professional dimension. In C. M.
    Norris (Ed.), *Proceedings of the first nursing theory conference* (pp. 33–
    46). Kansas City, KS: University of Kansas Medical Center.
Peplau, H. E. (1975). *Theoretical issues in nursing.* Lecture at University of
    Leuven, Belgium. Schlesinger Library, Radcliffe College, Cambridge,
    MA. No. 84-M107, Hildegard E. Peplau Archives, carton 29, volume
    1088.
Peplau, H. E. (1978, March/April). Psychiatric nursing: Role of nurses
    and psychiatric nurses. *International Nursing Review, 25:* 41–47.
Peplau, H. E. (Speaker). (1981). *Peplau on Peplau.* Cassette Recording.
    Schlesinger Library, Radcliffe College, Cambridge, MA. No. 84-M107,
    Hildegard E. Peplau Archives, carton 31, volume 1151.
Peplau, H. E. (1982, March). *Anxiety in the nurse and within the patient.* Pa-
    per presented at a nursing symposium, School of Nursing, University
    of Kansas, Kansas City, KS.
Peplau, H. E. (1983, June). *Written response to J. Turner interview.*
    Schlesinger Library, Radcliffe College, Cambridge, MA. No. 84-M107,
    Hildegard E. Peplau Archives, carton 32, volume 1168.
Peplau, H. E. (1984, April). *Therapeutic nurse–patient interaction.* Paper
    presented at Hamilton Psychiatric Hospital, Hamilton, Ontario,
    Canada.
Peplau, H. E. (1985a, November). *Interpersonal relations: constructs for
    nursing practice.* Paper presented at the University of Kansas, Con-
    ference on Issues in Nurse-Patient Relationship, Kansas City, KS.
Peplau, H. E. (1985b, November). *Pattern interactions at the unit level.*
    Paper presented at the Menninger Foundation, Topeka, KA.
Peplau, H. E. (1987). Nursing science: A historical perspective. In
    R. R. Parse, (Ed.) *Nursing science: Major paradigms, theories, and cri-
    tiques* (pp. 13–29). Philadelphia: Saunders.

Index

A

Acting-out, 358
Adaptation, 141, 143
  definition, 286
  steps of, 144
Alpenfels, E. J., 237
American Nurses' Association, xix,
  193, 271, 294, 357
Anger, 47, 68, 90, 94
Anxiety, 12, 13, 14, 24–25, 51, 68,
  88, 90, 104, 105, 112, 118, 125,
  142, 143, 144, 178, 180, 186,
  195, 199, 200, 201, 240, 270,
  271, 273, 278, 281, 283, 285,
  287, 289, 290, 307, 319, 322,
  329, 335, 336, 343, 347,
  357–359
  avoidance of, 323
  causes of, 105
  characteristics of, 279–280, 281
  definition, 269, 279, 281, 286
  degree of, 52, 67, 280, 283, 284,
    285, 287, 292, 293, 307, 310
  development of, 281
  and hallucinations, 324
  and learning, 292
  and mental illness, 290
  and nursing intervention,
    282, 292
  prevention of, 106, 107, 297,
    299, 303, 307, 312, 328
  and relief behavior, 280, 281,
    282, 286, 287, 289, 290,
    294, 297
  and self-system, 280, 287
  staff, 87, 89, 94
  transmission of, 60
  and victim expectation, 285
Arieti, S., 311
Attribution, definition, 275
Autistic inventions, 64, 110, 151,
  157, 160, 161, 162, 196,
  257–258, 320, 321, 323, 334
  problems of, 64
Avoidance, 188, 319

B

Barber, B., 235, 236
Bateson, G., 61, 244
Beck, C. K., 311
Becker, H. S., 237
Behavior,
  definition of, 201
  perpetuation of, 115–116, 119,
    195, 198–199, 327, 364
  relief, see Relief behavior
  replication of, 186, 187, 191
Behavior energizers, 66–68
Behavior modification, 130
Benjamin, R., 81
Bergman, G., 149
Birdwhistle, R., 60

Body language theory, 61
Bouwsma, W. J., 278
Bozian, M. W., 242
Bruner, J. S., 232, 233
Buerl, A., 120
Bullough, B., 23
Bullough, V., 23
Burd, S. F., 28, 29

C

Cannon, W., 8
Catharsis, 101
Caudill, W. A., 75, 83, 268
Chronicity, 84, 87, 89, 94, 98, 186,
    312, 320, 322, 323, 333, 364
  characteristics of, 86–87
  competency building, 85, 87
  definition, 81, 82
  development of, 89, 202
  disuse, 89
  and educational systems, 85
  and power struggles, 88, 90
  prevention of, 81–82
  testing, 90, 91, 93, 97
Circumstantiality, 344
Communication, 11, 14, 126, 194,
    196, 201, 202, 231, 239
  empathic linkages, 60, 231
  gestural messages, 60–61
  nonverbal gestures, 231
Community mental health centers,
    127, 129, 130
Concepts,
  application, 24–25
  definition, 23, 24–25, 154
  explanatory, 50
  function, 51
  naming of, 22, 23, 89, 359
  structure, 50–51
Conflict, 51, 155–156
Control, loss of, 345
Coping behavior, 233, 286, 288.
  See also Anxiety, and relief
  behavior

Cormack, D., 69
Counseling, 17, 129, 131, 133, 171,
    361. *See also* Investigative
    counseling; Psychotherapy
Counselor,
  behavior of, 210, 215–216
  role of, 206, 208–215

D

Daniels, M. J., 237
Data collection, 9, 16, 17, 23, 47,
    49, 85, 101, 107, 111, 115, 138,
    142, 144, 181, 235, 274, 355
  analysis, 138, 142, 144, 150, 158
  formulation of, 143
  interpretation, *see* Data
    interpretation
  objectivity, 49
Data interpretation, 150
  autistic invention, 151, 157, 160,
    161, 162
  categorizing, 153
  conceptual, 154–156
  decoding, 50, 151–152
  definition, 149
  frame of reference, 160–162
  generalization, 156–160
  methods of, 150–162
  problems with, 153
  purpose of, 161
  subdivision, 153
Davis, F., 27
Defense mechanisms, 286, 288.
  See also Anxiety, and relief
  behavior
Delusions, 66
  definition, 289
Denial, 105
DeShouwer, P., 120
Detachment, 101, 180, 202, 207,
    237, 238
  clinical, 92
Development processes, 26
Dickoff, J., 22

Disassociation, 53, 101, 307, 328, 332, 334
Dolan, M., xvi

E

Erickson, G. D., 311
Experiential teaching, 139, 145, 146, 147, 148
components of, 140
teacher's role, 145–146
vs. traditional education, 140

F

Family,
role of, 130
therapy, *see* Psychotherapy, family
Field, W. E., Jr., 275, 290, 322
Fitzpatrick, J. J., 353
Focal attention, 338–347
definition, 339
development of, 339–341
dysfunctions of, 343–345.
See also specific types of dysfunctions
and nursing actions, 346–347
Fraser, C. L., xvi
Freedman, J. L., 274
Freidson, E., 236
Freud, S., 8, 161, 288
Fromm, E., 255

G

Gecas, V., 294
Geriatric Nursing, xvii
Goffman, E., 75
Goldfarb, A. I., 232
Gordon, M., 274
Gould, L. N., 311
Greenblatt, M., 75
Gregg, D., 28
Gustafson, G., 311

H

Haber, J., 76
Habit training, 16
Hallucinations, 14, 15, 17, 26, 63, 66, 110, 270, 273, 300, 323
and adults, 318
and anxiety, 324
and autistic invention, 320, 323
and children, 317, 318, 319
and chronicity, 322, 323
definition, 12, 311, 312
development of, 311, 312–316, 317–323, 336
and illusory figures, 323
interpretation of, 13
and loneliness, 319, 323, 324
and nursing intervention, 312–316, 321, 322, 323–324
phases of, 319–323
and relief behavior, 319, 322
and therapy, 320, 322
types of, 311
see also Autistic invention; Illusory figures; Supervisory personification
Hardin, G., 153
Hays, D., 178
Health care,
cost of, 133
planning, 57, 58
Hochschild, A., 304
Home-care, 130
Hospitalization, 83, 322, 323
chronic wards, 131
discharge, 19, 77, 130
Hughes, E. C., 193, 235, 238

I

Identification process, 198, 209, 267
Illness-maintenance, 126, 127, 273, 323
Illusory figures, 92, 110, 196, 267, 300, 305, 311, 312, 321, 323

Inferences, 51, 59, 93, 111, 115,
    141, 145, 208, 234, 247,
    248
  definition, 50
  validation of, 50, 118, 143,
    360
Instances, 26
International Council of Nurses,
    xix
Interpersonal relations, 9, 58
  function, 59
  integrations, 59, 91–92
  origin, 58
  problematic, 184
  and psychotherapy, 10
  quality of, 5, 6–8
  theme of, 6
  theory of, 272, 273
Interpersonal Relations in Nursing,
    xi, xv, xviii
Interpersonal theory, 42, 77
  definition, 7
Intervention, *see specific types*
  of intervention
Interviewing, 3, 17, 23, 112, 156,
    162, 171–172, 178, 180, 185,
    203, 207, 275, 362
  techniques, 220–229
Investigative counseling, 205-229,
    362
  assumptions, 207–208
  counselor-patient relationship,
    206, 207
  definition, 205, 206
  detachment, 207
  guidelines, 215
  interview techniques, 207,
    220–229
  outcome, 205, 206, 235
  process of, 209, 217–218
  purpose of, 210
  session description, 210, 211
  session orientation, 211–214
  and trust, 209
  see also Counselor

J

James, P., 22
Jeffries, J., 240
Johns, E., 76
Johnson, F. H., 311
Jones, M., 75

K

Kaplan, A., x, xi
Kim, M. J., 274
King, I. M., 295
King, S., xvi
Kneisl, C. R., 76
Knowles, J. S., xvi, xvii, xix
Kübler-Ross, E., 63

L

Labeling, 8, 180, 244
Language, body, *see* Body language
  theory
Language behavior, 277, 290, 309,
    362
  and anxiety, 336
  and autistic invention, 334
  and chronicity, 333
  development of, 187
  generalizations, 200, 331
  impact of, 25, 49, 92–93, 327
  and inadequate classification,
    332–333
  and nursing, 197, 198, 199, 200,
    202, 323, 327–336
  overgeneralization, 200, 331, 333
  problematic, 188
  and pronoun usage, 188, 189,
    199, 332–334
  and psychotherapy, 188, 189,
    190, 191
  of schizophrenics, 327–337
  and self-system, 302, 307
Language-thought disorder, 290.
    See also Schizophrenia

Leach, A., 76
Learning, 26, 88, 106, 138, 141,
    143, 233, 235, 358, 359, 360
  vs. adaptation, 144
  and anxiety, 292
  definition of, 142, 286, 287, 348
  and nurse-patient relationship,
    147
  operations of, 142–143, 349–352
  process of, 349–352
Levinson, D. J., 75
Loneliness, 17, 319, 323, 324, 360
  vs. aloneness, 255–256, 360
  and autistic inventions, 257–258
  avoidance of, 264–267
  and contacts, 261–264
  and defense patterns, 258–261
  definition of, 256
  and dependency, 268–269
  development of, 256–257
  and emptiness, 266–267
  vs. lonesomeness, 255, 360

M

Marginal thought, 344
Marshall, M. A., 28, 29
Maser, J. D., 279
Mauksch, H. O., 239
McFarland, G. K., 274
McLane, A. M., 274
McQuade, A., 232
Mead, G. H., 299
Mechanistic theory, 8, 9
Meleis, A. I., 353
Mental health care,
  focus teams, 127–128
  team meeting, 129
  see also Psychiatric nursing
Mental illness, 82, 106, 121, 126,
    130, 183, 193, 194, 196, 290,
    291, 295, 323, 327
  and chronicity, 84, 94–98
  definition of, 121, 122–124, 126,
    128–129, 131

history of treatment, 194
  origin of, 82
  prevention of, 83–86
  and role reversal, 103, 266
  theories of, 121, 122–124
  see also Community mental
    health centers; Paranoid;
    Schizophrenia
Mental retardation, 130
Mereness, D., 23, 28, 76
Merton, R. K., 21, 354
Milieu, 111, 113
  history of, 75–78
  and nurse-patient interactions, 78
  and people-system, 77
  and ward government, 77, 125
Milieu therapy, 75, 77, 186, 187,
    363–364
Modes of experiencing, 53
  parataxic, 53, 54
  prototaxic, 53, 54
  syntaxic, 53
Moreno, J. L., 58, 77

N

Needs,
  biological, 67
  of nurse, 234
  security, 67
  sociocultural, 67
Noyes, A. P., 16
Nurse,
  needs of, 234
  role of, 16, 20, 22, 47, 78, 119,
    120–121, 126, 131–132, 146,
    171, 173, 192, 237
  see also Psychiatric nurse
Nurse-counselor, *see* Counselor
Nurse-patient relationships, 42, 43,
    83, 192, 193, 196, 197, 233,
    234, 248, 273, 295, 327, 361
  affective involvement, 237, 238
  barriers to, 15, 203
  detachment, 180, 202, 237

Nurse-patient relationships *(cont.)*
    interpersonal intimacy, 44, 231
    investigative approach, 197, 198,
        203, 277–278, 293, 362
    and learning, 147
    orientation, 57
    professional closeness, *see*
        Professional closeness
    pseudo-closeness, 231, 234
    purpose of, 57
    stimulus behavior, 241
    termination of, 57
    working, 57
Nursing,
    competence, 49, 112, 147, 202,
        239, 275
    and counseling, *see* Investigative
        counseling
    definition of, 193, 270–271, 274,
        356, 357
    development programs, 97–98
    focus on patient, 45–46
    and follow-up care, 130
    general duty *vs.* psychiatric, 174,
        175
    goal of, 15
    investigations, 47–49
    and language behavior, *see*
        Language behavior, and
        nursing
    and milieu function, 76
    and need-meeting behavior,
        67
    purposes of, 232
    and theory, 49
Nursing actions, 25, 28, 125, 232,
    238, 273, 346–347. *See also*
    Nursing intervention
Nursing care plans, 120–121, 274
Nursing concepts, 28, 29. *See also*
    Concepts
Nursing education, 7, 49, 51–52,
    126, 137, 157, 174, 177–178,
    248. *See also* Experiential
    teaching

Nursing history, 58, 113
Nursing intervention, 49, 63, 82,
    83, 93, 101–103, 116, 119,
    130, 163, 208, 236, 276, 295,
    296
    aim of, 63, 111
    and anxiety, 282, 292
    evaluation of, 23
    and focal attention, 338–347
    and hallucinations, 312–316,
        321, 322, 323–324
    and self-system, 309, 311
    see also Professional closeness
Nursing intervention strategies,
    115, 182, 183
    and psychotherapy, 184, 187, 191
Nursing literature, 76, 204, 294,
    311
Nursing practice manuals, 23
Nursing research, 271, 272
Nursing supervisor,
    aim of, 165–166
    future role of, 167
    profile, 166–167
    role of, 166
Nursing supervision, 164, 204
    conference, 165–166, 204
Nursing team, 248

O

Observation, 22, 23, 49, 50, 58, 59,
    101, 111–113, 117, 118, 138,
    142, 157, 179, 232, 236, 238,
    247–248, 273, 331
    empathic, 158, 301, 302, 329
    interpretation of, 23
    methods of, 118
    participant, 46, 47, 362
    participant *vs.* spectator, 46
    spectator, 46
Occupational therapy, 87
Operational concepts, 10
    four levels of, 10
Overprotection, 103

P

Panic, 17, 67, 126, 131, 194, 285, 289, 290, 292, 293, 297, 307, 322, 343
 transmission of, 60
Paranoid, 188, 189, 199
Parataxic distortions, 64–65, 142, 162
 problems of, 65
Parataxis, 53, 54, 342
Parsons, T., 297
Pattern integration, 83, 112, 115, 117, 186, 194, 208, 304, 364
 definition, 109
 need-, 109–110
 types of, 62, 110
Pattern interaction, 108
Patterns, 61–63, 100, 118
 definition of, 61, 108–109, 111
 exemplars, 61
 naming, 109
 observation of, 101, 111–113
 overgeneralization, 290
 problematic, 113–118, 119
Peplau, H. E., ix, xviii, 3, 22, 23, 26, 28, 63, 73, 76, 137, 138, 160, 171, 172, 234, 235, 270, 273, 274, 245, 286, 319, 339, 345
 development of theory, 353–356
 personal history, xvii–xix
Peplau, L. A., 274, 275
Perlman, D., 319
Pfefferkorn, B., 76
Process,
 application, 26
 definition, 26, 63
Professional closeness, 232, 233, 234, 235, 236, 238
 definition of, 230
 detachment, 238
 stimulus behavior, 235
Prototaxis, 53, 54, 343
 definition of, 335

Psychiatric literature, 126
Psychiatric nurses, 80, 148
 competence of, 121, 131, 192, 193
 and concepts, 273–275
 and counseling, 178, 179
 education of, 131, 193
 and health teaching, 178
 role of, 11, 13, 120, 121, 131–132, 147, 174, 271
 and self-system development, 300
Psychiatric nursing, 92, 171, 271, 275
 definition of, 193, 360
 and interpersonal techniques, 178, 179, 181
 and managerial activities, 177
 and mother-surrogate role, 175–176
 research, 138
 and socializing-agent activities, 177–178
 and technical expertise, 176–177
Psychiatry,
 descriptive, 8, 9, 244
 thematic, 244–248
 typological, 8, 9, 244
Psychogeriatrics, 130
Psycholinguistics, *see* Language behavior
Psychosis, 144, 290, 297, 343
Psychotherapy, 10, 99, 100, 129, 131, 133, 171, 320, 322, 360–363
 family, 77, 129, 130, 194
 group, 129, 130, 184, 194
 individual, 130, 194
 and workshops, 129

R

Rawlings, R. P., 311
Recovery, 126, 128–129, 141, 147, 197, 232, 241
Relatedness, 9, 11

Relationship, 192
  counseling, 54–55
  doctor-patient, 43
  experiential, 17
  illusionary, see Autistic
    intervention; Illusory
    figures; Parataxic
    distortions; Supervisory
    personifications
  mind-body, 8
  nurse-doctor, 43
  nurse-patient, see Nurse-patient
    relationship
  parent-patient, 94–95, 96
  parent-therapist, 95–96, 97
  therapist-patient, 95
Relief behavior, 68, 88, 89, 90, 105,
    106, 112, 199, 202, 215, 280,
    281, 282, 286, 287–288, 289,
    290, 291, 294, 297, 319, 322,
    357, 358, 361
  and anxiety, 294, 297
  failure of, 290
Remotivation groups, 130
Render, H. W., 76
Reynolds, W., 60, 69
Riesman, D., 267
Role-reversal, 103, 266
Rouslin, S., 76, 77, 93
Roy, C., 295
Ruesch, J., 244
Ruminative thought, 345

S

Scattered thinking, 199, 341, 344
Schachtel, E. G., 338
Schizophrenia, 112, 141, 151, 152,
    157, 161, 184, 185, 187, 188,
    190, 247, 256, 290, 311
  automatic knowing, 329–330,
    332
  language behavior of, 327–337
Schudy, S. M., 76
Schwartz, M. S., 75, 126

Sears, D. O., 274, 275, 295
Self, 51, 270, 294
  definition of, 296, 297
  dimensions of, 298
Self-awareness, 43, 49
Self-disclosure, 295
Self-system, 53, 66, 67–68, 69, 85,
    98, 103–104, 112, 119, 195,
    196, 209, 210, 280, 287, 289,
    291, 294, 295, 296, 297,
    300–311, 322, 346, 358
  components of, 299
  development, see Self-system
    development
  and language behavior, 307
  maintenance, 297, 301, 303, 307,
    310, 312, 319
  self-control, 308
  self-esteem, 308–309
  self-images, 308
  self-views, 301, 303, 304, 307,
    308, 309, 310
  self-worth, 308
Self-system development, 104,
    300–307, 340, 341–342
  adult behavior, 303, 304
  and anxiety, 302
  empathic observation, 301, 302
  felt relations, 301, 302
  and hallucinations, 305
  input appraisals, 301, 306
  and language behavior, 302
  and peers, 306, 307
  and psychiatric nursing, 300
  supervisory personifications,
    301, 305
Selye, H., 233
Sidelaeau, B. F., 76
Sills, G. M., 76, 192, 193
Skipper, J. S., Jr., 239
Socialization process, 26
Somatization, 358
Stainbrook, E., 27, 268
Stanton, A. H., 75, 126
Steele, K. McL., 16

Stress, 233, 357
Sullivan, H. S., 9, 52, 53, 58, 59,
    64, 66, 68, 75, 77, 142, 151,
    233, 257, 266, 272, 295, 297,
    300, 302, 305, 327, 340, 353,
    355
Supervisory personifications, 65,
    110, 301, 305
Systems theory, 77

T

Tagliacozzo, D. L., 239
Taylor, S. E., 274
Teaching methods, experiential, *see*
    Experiential teaching
Terror, 17, 271
    development, 297
Thematic apperception test, 245
Theme, definition of, 245
Theorem of Reciprocal Emotion,
    233–234
Theory,
    definition of, 27
    development of, 50
    validation of, 21–22
Therapist, role, 100, 103
"Tools and Tasks of Personality
    Development," 31–41, 160

Tudor, G. E., 76, 247
Tuma, H., 279

U

Ullman, M., 236

V

Von Bertalanffy, L., 77

W

Ward atmosphere, 73. *See also*
    Milieu
Ward government, 125
Whall, A. L., 353
Whorf, B., 25, 187, 327
Williams, R. H., 75
Williams, S. R., 311
Wilson, H. S., 76
Withdrawal, 17, 68, 76, 92, 179,
    195–197, 199, 200, 276–277,
    288, 304, 319, 321, 322, 342,
    358
    development of, 196
Wylie, R., 294